# PATIENT
# & PERSON

*To Charles and the person you are*

**6TH EDITION**

# PATIENT & PERSON

## INTERPERSONAL SKILLS IN NURSING

### JANE STEIN-PARBURY

ELSEVIER

# ELSEVIER

Elsevier Australia. ACN 001 002 357
(a division of Reed International Books Australia Pty Ltd)
Tower 1, 475 Victoria Avenue, Chatswood, NSW 2067

**National Library of Australia Cataloging-in-Publication Data**

Stein-Parbury, Jane, author.
Patient and person: interpersonal skills in nursing / Jane Stein-Parbury.
Sixth edition.
9780729542562 (paperback)
Includes index.
Nurse and patient.
    Interpersonal relations.
    Communication in nursing.

Senior Content Strategist: Libby Houston
Senior Content Development Specialist: Tamsin Curtis
Senior Project Manager: Anitha Rajarathnam
Edited by Matt Davies
Proofread by Tim Learner
Design by Simon Rattray
Index by Innodata Indexing
Typeset by Toppan Best-set Premedia Limited
Printed in China

# CONTENTS

# FOREWORD

*Patient & Person* is a 'must-have' for any student, practitioner or teacher of nursing or any health-related discipline. Throughout the world, where there have been government inquiries into poor healthcare, the reports inevitably have noted that patient care had been compromised through poor communication, whether between health professionals or between health professionals and their patients and families. Once regarded by some as a 'feel good' or 'touchy-feely' part of a curriculum, it has become clear now that interpersonal communication is at the heart of safe and effective practice, and is the critical underpinning of quality care. Used well, the nurse–patient interaction is in itself a potent therapy.

This 6th edition of *Patient & Person* embodies the very best of educational practice. It is research-based, theoretically grounded and always practice- and person-focused. Such an undertaking requires a great and uncommon skill but one that Professor Emerita Jane Stein-Parbury has developed over many years of bridging excellence in both academic and clinical practice. A dedicated mental health nurse, Jane has a deep understanding of the nature and power of good communication.

This edition is constructed in three meaningful sections. The first introduces the reader to the nurse–patient relationship, its evidence base and the importance of understanding oneself in any interaction; the second delves deeply into the development of the skill components of a nurse–patient relationship; and the third takes the reader into the realities of practice, of using these skills in therapeutic ways to help those experiencing loss, vulnerability and the need to cope. This third section builds skills in dealing with difficult encounters and, with great practicality, takes the conversation into the complexity of the healthcare work environment, looking at the skills of building a supportive workplace and developing personal resilience.

The book is infused with the voices of patients and their families through the use of 'patient stories'. This brings life and relevance to every aspect of the interpersonal skill development. The practical exercises throughout enable reflection on this development and allow the participant to focus on areas in which they need further refinement in their communication. This enables this refinement to occur in a safe and non-threatening environment. The support for students undergoing this learning is enhanced by the extremely useful appendix, which provides detailed 'tips' for facilitators.

This book is the product of a professional lifetime of dedicated practice and reflection by Jane. I wholeheartedly recommend it to anyone interested in improving their interpersonal interactions for the benefit of patients and their families. My congratulations to Jane and my thanks for this wonderful contribution.

*Professor Jill White AM RN, RM, MEd, PhD, MHPol*
*Faculty of Nursing and Midwifery*
*University of Sydney*

# PREFACE

To some readers, the use of the term 'patient' in the title of this book may be interpreted as a reinforcement of the 'sick role' in which ill people wait passively to be directed as to what to do next. Such an interpretation is in direct contrast to the meaning of the title. The title *Patient & Person* is intended to mean that patients should be treated as individual people who play an active role in their healthcare. The basic tenet of the book is that patients should be treated as people whose unique experiences are significant to their nursing care.

In addition to updating references and research highlights, this edition of *Patient & Person* includes changes to structure and content. Chapter 1 has been restructured in order to orient the focus on patient-centred care. While the concept of caring in nursing is still discussed, the historical background as to its development and refinement has been deleted. Reflection and reflective practice has been substantially revised in Chapter 3. The focus of Chapter 4 is now on how healthcare environments and culture are often at odds with people whose cultural beliefs do not match these environments. Thus the emphasis is now on the influence of culture in relation to healthcare quality and safety. The section on empathy in Chapter 6 has been completely revised and includes contemporary neuroscientific research about how empathy develops. In addition, the concept of compassion is also discussed in relation to empathy. Chapter 11 has been substantially revised. There is now an emphasis on the importance of interprofessional communication. There is less focus on the causes of stress in nursing and more emphasis on caring for self, including mindfulness, resilience and self-compassion.

A major challenge in writing a book about interpersonal aspects of nursing is the tension between capturing the complexity of interpersonal connections and presenting concrete guidelines and general rules for beginning nurses. Beginning nurses, like novices in any discipline, rely on guidelines and rules. In presenting rules and guidelines, there is an inherent danger of a 'cookbook' approach. Such an approach assumes there is a rational, objective, 'right' way for nurses to interact with patients. Recipes such as 'Combine three open-ended questions with two empathic statements, add one large tablespoon of support and reassurance, then mix well for 10 minutes during an interaction with a patient' are simple to understand but inadequate in addressing the intricacy of patient–nurse interactions.

In meeting this challenge, I have tried to avoid an oversimplified approach to using interpersonal skills by including a discussion of the contextual variables that need to be considered. I have done so in the hope that the guidelines and rules presented in this book will not be interpreted as prescriptions or recipes.

Finally, I want to emphasise that I realise that skills are not learnt simply by reading about them in a book. While this book offers guidelines and suggestions for developing interpersonal skills in nursing, the best way to learn them is by interacting with patients. In listening to and understanding patients' experiences of health and illness, nurses will come to appreciate that their real teachers are the people who happen to be patients.

*Jane Stein-Parbury*
*Sydney, 2017*

# ACKNOWLEDGEMENT

The author acknowledges and thanks Professor Juanita Sherwood, The University of Sydney, for her review of Chapter 4 *Considering culture*.

# HOW TO USE THIS BOOK

*Patient & Person* is a textbook about the practice and theory of developing interpersonal skills in nursing. Incorporated throughout Chapters 3–8 and 10 are various learning activities designed to provide a means by which skills can be developed and theoretical concepts understood. The text that precedes and follows each activity reinforces the point of that activity. For this reason, it is essential that the activities be used in their context (i.e. that they *not* be separated from the text).

Activities throughout the text adhere to a standard format. Importantly, this serves to develop a working pattern of reflection and enquiry. The activity structure comprises two major sections: *process* and *discussion*. The process includes detailed instructions for completing the activity, setting the parameters of the learning experience. The discussion contains exploratory statements and questions designed to encourage reflection on and dialogue about the learning experience, focusing attention on the theoretical concepts highlighted in the learning experience.

Activities are characterised by symbols as follows:

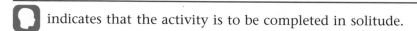 indicates that the activity is to be completed in solitude.

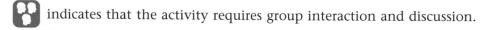 indicates that the activity requires group interaction and discussion.

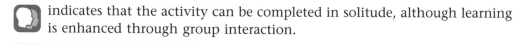 indicates that the activity can be completed in solitude, although learning is enhanced through group interaction.

Some activities are identified with the symbol ↻, followed by a page number, which indicates there is further material in the appendix, primarily intended for instructors who are using the activity to facilitate learning. It is useful to note that the appendix is organised on a chapter-by-chapter basis, preceded by some very useful information to assist facilitators conducting practical sessions.

# ONLINE VIDEOS – SCENARIOS AND INTERVIEWS

For this edition of *Patient & Person* a suite of videos have been created and are available on the Evolve site: http://evolve.elsevier.com/AU/Stein-Parbury/patient/.

The videos further explore the themes and content within the chapters on topics such as empathy, cultural diversity, interviewing skills, active listening, nursing presence and many more, which are outlined below under each video as well as the chapters where those topics are discussed. All of the scenarios feature reflection and reflective practice.

There are two sets of videos, a series of interviews with people from diverse cultural backgrounds and scenario-based interactions that a nurse might experience.

In the interviews three people discuss their belief systems, especially in relation to health and illness. The purpose of these interviews is to provide insight into and understanding about how cultural belief systems influence the delivery of healthcare. Their experiences with the healthcare system are explored, as well as how their cultural background may have affected that experience. They elaborate on how their dealings with the healthcare system could have been improved. These videos pertain to content in Chapter 4, *Considering culture*.

The second set of videos are scenarios that depict typical interpersonal interactions that nurses experience in their clinical work. The skills that are demonstrated and their links to chapters are outlined below.

| Scenario | Skills | Chapter links |
|---|---|---|
| Admitting a patient: initial interview | Listening and attending:<br>• Active listening<br>• Attending behaviour<br>• Nursing presence<br>• Silence<br>• Non-verbal communication<br>Exploring:<br>• Planned exploration: taking the lead<br>• Spontaneous exploration: following the patient's lead<br>• Prompting skills: exploring with statements<br>• Probing skills: open and closed questions<br>• Focused exploration<br>• Cue recognition and exploration<br>• Sharing perceptions | • Chapter 3: Nurse as therapeutic agent<br>• Chapter 5: Encouraging interaction: listening<br>• Chapter 7: Collecting information: exploring |

| Scenario | Skills | Chapter links |
|---|---|---|
| Dealing with challenging behaviours/ conflict | • Interpersonal conflict<br>• Conflict resolution strategies<br>• Negotiation in conflict<br>• Assertive communication<br>• Responding to anger | • Chapter 3: Nurse as therapeutic agent<br>• Chapter 10: Challenging interpersonal encounters |
| Advocating for a patient | • Assertive communication<br>• Demonstration of 'knowing the patient' | • Chapters 10: Challenging interpersonal encounters<br>• Chapter 11: Building a supportive workplace |
| Empathy expression | • Spontaneous exploration: following the patient's lead<br>• Cue recognition and exploration<br>• Empathy<br>• Sympathy<br>• Paraphrasing<br>• Seeking clarification<br>• Reflecting feelings | • Chapter 5: Encouraging interaction: listening<br>• Chapter 6: Building meaning: understanding<br>• Chapter 7: Collecting information: exploring |

**Please see the inside front cover for the access instructions for these online resources.**

# ACTIVITIES

# AUTHOR

**Jane Stein-Parbury RN, BSN, MEd (Pittsburgh), PhD (Adelaide)**
Emeritus Professor, Faculty of Health, University of Technology Sydney,
New South Wales

# REVIEWERS

**Sue Dean RN, MA**
Lecturer, Faculty of Health, University of Technology Sydney, New South Wales

**Diana Jefferies RN, BA, PhD, ACMHN**
Lecturer, School of Nursing and Midwifery, Western Sydney University,
New South Wales

**Denise McGarry RN, CMHN, GradCertHEd, BA, MPM, MACN, FACMHN**
Lecturer, School of Nursing, Midwifery and Paramedicine, Australian Catholic
University, New South Wales

**Yvette M Salamon RN, GradCertPeriopNurs, GradCertOnlineEd,
GradDipNursMang, BEd, MPeriopNurs**
Lecturer, Adelaide Nursing School, The University of Adelaide, South Australia

# PART

# 1

# INTRODUCTION

The four chapters in Part 1 reinforce each other by pursuing the same intention – to distil the overall significance of interpersonal relationships in nursing, especially in relation to the potential for nurses to realise their therapeutic agency in helping others. Although similar in intent, each chapter realises its aim through different means. The stories in Chapter 1 engage the reader through identification and serve as illustrations that reassert the subject of this book. The stories are reinforced with relevant research that provides evidence about the importance of interpersonal connections between nurses and patients.

Chapter 2 presents theoretical evidence that reinforces the importance of interpersonal communication, which builds and maintains therapeutic relationships between nurses and patients. The evidence is a synthesis of relevant and meaningful research into the nature of basic psychosocial care in nursing and healthcare. Of particular relevance is the variability in each relationship.

Chapter 3 explores nurses' therapeutic use of self and the development of therapeutic agency through reflective learning that promotes self-understanding and acceptance.

The importance of culture is discussed in Chapter 4, with an emphasis on promoting culturally congruent care in order to address inequities in healthcare. The system of healthcare as a culture itself is considered. The presentation of stories juxtaposed with discussion of research sets a scene that is carried throughout the remaining chapters in this book.

# Why interpersonal skills?

## CHAPTER OVERVIEW

- Interpersonal communication and relationship building are essential in delivering patient-centred care.
- Patient-centred care involves active patient participation.
- Current healthcare systems need to be reformed in order to become more patient-centred.
- Interpersonal relationships are central to patient-centred care.
- Nurses need to understand the subjective human health experience and come to know the patient as a person.
- Nurses are morally bound to relate to patients in a caring manner.

# INTRODUCTION

Throughout the course of their professional lives, nurses interact with a variety of people in a variety of contexts, and for a variety of reasons. During these social interactions they need to be able to effectively communicate with and relate to other people. As such, nursing is a social activity, and nurses need to be socially competent. They must be skilled in the art of interpersonal communication and human relationship building.

There are professional mandates for nurses to communicate competently with patients in order to gather relevant and useful data for clinical assessment (Nursing and Midwifery Board of Australia 2016; Nursing Council of New Zealand 2007). Furthermore, nurses need to relate to patients as more than simply a source of data. Professional codes of conduct (Nursing and Midwifery Board of Australia 2008; Nursing Council of New Zealand 2009) dictate that nurses are capable of relating therapeutically with patients as more than passive recipients of care; that is, engaging the patient through communicating and relating are necessary to professional nursing practice.

The interpersonal skills of communicating and relating described throughout this book are central to developing the social competence nurses need to demonstrate in their professional role. This is especially true in relation to the people nurses call patients. The word 'patient' is used purposely throughout this book. This is not done to perpetuate the problems of treating patients as passive recipients of nursing care, but rather to emphasise that patients should be treated *as a person*. This is based on a humanistic philosophical belief that humans are capable and competent.

The central premise of this book is that human connection, in the form of a patient–nurse relationship, is vital to nursing. Along with technical capability, the capacity to establish human connection is required for clinical competence in nursing practice. The connection is created by the way nurses and patients interact, and every interaction between a nurse and a patient is placed within the overall context of a relationship. For example, listening without judging and responding with understanding help to create a therapeutic relationship that is based on acceptance and respect.

Interpersonal relationships between patients and nurses humanise healthcare because they are the vehicles through which nurses are responsive to patients' subjective experiences. The relationship meshes the nurse's compassion and knowledge with the patient's experience of health events. Through their relationships with patients, nurses express concern, care and commitment. In the absence of interpersonal relationships with nurses, patients can be viewed as objects, clinical conditions or a set of problems to be solved. Nursing care that is offered without a human connection is impoverished. It lacks a caring connection.

The significance of interpersonal skills in nursing practice is sometimes difficult for beginning nurses to fully appreciate. Completing skill-based tasks often comes to the foreground, as technical proficiency is required for clinical competence. Interpersonal contact may seem like something that happens after tasks are completed. Focusing on interpersonal aspects of nursing does not mean that attention to task-related nursing functions is diminished. In fact, interpersonal contact increases the therapeutic effectiveness of nursing activities. For example, the restful state of feeling reassured by knowing what to expect and through explanations about details of an upcoming procedure benefits patients. Nurses are often in a prime position to establish interpersonal contact in order to provide such explanations. Nursing care involves making contact with the person who is the patient.

# PATIENT-CENTRED CARE

There are current efforts in healthcare to reform existing systems in order to make care more patient-centred (Constand et al 2014; Kitson et al 2013; Newell & Jordan 2015; Pelletier & Stichler 2013; Sharma et al 2015). Patient-centred care, also referred to as person-centred care, means that care is not only individualised but also that patients are actively involved in decision making. In order to do so, it is essential that patients' views, desires, needs and values are at the heart of healthcare. Patients value care that is focused on their individual needs and facilitates their involvement in care (Sidani & Fox 2014).

In a recent analysis of existing reviews of patient-centred care, Sharma et al (2015) identified six key components of this type of care: the establishment of a therapeutic relationship; building trust and respect; knowing the patient as a person, as well as families; shared power and decision making; empowering the patient; and effective communication between the patient and healthcare providers, especially in relation to the provision of meaningful information about their health status and treatment. While the authors concluded that there is no universal definition of person-centred care, there was an overriding theme of the importance of establishing relationships built on partnerships.

The focus on patient-centred care has come to the foreground as a result of increasing evidence that healthcare quality and safety can be improved when patients are included as partners in care (Australian Commission on Safety and Quality in Health Care 2011). There are better outcomes and fewer adverse events for patients when they experience care that is emotionally supportive, respectful and understanding of their preferences, is informative and involves them in decisions (Doyle et al 2013). From a patient's point of view, emotional support and the relief of distress and anxiety is most associated with care quality (Rathert, Williams et al 2012). This indicates that interactional and interpersonal aspects of care are central to the quality of that care (Dierckx de Casterlé 2015). In addition, patients are more satisfied and experience a sense of wellbeing when care is patient-centred (Rathert, Wyrwich et al 2012). In a review of controlled trials investigating the efficacy of person-centred care, it was found that this type of care not only improves patient satisfaction, wellbeing and quality of care but also objective measures such as reduced cost of care and length of hospital stay, as well as physiological improvements (Olsson et al 2013).

# Patient participation in healthcare

The central aspect of patient-centred care that is identified in the literature is that patients need to actively participate in their own healthcare. The notion of patients as active participants in healthcare challenges the traditional 'sick role' (Parsons 1951/1987) in which patients are expected to be passive, relinquish their responsibilities and follow the advice of healthcare experts. Such a role prevents people from assuming responsibility for their own health and places decision-making authority in the hands of healthcare practitioners because 'they know best'. As such, the sick role can disempower patients, thus rendering them more vulnerable. Patient participation alters the power balance such that patients are encouraged to engage in partnerships with healthcare practitioners, with increased capacity to act on their own behalf as a result. It shifts the roles of patients from passive participants to active agents and the nurse from provider of care to partner in care. This requires a change in the traditional culture of healthcare that is characterised by authoritarian and paternalistic attitudes (Snyder & Engström 2016).

Patient participation has its roots in the consumer movement, through which people have rights to be informed, be heard and have choice in matters not only pertaining to their own healthcare but also in the re-design of healthcare processes and systems. Having patients participate in their healthcare is both an ethical ideal and a practical reality. From an ethical point of view, all patients should have a say in their care (i.e. having a legitimate voice in care is a recognised patient right). From a practical standpoint, patients who participate in their healthcare are more likely to commit to that care because the care takes into account their particular circumstances. In this regard, health outcomes are more likely to be successful when patients have input into that care.

In the contemporary world of healthcare there is an international movement to increase patient participation that has been sparked by the recognition that patient participation is not only related to patient satisfaction but also increased care quality and safety (Castro et al 2016; Hudon et al 2011; Mavis et al 2015). Lack of patient participation can result in patients being harmed (Andersson, Frank et al 2015). Furthermore, patients believe they can help to prevent errors by being involved and participating in their care (Tobiano et al 2015). The concept of patient participation is fully explored in Chapter 8.

# The challenge ahead: reforming healthcare systems

If the interpersonal skills in this book are to be employed to their best advantage in patient care, then existing healthcare systems need to be reformed. Patient-centred care is only possible when nurses and other healthcare professionals not only have a commitment to such care but also operate in a system that is supportive of such care. At present, healthcare systems in the Western world are driven by

*Wiechula, R., Conroy, T., Kitson, A.L., et al., 2016. Umbrella review of the evidence: what factors influence the caring relationship between a nurse and patient? J. Adv. Nurs. 72 (4), 723–734.*

## Background

Forming productive and caring relationships with patients is essential to achieving person-centred care. Nurses need to attend to the development of these relationships through effective and helpful communication that establishes a meaningful interpersonal connection with patients. Research evidence that provides an understanding of the factors influencing this connection helps to enlighten nurses as to what patients expect and how they can approach establishing a productive and caring relationship with patients.

## Purpose of the study

The aim of this study was to examine published literature reviews of research related to the factors that influence the development of caring relationships between patients and the nurses who care for them.

## Method

This study was termed an 'umbrella review' – an overall examination of the body of published literature reviews that provide evidence about the factors that influence the formation of caring relationships between nurses and patients. Twelve previous reviews of both patients' and nurses' perspectives were included in this review. Findings from each of these reviews were categorised then synthesised into six groups.

## Key findings

The first group that was identified pertained to the expectation of the relationship. Nurses expected that the relationship would involve knowledge about the patient that was both deep and intimate. Both nurses and patients expected there to be trust in the relationship. The next group related to the values that nurses demonstrated, including being interested, kind and friendly, and acting like themselves (as opposed to acting in a role). The third group highlighted the knowledge and clinical competence of nurses, including their availability and accessibility to patients and their ability to support them. The centrality of communication to the building of relationships was the fourth group, underscoring the importance of it being both ordinary and technical. The fifth group was the organisational culture that was influential on the relationship, for better or worse; for example, a task-focused environment negatively impacted on the relationship. Finally, the impact of the relationship on both nurses and patients was reported, with nurses experiencing satisfaction and patients feeling satisfied, comfortable and safe when relating effectively with nurses.

## Implications for nursing practice

This extensive review of the literature demonstrates that both nurses and patients value the relationships that form between them. Nurses need to appreciate that patients want to make interpersonal connections and place their trust in nurses. Focusing on tasks, or behaving in a mechanical, impersonal manner, negatively impacts on making these connections. Technical and compassionate care needs to be blended in order for nursing care to be effective in helping patients.

managerialism and the meeting of target goals (Andersson, Willman et al 2015; Feo & Kitson 2016). These goals are not necessarily based on patients' needs and desires but rather to make healthcare systems operate in a manner that is efficient and keeps costs contained.

The healthcare system is based on a biomedical model in which patients are reduced to their illness and the focus is on their physical care, thus ignoring the relational aspects of care (Feo & Kitson 2016). While nurses recognise the importance of patient-centred care, they feel frustrated and challenged by a healthcare system that is task-oriented and focused on the physical and technical aspects of care (Bridges et al 2013; Ross et al 2014). When they experience time pressures to complete tasks, relational care such as providing emotional support, considered to be fundamental to nursing care, is omitted (Feo & Kitson 2016; Roch et al 2014). In contemporary, efficiency-driven healthcare systems the work of relating to patients is often not even perceived as 'work' (DeFrino 2009) (see *Research highlight*).

The social power structures of healthcare systems need to be altered if patient-centred care and patient participation in care is to become a reality. Professional dominance restricts care that truly involves patients (Angel & Frederiksen 2015; Mavis et al 2015), and patients feel powerless as a result (Sheridan et al 2015). When they feel disempowered they simply comply with healthcare professionals (Tobiano et al 2016), thus reverting to the classic sick role.

What is clear from the literature is that sound working relationships between patients and healthcare providers are the key to making patient-centred care and patient participation a reality (Angel & Frederiksen 2015; Kitson et al 2013; Mavis et al 2015). And, caring relationships and connecting with patients is what nurses find meaningful and satisfying in their work (Bridges et al 2013; Pavlish & Hunt 2012; Wiechula et al 2016). Nurses bring a unique perspective to this relationship, so understanding the nature of that relationship enables nurses to promote such care.

# PATIENT-NURSE RELATIONSHIPS IN NURSING PRACTICE

It was in the early 1950s that Peplau wrote what was to become the seminal work that specifically addressed patient–nurse relationships. *Interpersonal Relations in Nursing* (Peplau 1952/1988) outlined a theoretical framework and structure for therapeutic patient–nurse relationships, articulating how the nursing relationship could be a vehicle for a corrective human experience for patients. This framework was considered revolutionary at the time and continues to have relevance in nursing practice, scholarship and research (Peterson 2017). In keeping with Peplau, Travelbee (1971) expanded the interpersonal aspects of relating to patients, referring to such activities as therapeutic use of self as an art.

This relationship is dependent on both the clinical context and the level of interpersonal involvement that is negotiated between them. Patients will reveal themselves to nurses selectively, and some relationships will progress to deeply moving levels, while others remain therapeutically superficial. Some patients will require direct aid and assistance with managing their lives, while others will need information and advice in order to cope with and problem-solve challenges related to their health. Still others may simply need the supportive and comforting understanding of another human being. Each has a different level of involvement and commitment that is negotiated. The negotiation process is fully described in Chapter 2.

What makes the relationship therapeutic in nursing spans a range of possibilities, and this is why context-free rules cannot be applied. There are many ways that nurses help through their interactions with patients. According to Benner (1984, p. 48), 'helping [in the nursing context] encompasses transformative changes in meanings, and sometimes simply the courage to be with the patient, offering whatever comfort the situation allows'. This description provides useful guidance in understanding the range of form and purpose patient–nurse relationships can encompass. It reinforces the notion that 'being with' a patient, fully present and involved, is helpful in itself.

Consider the following story, told by a nurse.

## A Nurse's Story

Tony, aged five, was hospitalised as a result of serious injuries he sustained in a car accident. He was a passenger in the car driven by his mother, who also sustained injuries and required hospitalisation in a different facility. Although Tony's mother was in hospital, her injuries were minor. Because Tony's injuries were to his head and spine, he was initially admitted to the intensive care unit of the hospital but was eventually transferred to a general medical ward. This is when we first met.

Tony's father remained by his son's side day and night throughout the entire hospitalisation. He didn't say much, and most of our interactions were either non-verbal or limited to brief and factual information about Tony's condition. I noticed that Tony's father looked increasingly tired and drained as the days went by. The dark circles under his eyes were noticeable. He walked with a slumped posture.

After five days on the ward, Tony's condition deteriorated, necessitating a transfer back to the intensive care unit. This setback was overwhelming for Tony's father. I could see it in his face. Initially, I concerned myself with the details of getting the transfer underway. After the transfer was complete, Tony's father returned to the ward area to collect his son's belongings. He didn't look at me and seemed quite distant. I wanted to say something to him in an effort to offer some degree of comfort but knew better than to deliver a trite cliché such as 'It will be all right'. After all, how was I to know it would be? Instead, I approached him in the hallway as he was about to leave the ward area and told him how sorry I was that his son had to be transferred back to intensive care. I expressed my genuine sympathy for the turn of events that led to the transfer. He didn't respond but rather looked at me with a vacant stare, as if he was looking through and past me. I wanted to say more. I couldn't leave it at just that. So I said: 'I can only imagine one-hundredth of what you must be feeling. It seems like Tony has taken two steps forward and three steps back.'

Tears welled in his eyes and he said, 'I keep hoping ... but something always happens.' He began to cry and talk about how much he loved his son and how helpless he felt in this situation. I placed my hand on his shoulder and guided him to a private area of the ward. He expressed his thoughts and feelings about what was happening to his son, describing his condition in detail and expressing feelings of despair. Although I, too, felt extremely sad for Tony and his father, I maintained control over my emotions at that moment because I wanted to focus on him, not me (although I did cry later). I said nothing but simply placed my hand on his hand and squeezed it. It seemed enough. After a few minutes he composed himself, told me how much he appreciated my concern, thanked me and left the ward. I recall how helpless I felt about Tony's situation. It was likely that he would not walk again.

Although I felt helpless, I focused my energy on making contact with Tony's father. I had to make contact and was glad I found the courage to do so. In some small way I knew my concern for him and his son helped Tony's father. I could not change the situation, but I was there for him. I demonstrated that I cared and that I wanted to understand how he felt, no matter how helpless it made me feel.

The situations that nurses encounter often create feelings of helplessness within them when the patient's circumstances cannot be changed. Nurses may fear that because they cannot change the situation, there is nothing else that can be done. When this happens, nurses may avoid interaction and interpersonal contact, or limit contact with patients to those times when physical aspects of care require attention.

This story illustrates how conveying concern and understanding enables nurses to connect with patients and their families. It also demonstrates that the helpless feelings nurses sometimes experience as a result of clinical realities that are devastating and sad do not mean that *they* are helpless. Such feelings do not mean that nothing more can be done. The clinical reality of Tony's injuries was not altered, but the emotional pain that Tony's father was experiencing was shared by this nurse. The fact that nurses do encounter situations of human suffering means they cannot avoid it. Not only must nurses face such realities but also, on a personal and professional level, they need to learn how to make contact with people who are experiencing human pain and suffering. Being with patients in a manner that is wholly human and caring is more than just something that can be done. It may be everything.

## The nature of the patient–nurse relationship

Many professions involve the ability to interact with and relate to people. In fact, good interpersonal skills are needed for successful employment across a range of disciplines. In this respect, nursing is not unique. What differs in the nursing context is what qualifies as 'effective' within the sphere of patient interaction. 'Effective' in the nursing care context refers to interpersonal interactions between nurses and patients that are helpful to patients. In effective patient–nurse interactions, there is an orientation on the part of the nurse to be of benefit to the patient and, more importantly, the patient feels assisted in some way by the interaction.

The helpful nature of effective patient–nurse interactions is important to bear in mind because effective interaction in other contexts would have other meanings and orientations. For example, an effective interaction in the world of business sales is oriented towards company profit. While assisting the customer is important to successful ongoing interactions, the intention of the sales interaction is the exchange of money for goods and services. Furthermore, customers in a sales transaction are not vulnerable; they are not dependent on the salesperson for their wellbeing. People in need of healthcare are often not in such a position – they are vulnerable. Nurses are in a prime position to reduce patient vulnerability.

Nurses are able to reduce patient vulnerability when they operate from a position of 'being for' the patient; that is, they need to function as a useful resource in reducing distress and suffering. 'Being for' patients reflects an attitude and a value; it is a moral positioning on the part of the nurse, a commitment and a promise to embody caring. Such positioning is an imperative in nursing practice (Watson 2011). An attitude of 'being for' patients is how nurses demonstrate they care.

The act of aligning oneself alongside another person in an attempt to help or be of assistance – in this case, to nurse – helps to distinguish that interpersonal relationship from other social relationships such as friendships. True friends meet each other's needs on a regular basis and reciprocate in giving and receiving. In addition, they expect to remain friends for life. The patient–nurse relationship is usually time-limited and more one-way, with the nurse being there 'for' the patient. The focus of the nurse's interest in the person who is the patient is for the sake of the patient's wellbeing. While nursing can be an extremely rewarding profession, professional nurses do not use their relationships with patients to meet their own needs.

Making explicit the beneficial aspects of the interpersonal interventions (i.e. helping patients by talking and relating to them) is an attempt to move away from nursing care that is predominantly task-oriented to that which is holistic, personalised care. Such care is contingent on knowing more about a patient than simply a diagnostic category or an anticipated clinical pathway.

Sometimes nurses become so accustomed to the routine of healthcare that they treat patients in a routine manner. They treat patients as objects and fail to demonstrate an appreciation that, to patients, illness and health are not routine matters – they are highly personal and often significant. When nurses demonstrate understanding of the personal and unique experiences of patients, they are therapeutically connecting on an interpersonal level.

Consider the following story, told by a patient.

## A Patient's Story

As I awaited my coronary bypass surgery I was filled with mixed emotions. I was pleased that technological advances in healthcare enabled such surgery to be performed, but at the same time I was worried about the outcome. When the surgeons explained the surgical procedure, they did so with a detail that I appreciated. Everything I wanted to know had been covered, and they answered each of my questions with patience and complete explanations. But I could still see that to them the procedure was routine. They had successfully completed hundreds, even thousands, of these procedures and approached the explanations with a matter-of-fact manner that would be expected with such familiarity. But, to me, the surgery could never be routine.

After they left my hospital room, the nurse who was caring for me that day, Jan, came in to see me. I had come to know and trust Jan during my stay in hospital. She had been present as the surgical team explained what was to happen during the bypass procedure. Jan also had many years of experience in caring for patients who were undergoing coronary bypass surgery.

I had a few more questions that Jan answered with knowledge and detail. She then sat down next to my bed and explained that sometimes patients need more than factual details. Sometimes, she said, they also have fears related to the surgery that cannot be allayed through information alone. She asked me if I had any fears.

Because I knew and trusted Jan, I told her my greatest fear was becoming a cripple, unable to care for myself and function as an independent person. Some of the possible complications that the surgeons reviewed led me to believe that this was a possibility. I was surprised at how freely the words came out, because I am not a person who discusses feelings easily, especially when these feelings are related to my fears. Obviously, I had some fears and Jan's concern and interest helped me to express them. I told her that I was not afraid of dying, only afraid of living half a life following the surgery.

She understood what I was telling her. She didn't try to alleviate my fears by offering me statistics about the probability of my becoming a cripple. The surgeons had already presented the statistics. There is not much consolation in knowing that there is a 10 per cent chance of this complication or a five per cent chance of that complication. Although I was somewhat reassured in hearing these facts, how was I to know whether I'd be the 90 per cent or the 10 per cent?

Instead of focusing on further details, Jan just listened to me. And she demonstrated to me that she understood. When my daughter came to visit me that evening I relayed my conversation with Jan to her. I told my daughter how impressed I was with the fact that Jan initiated this discussion with me. Talking about my interaction with Jan provided an opportunity for me to discuss my fears with my daughter, who also listened and understood. Without the trigger from Jan, I'm not sure I would have discussed my feelings with my daughter. My daughter demonstrated the same level of supportive understanding as Jan. We both felt relieved and a bit closer that evening.

Contrast the above story with the following, also told by a patient.

## A Patient's Story

When Therese entered my hospital room that morning I had the feeling the day wasn't going to be all that pleasant. She had the manner of an army drill sergeant, moving quickly from patient to patient, not asking how our night had been or how we were feeling. She was one of those nurses who was focused on what she was doing as if we, the patients in that room, were superfluous to her mission. Had she bothered to ask, or even notice the expression on my face, she would have realised how awful the previous night had been for me. I had not slept or even rested for that matter. I could not find a comfortable position in bed because the pain in my hip seemed to be getting worse.

My hip had been badly broken in a car accident six days earlier. When the surgeons described how they repaired my hip, it sounded like carpentry work to me. There were metal pins, screws and plates used to repair and strengthen what would now be a weak part of my body. The pain in my hip was excruciating. During the 21 years of my life, I had not experienced anything like it. In fact, I can hardly recall ever being sick.

The nurses in hospital seemed to come in two varieties – the ones who were sympathetic and understanding about my pain, and the ones who treated me like a sook when I complained. Therese seemed like the latter type. She briskly attended to the other patients in the room before coming to me. I had the feeling she was going to make a big deal about having a shower right now. She did. As she approached me she said, 'Now it's your turn, young man. Time to get up. Let's go.'

I tried to be pleasant when I asked her to let me have my shower after morning tea. I explained that the pain medication I had received earlier was starting to take effect and I wanted to relax and rest awhile before getting out of bed. But Therese was not open to any negotiation on the shower time. She told me that I had to get up and get going now. 'Part of the treatment,' she said. She offered no explanation about why the shower had to be now, only that now is what she expected. I felt angry and frustrated but knew better than to try to talk her out of her plans for me. She was in control. She did not seem to care about me.

In the first patient story, Jan demonstrated that she understood what her patient was experiencing in relation to his impending surgery. Jan showed that she knew his impending surgery was more than just another statistic or a routine event. He was facing a major event in his life, and she was there to understand what this event might mean to him. She was concerned about the patient as a person.

In the second story, Therese failed to take an individual patient's needs into account. Had Therese listened to this patient and explored his reasons for wanting to delay the shower, she might have understood his request. Instead she alienated him and gave the impression of only caring about what *she* believed was best.

Not only did she fail to negotiate care with the patient but she also contributed to his distress and suffering. In doing so, she increased his vulnerability.

An attitude of 'being for' the patient means that nurses will take time to listen and understand the patient's experience. In addition to such empathic understanding, this type of relationship will reduce or resolve difficulties being experienced by those in need of help. Finally, a helping relationship will enable the person in need to cope with the demands placed on them by difficult situations.

As such, a helping relationship between a nurse and a patient is based on shared understanding – alignment that enables them to engage in mutual endeavours. In this sense, relating to patients assists nurses in their clinical decision making because of the importance of 'knowing the patient', a central aspect of sound clinical judgments that are *in the interest* of the patient.

## Knowing the patient

In making clinical decisions about care, nurses take into account different sources of knowledge and different ways of knowing. For example, knowledge about pathophysiology assists nurses in knowing what to do when patients are recovering from abdominal surgery. In addition to knowledge in areas such as anatomy and physiology, nurses need to take into account how individual patients are responding as they recover from surgery. In synthesising results of field studies in a variety of nursing care settings, Liaschenko and Fisher (1999) have differentiated three different types of knowledge that nurses use in their work. These knowledge types assist in understanding the importance of relating to patients.

The first of these knowledge types is 'case knowledge'. This knowledge is generalised and objective and includes areas such as the knowledge of anatomy, physiology, physical disease processes and pharmacology. Such knowledge is based on statistics and probabilities of the clinical situation. Nurses need not necessarily interact with patients in order to use this knowledge. They can understand the biomechanics of a myocardial infarction without ever seeing a patient who has experienced one.

The second type of knowledge in Liaschenko and Fisher's schema is central to nursing work. Referred to as 'patient knowledge', it is the knowledge of how individual patients are responding to their clinical situations. This knowledge enables nurses to negotiate the care of patients within a healthcare system. This type of knowing is based on understanding what individual patients are experiencing and therefore requires interaction between the nurse and the patient. That is, nurses need interpersonal skills to understand a patient's response to the clinical situation at hand.

A third type of knowledge identified by Liaschenko and Fisher involves an understanding of the unique individuality of the patient, knowing the patient's personal and private biography and understanding how that person's actions make sense for them. It is 'person knowledge'.

The types of knowledge that are used in nursing will vary with clinical contexts. For instance, therapeutic relationships formed in a palliative care setting will often bring *person knowledge* to the foreground. In an outpatient context where patients are being seen for a routine screening test, *person knowledge* might not be necessary. For example, in a study conducted in an outpatient endoscopy clinic, nurses identified knowing the patient in a practical sense such as their immediate concerns about the procedure they were about to undergo (Bundgaard et al 2012). It is not always desirable or necessary for nurses to enter into the personal and intimate aspects of a patient's life (i.e. to have *person knowledge*). Such entry may even be intrusive or coercive. However, knowing how individual patients are responding to their state of health and healthcare (*patient knowledge*) is essential in all clinical contexts of nursing.

A combination of *patient knowledge* and *person knowledge* encompass what is identified in the nursing literature as the concept of 'knowing the patient' (Bundgaard et al 2012; Mantzorou & Mastrogiannis 2011; Zolnierek 2014). Broadly speaking, the concept refers to a process whereby nurses are able to treat a patient as an individual person because they know something about them. 'Knowing the patient' means that nurses are able to create relationships based on understanding of the patient's point of view and therefore is central to patient-centred care.

## Caring and the patient–nurse relationship

Much of what is said and written about the patient–nurse relationship rests on the assumption that the nature of the relationship is helpful – that is, patients are assisted in some way through their interpersonal interactions with nurses. One explanation of the notion of 'being helpful' is found in the concept of caring.

Since the time of Nightingale (1859) caring has been characterised as the essence of nursing (Andersson, Willman et al 2015). Understanding the theoretical construct of caring is akin to understanding nursing itself. This raises a number of questions, not the least of which is the meaning of the word 'caring' in the context of nursing. Quite simply, caring means 'it matters' (Benner & Wrubel 1989).

If a person cares about their car, then what happens to the vehicle matters to them. In the process of caring *about* the vehicle, they will also care *for* it (e.g. by keeping it tuned and running smoothly). To understand a person's care, it is useful to consider *why* they care (i.e. the motivation to care). The motivation to care may be because the machine is their sole means of transportation, or it may be because the car is a symbol that boosts the owner's sense of self and identity. Attention to the motivation to care in nursing is important to consider, especially in relation to the need for reflection and self-understanding (see Ch 3). Nurses who care because it helps them to increase their self-concept run the risk of harming others by confusing their own needs with the needs of patients. The self-awareness required to understand this motivation is considered a requisite for caring.

According to Watson (2011), who was one of the first nursing scholars to explore the essence of caring, caring is both instrumental or action-oriented and expressive or feeling-oriented. Instrumental actions include meeting basic needs and providing physical care, while expressive caring is related to recognising and acknowledging the 'personhood' of the patient.

Patients place value on instrumental actions – for example, giving medications on time, notifying medical staff when necessary and explaining what is physically wrong with the patient (Papastavrou et al 2011; Wiechula et al 2016). They consider that nurses' technical competence indicates that they care.

## A Patient's Story

At 20 years of age, I was shocked when I received a diagnosis of cancer. Cancer was something that happened to old people, not young uni students like me. The diagnosis did provide an explanation for my fatigue and lack of usual enthusiasm for life but was one that I was not at all prepared to hear. The good news was that the medical staff thought that the diagnosis had been made early enough in the progress of the disease for there to be a good likelihood of remission. But getting to remission required a series of chemotherapy treatments that not only made me feel incredibly sick and very tired but that also resulted in losing my hair.

My family and friends were incredibly supportive throughout the whole ordeal. So were the majority of the nursing staff. It was one nurse who really upset me by her lack of caring concern for my welfare.

Donna worked in the chemo clinic, and I had only met her fleetingly on previous visits to the clinic. Having chemo required daily visits during each course of treatment. When Donna approached me that morning in order to prepare the intravenous line that would deliver the medication, I noticed that she looked very tired and not 100 per cent well. I overheard her talking to one of her colleagues about her big night the previous evening, as she relayed having too much to drink with her friends in the pub. She was complaining of feeling hungover but came to work nevertheless. She didn't say much to me personally, although she kept talking to her colleagues as she prepared the equipment for me.

It was when she tried to insert the needle that I began to get distressed. Her hands were not that steady as she went about her work. She was fumbling with the equipment. She did not seem to know what she was doing, although I had every reason to believe she was usually a competent nurse. Each attempt to insert the needle was creating more pain and anxiety in me. Side effects of the medications were bad enough. Why did I have to suffer because of this nurse's lack of skill? After three attempts to insert the needle, she called for assistance. My mum and I just looked on in fear. Another nurse came over to the bedside and assisted. Donna laughed about her inability to insert the needle. I didn't see the humour in the situation.

Donna's actions that morning indicated to me that she didn't care. How could she when she did not arrive for work prepared to focus her energy on her patients? I thought to myself that she should have called in sick, rather than expose vulnerable patients to herself that morning. I received my chemo okay that morning but am still angry about Donna's actions. Her behaviour seemed like a lack of caring, and I was not impressed. It's not that I'm a prude; my friends and I enjoy our evenings in the pub. It was that Donna should've realised that she had responsibilities to her patients that morning, and she failed to meet them to the best of her capability.

This story demonstrates that caring involves technical competence; the patient's distress was created by a lack of demonstration of this. But the real reason for the patient's distress in this story was that Donna's technical capacity was compromised that morning by her own state of health and behaviour. In effect, she was not really 'available' to patients that day. To this patient, that meant that she did not care.

Caring cannot be understood as compassion and concern while ignoring physical aspects of nursing. This sentiment was expressed well many years ago by Roach (1985, p. 172), who said:

> *While competence without compassion can be brutal and inhumane, compassion without competence may be no more than meaningless, if not harmful, intrusion into the life of a person or persons needing help.*

## Interpersonal skills and caring

The material in this book is concerned with the expressive aspect of caring and the interpersonal skills that are needed for this aspect of nursing to be fully realised. Swanson's (1993) theory of nursing as 'informed caring' provides a useful framework for these interpersonal skills. Swanson claimed that caring occurs in every patient–nurse relationship when that nurse is committed to the wellbeing of the patient (Wojnar 2017). She outlined five processes that are involved in this relationship. The patient–nurse relationship is discussed in full in Chapter 2, and each process of Swanson's theory directly relates to the interpersonal skills outlined in other chapters of this book, as illustrated in Table 1.1.

The first of these processes is a philosophical grounding of nursing in an inherent belief in people. This is enhanced through self-awareness and reflection, which is emphasised in Chapter 3. Once 'grounded' in this philosophical stance, nurses 'anchor' their caring through striving to know patients and understand the meaning that they attach to health events, the second process. This is achieved by

### TABLE 1.1 Processes of informed caring and related interpersonal skills

| PROCESSES OF INFORMED CARING (SWANSON 1993) | INTERPERSONAL SKILLS | RELEVANT CHAPTER |
|---|---|---|
| Maintaining belief in people | Self-understanding | Chapter 3 |
| Appreciating personal meanings of health events | Understanding | Chapter 6 |
| | Exploring | Chapter 7 |
| Being with patients | Attending and listening | Chapter 5 |
| Doing for patients | Comforting and supporting | Chapter 8 |
| Enabling patients | Encouraging participation by sharing information and challenging | |

'knowing the patient', introduced in this chapter and fully explored in Chapter 2, and is brought to life through the interpersonal skills of understanding and exploring in Chapters 6 and 7. The third process in the theory of informed caring is enacted by nurses when they are fully present and available to patients through attending and listening. Referred to by Swanson (1993) as 'being with' patients, this process is reviewed in Chapter 5 in the form of attending and listening skills.

Once they are 'with' patients and understand their situation, nurses express their caring through actions that pertain to the final two processes in Swanson's theory, termed 'doing for' patients and 'enabling' patients to do for themselves. Although the process of 'doing for' is predominantly expressed through physical care and skilled clinical performance of nursing care, 'doing for' also includes comforting measures that are achieved through interacting with and relating to patients. Comforting measures and supporting actions are discussed in Chapter 8. Swanson's process of 'enabling' includes having patients participate in their healthcare. Such participation, introduced in this chapter, is contingent on patients' knowledge and understanding of their health status and care. The interpersonal skills needed to inform and assist patients in obtaining this knowledge are also reviewed in Chapter 8.

Although not rigid in the sense that the processes are passed through as stages and phases, there is a sequential aspect to them. For example, 'doing for' requires nurses to understand what must be done (i.e. to understand a patient's frame of reference before attempting to provide psychosocial help).

## Practical know-how in relating to patients

The skills described throughout this book are designed to enable nurses to develop practical know-how in relating to patients. While it is important for nurses to *know that* it is important to communicate with patients, they also must *know how* to do so. The theory of how to relate serves little purpose in the absence of interpersonal skills that promote therapeutic relationships. The skills are techniques that will enable the type of relationships that have been described in this chapter as 'helpful' and 'caring' to develop.

The techniques are presented in a 'micro-skills' manner, meaning they are broken down into component parts. Learning the techniques is supported by experiential activities interspersed throughout the text. This style of presentation has been influenced by writers in the counselling field such as Egan (2014) and Ivey and Ivey (2010). Describing skills in this way runs the risk of it appearing that they can be applied mechanistically. However, the skills cannot be used in such a prescriptive manner.

*There are no context-free rules about interacting with patients.* Nurses must consider a host of variables when they make contact with patients. Sometimes a discussion about feelings is suitable to the context, while at other times such discussions are inappropriate. Throughout this book, guidelines and theory about how to establish interpersonal contact with patients are presented. However, each interaction, like each patient and each nurse, will be unique and dynamic in its own right.

# SUMMARY

Taking the time and expending the effort to understand the world as the patient experiences it results in nursing care that integrates the patient's experiences. The most effective way to review the material that has been presented in this chapter is through the following nurse's story, which illustrates the art and science of nursing relationships. It was told by an experienced nurse who was recollecting her time as a student of nursing.

## A Nurse's Story

I was in my second undergraduate year at university when I met Margaret. We met during my clinical placement at a large public healthcare facility that was established to provide rehabilitation services for people with a disability or who were chronically ill. There were more than a thousand patients in this facility, and the sheer mass of this humanity hit me like a tonne of bricks on the first day. We were taken on a grand tour of the entire facility on that day and told that the average age of the residents was 72. It was 'so young', we were told, because there were a few patients in their 30s and 40s who were suffering from progressive conditions such as multiple sclerosis. To me the place looked like an enormous nursing home.

Although I had an overview of all patients who lived in this facility, I only came to recognise the 50 who lived in the ward to which I was assigned, and one of these patients became well known to me.

Margaret caught my attention on that first day I was on the ward. She was a frail-looking lady who sat in a wheelchair the entire day, being transported from bed to dining table and back to bed at various times during the day. Margaret captured my attention because she kept repeating the same phrase over and over again. 'Why am I being chastised?' she kept saying. The word 'chastise' struck me as quaint and curious, as if it was a relic from a bygone era. I had to look in a dictionary to find its meaning. Once I discovered the meaning of the word, I became intrigued by Margaret's thought that she was being punished. 'Punished for what?' I thought. What is making Margaret feel she is being punished? I thought to myself that being a permanent resident of this facility could be perceived as punishment, but there was more than this in Margaret's experience.

I set out to learn more about Margaret. It didn't take long for me to get to know her. The fact that I was willing to sit and listen to her was sufficient to establish a rapport. During the two days a week I spent on the ward, I sat next to her and listened, mostly to her thoughts about being punished. For what, I still did not know. I accepted her feelings, although in the back of my mind there were nagging thoughts about the reason for them.

Whenever we talked, I couldn't get past her expression of the feeling that she was being chastised, so I went to the records to learn more about her. There I saw the words 'legally blind' and 'nearly deaf'. I began to wonder how much sensory input Margaret was receiving and how much this was contributing to her feelings. I located material in my textbooks that described the possible effects of reduced sensory input (in Margaret's case, near blindness and near deafness). I learnt that one of these effects is suspicious feelings.

I also discussed Margaret with the regular staff working in the ward. They told me that Margaret was a 'bit crazy' and 'definitely paranoid'. Because I thought there was more to Margaret than her suspicion, labelling her as paranoid didn't satisfy me. Although the label of 'paranoid' seemed insufficient to me, I could see how easily such a label could dismiss Margaret's reality. I still wanted to learn more about Margaret and only she could help me to do so. Week after week I came to Margaret, sat next to her, expressed my interest in her and then just listened.

Eventually, Margaret began to share with me more than just her feelings of being punished. We talked about her family and discussed other things. I learnt more about Margaret, beyond her paranoia. I think me just being there – showing interest in her and listening to her – was enough to enable her to open up and share her thoughts. As I listened to Margaret's story, I began to piece together bits of what she said.

She mentioned that when she entered the facility her handbag had been taken away and put into a room somewhere. She often spoke of the handbag and the room where it was held. I began to realise that the handbag was significant. I asked, 'What's in the handbag?' She told me it contained a card that had her nephew's address written on it. Her nephew, who lived in the next state, was her only living relative. Margaret's husband had died and so had all her brothers and sisters. She had no children. Her nephew was her only link with her family and she didn't have his address! Margaret wanted desperately to write to this nephew but couldn't.

Through my perseverance and with the aid of my clinical instructor, I located the room that held Margaret's possessions. They had been taken from her when she was admitted and placed for 'safe keeping' in this room. Fortunately, I was able to retrieve the handbag and, sure enough, inside was a card from her nephew that was sent to her shortly before Margaret entered the facility. Margaret was ecstatic about the find. With it came the possibility of re-establishing contact with her family. I penned Margaret's words to her nephew and made sure the letter was posted to him. Margaret seemed to settle after this, although she continued to complain about being punished and I continued to wonder why this feeling persisted.

While the contact with her nephew had helped to calm Margaret, she remained quite anxious about being in this facility. So I kept listening. One day she mentioned that sitting near the window hurt her eyes. Her diminishing eyesight was the result of cataracts and the bright summer sun through the window created discomfort for her. Each day after lunch she was wheeled to the window to 'enjoy the sunshine'. But instead of enjoying this afternoon ritual, Margaret found the experience quite uncomfortable. Could this be perceived by Margaret as punishment? I explored my hunch with Margaret, directing my questions towards the subject of her daily seating near the window. She confirmed my hunch. In Margaret's mind, the afternoon ritual of being placed in the sun was equivalent to a daily punishment. For what reason, she was not certain. But in her mind she thought it was because she had done something wrong and this was punishment for the transgression. With this revelation came my understanding of Margaret's reality. Her feelings of being punished made more sense to me.

My next plan of action was to try to get the other staff on the ward to appreciate Margaret's experience. I spoke with the nursing staff and they realised what was happening to her. They agreed that placing her in direct contact with the sunshine was counterproductive to what was intended by the move. Placing her near the sun, but not in its direct path, would still help her. No longer would Margaret be placed in the direct sunlight.

When it came close to the time that I would be leaving the placement, I could hardly contain my feelings of sadness. Saying goodbye to Margaret was going to be difficult for me. When the time finally came to do so, Margaret reached into her 'newly found' handbag, pulled out an embroidered handkerchief and placed it in my hand. 'Here,' she said, 'this is for you.' In the back of my mind I recalled the warnings I had heard about accepting gifts from patients. I ignored the warnings, placed the handkerchief in the pocket of my uniform and thanked Margaret. We had shared a special understanding and the handkerchief became a symbol of this understanding. I cherished this gift because it served as a reminder of the importance of being interested in patients, listening to and accepting their reality and, most importantly, understanding their experiences.

The nurse in this story demonstrated concern and compassion for Margaret. In addition, she came to know Margaret as a case, a patient and a person. She used understanding that generated from case knowledge when she connected Margaret's feelings with her sensory deprivation through loss of vision. She had learnt in her studies that derogatory labels such as 'paranoid' could lead to nurses rejecting and ignoring patients. This is an example of patient knowledge because Margaret's behaviour is viewed in the social context of healthcare organisations. She came also to know the person who was Margaret. Through understanding that contact with her family mattered to Margaret, this nurse came to know something of Margaret's life value system.

Her relationship with Margaret enabled this nurse to feel the sadness that Margaret was experiencing in relation to the loss of contact with her family. She also felt empathic understanding of Margaret's feeling of being punished. She then went one step further and functioned, with the aid of her clinical supervisor, as a useful resource for Margaret in locating her family contact details.

In this final sense they both functioned as advocates for Margaret by working through an organisational system that disabled Margaret from contacting her relatives. Although still a student, this nurse functioned with professional autonomy and responsibility because she had come to know the person who is the patient. And she made a difference as a result.

# REFERENCES

Andersson, Å., Frank, C., Willman, A.M.L., et al., 2015. Adverse events in nursing: a retrospective study of reports of patient and relative experiences. Int. Nurs. Rev. 62, 377–385.

Andersson, E.K., Willman, A., Sjöström-Strand, A., 2015. Registered nurses' descriptions of caring: a phenomenographic interview study. BMC Nurs. 14, 16. (open access). doi:10.1186/s12912-015-0067-9.

Angel, S., Frederiksen, K.N., 2015. Challenges in achieving patient participation: a review of how patient participation is addressed in empirical studies. Int. J. Nurs. Stud. 52, 1525–1538.

Australian Commission on Safety and Quality in Health Care, 2011. Patient centred care: Improving quality and safety through partnerships with patients and consumers, ACSQHC, Sydney.

Benner, P., 1984. From Novice to Expert: Excellence and Power in Clinical Nursing Practice. Addison-Wesley, Menlo Park, CA.

Benner, P., Wrubel, J., 1989. The Primacy of Caring: Stress and Coping in Health and Illness. Addison-Wesley, Menlo Park, CA.

Bridges, J., Nicholson, C., Maben, J., et al., 2013. Capacity for care: meta-ethnography of acute care nurses' experiences of the nurse-patient relationship. J. Adv. Nurs. 69 (4), 760–772.

Bundgaard, D., Nielsen, K.B., Delmar, C., et al., 2012. What to know and how to get to know? A fieldwork study outlining the understanding of knowing the patient in facilities for short-term stay. J. Adv. Nurs. 68 (10), 2280–2288.

Castro, E.M., Van Regenmortel, T., Vanhaecht, K., et al., 2016. Patient empowerment, patient participation and patient-centeredness in hospital care: a concept analysis based on a literature review. Patient Educ. Couns. Online. Available at: http://dx.doi.org/10.1016/j.pec.2016.07.026. (Accessed 24 July 2016).

Constand, M.K., MacDermid, J.C., Dal Bello-Haas, V., 2014. Scoping review of patient-centered care approaches in healthcare. BMC Health Serv. Res. 14 (1), 271–280.

DeFrino, D., 2009. A theory of the relational work of nurses. Res. Theory Nurs. Pract. 23 (4), 294–311.

Dierckx de Casterlé, B., 2015. Realising skilled companionship in nursing: a utopian idea or difficult challenge? J. Clin. Nurs. 24, 3327–3335.

Doyle, C., Lennox, L., Bell, D., 2013. A systematic review of evidence on the links between patient experience and clinical safety and effectiveness. BMJ Open 3, e001570. doi:10.1136/bmjopen-2012001570.

Egan, G., 2014. The Skilled Helper, tenth ed. Brooks/Cole, Belmont CA.

Feo, R., Kitson, A., 2016. Promoting patient-centred fundamental care in acute healthcare systems. Int. J. Nurs. Stud. 57, 1–11.

Hudon, C., St-Cyr Tribble, D., Bravo, G., 2011. Enablement in health care context: a concept analysis. J. Eval. Clin. Pract. 17, 143–149.

Ivey, A., Ivey, M., 2010. Intentional Interviewing and Counselling, seventh ed. Brooks/Cole, Pacific Grove, CA.

Kitson, A., Marshall, A., Bassett, K., et al., 2013. What are the core elements of patient-centred care? A narrative review and synthesis of the literature from health policy, medicine and nursing. J. Adv. Nurs. 69 (1), 4–15.

Liaschenko, J., Fisher, A., 1999. Theorizing the knowledge that nurses use in the conduct of their work. Sch. Inq. Nurs. Pract. An International Journal 13 (1), 29–41.

Mantzorou, M., Mastrogiannis, D., 2011. The value and significance of knowing the patient for professional practice according to the Carper's pattern of knowing. Health Sci. J. 5 (4), 251–261.

Mavis, B., Rovner, M.H., Jorgenson, S., et al., 2015. Patient participation in clinical encounters: a systematic review to identify self-report measures. Health Expect. 18, 1827–1843.

Newell, S., Jordan, Z., 2015. The patient experience of patient-centered communication with nurses in the hospital setting: a qualitative systematic review protocol. JBI Database System. Rev. Implement. Rep. 13 (1), 76–87.

Nightingale, F., 1859. Notes on Nursing: What It Is and What It Is Not. Reprinted 1992. Lippincott, Philadelphia, PA. originally published by Harrison & Son, London.

Nursing and Midwifery Board of Australia, 2008. Code of professional conduct for nurses in Australia. Nursing and Midwifery Board of Australia, Melbourne. Online. Available at: www.nursingmidwiferyboard.gov.au/Codes-Guidelines-Statements/Codes-Guidelines.aspx#competencystandards. (Accessed 24 July 2016).

Nursing and Midwifery Board of Australia, 2016. Registered nurse standards for practice. Nursing and Midwifery Board of Australia, Melbourne. Online. Available at: http://www.nursingmidwiferyboard.gov.au/Codes-Guidelines-Statements/Professional-standards.aspx. (Accessed 24 July 2016).

Nursing Council of New Zealand, 2007. Competencies for registered nurses. Nursing Council of New Zealand, Wellington. Online. Available at: http://www.nursingcouncil.org.nz/Publications/Standards-and-guidelines-for-nurses. (Accessed 24 July 2016).

Nursing Council of New Zealand, 2009. Code of conduct for registered nurses. Nursing Council of New Zealand, Wellington. Online. Available at: http://www.nursingcouncil.org.nz/Publications/Standards-and-guidelines-for-nurses. (Accessed 24 July 2016).

Olsson, L., Jakobsson Ung, E., Swedberg, K., et al., 2013. Efficacy of person-centred care as an intervention in controlled trials – a systematic review. J. Clin. Nurs. 22, 456–465.

Papastavrou, E., Efstathiou, G., Charalambous, A., 2011. Nurses' and patients' perceptions of caring behaviours: quantitative systematic review of comparative studies. J. Adv. Nurs. 67 (6), 1191–1205.

Parsons, T., 1951/1987. Illness and the role of the physicians: a sociological perspective. In: Stoeckle, J.D. (Ed.), Encounters Between Patients and Doctors: An Anthology. MIT Press, Cambridge, MA, pp. 147–156.

Pavlish, C., Hunt, R., 2012. An exploratory study about meaningful work in acute care nursing. Nurs. Forum 47 (2), 113–122.

Pelletier, L.R., Stichler, J.F., 2013. Action brief: patient engagement and activation: a health reform imperative and improvement opportunity for nursing. Nurs. Outlook 61, 51–54.

Peplau, H., 1952/1988. Interpersonal Relations in Nursing. Macmillan, London. originally published by GP Putnam and Sons.

Peterson, S.J., 2017. Interpersonal relations. In: Peterson, S.A., Bredow, T.S. (Eds.), Middle Range Theories: Application to Nursing Research and Practice. Wolters Kluwer, Philadelphia PA, pp. 147–163.

Rathert, C., Williams, E.S., McCaughey, D., et al., 2012. Patient perceptions of patient-centred care: empirical test of a theoretical model. Health Expect. 18, 199–209.

Rathert, C., Wyrwich, M.D., Boren, S.A., 2012. Patient-centered care and outcomes: a systematic review of the literature. Med. Care Res. Rev. 70 (4), 351–379.

Roach, S.M., 1985. A foundation for nursing ethics. In: Carmi, A., Schneider, S. (Eds.), Nursing Law and Ethics. Springer-Verlag, Berlin, pp. 170–177.

Roch, G., Dubois, C., Clarke, S.P., 2014. Organizational climate and hospital nurses' caring practices: a mixed-methods study. Res. Nurs. Health 37, 229–240.

Ross, H., Tod, A.M., Clarke, A., 2014. Understanding and achieving person-centred care: the nurse perspective. J. Clin. Nurs. 24, 1223–1233.

Sharma, T., Bamford, M., Dodman, D., 2015. Person-centred care: an overview of reviews. Contemp. Nurse 51 (2–3), 107–120.

Sheridan, N.F., Kenealy, T.W., Kidd, J.D., 2015. Patients' engagement in primary care: powerlessness and compounding jeopardy: a qualitative study. Health Expect. 18, 32–43.

Sidani, S., Fox, M., 2014. Patient-centered care: clarification of its specific elements to facilitate interprofessional care. J. Interprof. Care 28 (2), 134–141.

Snyder, H., Engström, J., 2016. The antecedents, forms and consequences of patient involvement: a narrative review of the literature. Int. J. Nurs. Stud. 53, 351–378.

Swanson, K., 1993. Nursing as informed caring for the well-being of others. J. Nurs. Scholarsh. 25, 352–357.

Tobiano, G., Bucknall, T., Marshall, A., et al., 2015. Patient participation in nursing care on medical wards: an integrative review. Int. J. Nurs. Stud. 52, 1107–1120.

Tobiano, G., Bucknall, T., Marshall, A., et al., 2016. Patients' perceptions of participation in nursing care on medical wards. Scand. J. Caring Sci. 30, 260–270.

Travelbee, J., 1971. Interpersonal Aspects of Nursing, second ed. FA Davis, Philadelphia, PA.

Watson, J., 2011. Human Caring Science: A Theory of Nursing, second ed. Jones and Barlett Learning, Sudbury MA.

Wiechula, R., Conroy, T., Kitson, A.L., et al., 2016. Umbrella review of the evidence: what factors influence the caring relationship between a nurse and patient? J. Adv. Nurs. 72 (4), 723–734.

Wojnar, D.M., 2017. Caring. In: Peterson, S.A., Bredow, T.S. (Eds.), Middle Range Theories: Application to Nursing Research and Practice. Wolters Kluwer, Philadelphia PA, pp. 136–146.

Zolnierek, C.D., 2014. An integrative review of knowing the patient. J. Nurs. Scholarsh. 46 (1), 3–10.

# The patient–nurse relationship

## CHAPTER OVERVIEW

- Professional relationships in nursing are helpful to the person who is the patient when they are based on mutual understanding and collaboration.

- Professional relationships differ from social relationships.

- Central aspects of the professional relationships include interpersonal distance versus involvement, superficiality versus therapeutic intimacy, and mutuality and reciprocity.

- Professional relationships vary in their degree of commitment and involvement and are negotiated between a patient and a nurse.

- Trust between patients and nurses is essential.

- As professional relationships progress, there are critical issues in each stage of relationship development.

# INTRODUCTION

The skills described in the following chapters offer nurses a range of alternatives when interacting with patients. The skills of listening, understanding and exploring are not ends in themselves but useful ways to establish and build relationships between patients and nurses. Using such skills effectively increases the possibility that patients and nurses will connect and relate in meaningful ways. These skills enable nurses to understand patients' experiences. Operating from within patients' experiences enhances the possibility that nursing interventions will be individualised and context-specific, as opposed to mechanical, procedural or task-oriented.

Technical proficiency in skill use holds no guarantee that skills will be used in ways that are beneficial to patients. A view that skills can be used merely as techniques applied in a rational, objective manner loses an essential element – that the skills only make sense when viewed within the subjective reality of a relationship between two human beings: patient and nurse. When viewed as techniques, devoid of the subjective experience of the relationship, interpersonal skills lose their most crucial quality – that they are relational and context-bound.

General guidelines for appropriately using each skill are presented in the following chapters, but these guidelines may not provide enough direction for nurses as they try to determine which skill is most fitting under a given set of circumstances. This is because the 'best' approach can be determined only within the context of the relationship between a patient and a nurse. No single response is ever correct in itself; no magical formula can be applied out of this context.

Nurses' personal styles; personality factors of both patient and nurse; the patient's immediate situation and their perception of it; how patients are responding to nurses; and how nurses are responding to patients – these are but a few of the contextual variables that need to be considered when determining the 'best' way to respond helpfully to patients. It is through direct involvement in the relationship ('being there') that nurses can develop appropriate responses. There is no available blueprint for skill use.

# CHARACTERISTICS OF HELPFUL PATIENT-NURSE RELATIONSHIPS

A basic contribution that nurses make to positive patient outcomes is through engaging in responsive, trusting and helpful relationships with patients (Charalambous et al 2016; Lasiter & McLennon 2015). This is because the main intention of interacting with patients and forming helpful relationships is to influence the health status and wellbeing of patients (Evans 2016; Fleischer et al 2009). As such, relationships are therapeutic when they are beneficial to patients.

No single explanation could possibly capture the rich and complex nature of the relationships between patients and nurses. Each relationship is distinct because both patient and nurse are distinctive, and the way they interact and relate is unique. Each participant brings particular experiences to the relationship. Rather than imposing artificial limits by specifying a definition of the relationship, various facets of the patient–nurse relationship are described here.

## Social versus professional relationships

When the suggestion is made to beginning nurses that they are 'to be professional' in their relationships with patients, they sometimes state a preference 'to be friends' with patients. In saying this, these nurses could be revealing a desire to remain in the comfortable and familiar arena of social relationships, where the rules for relating are predictable. It may also be that an emphasis on problem solving and goal setting (two processes often considered to be 'professional') contributes to the preference for 'being friends'. A common distinction made between the social relationships of friendship and professional relationships is that the professional relationship is goal-directed. Fears of 'not knowing what to do' and anxieties about 'How can I help to solve patients' problems?', especially when such problems seem overwhelming, are logical responses to being asked to form professional relationships with patients.

The most likely reason for the expressed desire 'to be friends' with patients, as contrasted to being professional, probably emanates from a preconceived notion that 'to be professional' is to be distant, detached, aloof and cool. This aura of the professional stance – that of the detached observer who also has the answers – involves expectations that these nurses may be unwilling to accept. Being professional is sometimes equated with denying or abandoning the personal, human side of the nurse. These beginning nurses could be saying, 'How can I leave myself behind when I interact with patients?'.

Nurses do not, and cannot, leave themselves behind when they enter the healthcare setting, but neither are they there to be friends with patients, in the strictest sense of the word. This is not to say that nurses cannot be friendly, sociable and personable with patients, or that professional relationships do not have similarities with social relationships. Nevertheless, professional relationships are different from other types of personal relationships, such as friendship.

Some of the ways that social relationships differ from professional relationships include the following: the nurse usually initiates the professional relationship with patients; there are time and space limits to professional relationships, in that they do not go on for life; and interactions are confined to a particular setting, be it a hospital setting or a patient's home. The final, and perhaps the most significant, difference is that patient–nurse relationships are formed with a focus on the needs of one of the participants only – the patient. Nurses are expected to meet their own needs for social contact, inclusion and affection outside of their relationships with patients. This is not to say that these needs might not be met through relationships with patients but more to emphasise that the relationships are not used as the primary source of nurses' social-need fulfilment. These differences between social and professional relationships are summarised in Table 2.1.

| TABLE 2.1 Differences between social and professional relationships | | |
| --- | --- | --- |
| **DIMENSION** | **SOCIAL** | **PROFESSIONAL** |
| Length of time | Unlimited | Limited |
| Focus of concern | Two-way and equal Shared focus on both self and the other person | One-way and unilateral Nurse shifts focus from self to the patient |
| Intensity of emotion | Unlimited expression of emotions | Emotions may be felt but their expression is limited to concern about how to help |
| Perspective | Subjective personal feelings are expressed and shared | Objective personal feelings are not expressed but rather used as a means of reflecting how to help |

## Differences in focus, intensity and perspective

In a seminal work, Gadow (1980) offered a philosophical analysis that is useful in differentiating personal and professional relationships by describing these differences in terms of focus, intensity and perspective.

In professional relationships, the nurse's focus of concern is away from self and towards the other – the patient. Emotions are expressed and genuine feelings of distress for the patient's situation are felt (as in social relationships), but these emotions are not expressed by nurses for the purpose of obtaining relief or attention from patients. Nurses' concern and interest remain for the patient. There is no expectation that the patient is concerned about the nurse's wellbeing, as would be the case in a social relationship. In friendships, there is equal concern; in a professional relationship, the concern is one-sided and focused on the patient.

In addition, the intensity of the situation is experienced differently in personal and professional relationships. In professional relationships, nurses may become emotionally roused and feel the patient's concern, distress or sense of urgency. Therefore, nurses may experience emotional intensity along with the patient in a given situation, but they do so in a reflective manner rather than the immediate way that patients experience emotions (Gadow 1980). The reflective nature of nurses' experiences means that nurses use their experience of patients' distress as a way of considering what would be of help to patients. Nurses integrate the experience of feeling patients' distress with their knowledge of how to be of help. Helping to alleviate patients' distress is why nurses share and experience patients' distress. In personal relationships, more value is placed on sharing experiences than helping (Gadow 1980).

The final difference in Gadow's analysis is that of perspective. The professional maintains an objectivity that is impossible for friends to sustain. While objectivity does not equate with distance and lack of connection with the patient, it does relate to the one-sided nature or focus of these relationships. That is, in professional relationships, nurses remain focused on patients rather than on their own subjective experiences. This is not to say that nurses should disregard their own subjective experiences, but rather the significance of these experiences is placed in the context of how it affects the patient and the relationship.

Gadow's (1980) emphasis of shifting motivation from the self (the nurse) to the other (the patient) is consistent with the findings of a study into clinicians of various professional groups who are known to be capable of forming compassionate relationships with patients (Graber & Mitcham 2004). These clinicians described levels of interpersonal involvement, from superficial to intimate, on the basis of the degree to which they shifted focus and concern from themselves to the patient. Increasing focus of concern for the other, with decreasing concern for the self, was associated with greater levels of involvement and intimacy. This capacity to shift focus from the self, putting the interest of the other ahead of one's own, is considered a central aspect in caring relationships (Noddings 1984).

It is not the level of personal involvement that differentiates friendship from professional relationships but the form and direction of the involvement. The amount of personal involvement in the two types of relationship may be equal. Both types of relationship rely on active demonstration of personal qualities, so the notion that nurses' professional relationships are devoid of their personal selves is rejected. In fact, nurses rely on their personal qualities and style of relating.

This idea challenges the notion that to be professional is to maintain a distanced stance in which nurses share little of their personal selves. By sharing themselves, nurses share their humanity with patients. Experienced clinicians (Graber & Mitcham 2004) do judge the 'correct' level of engagement with each patient because not all relationships will reach the same degree of personal involvement. This brings forward the next facet of patient–nurse relationships: interpersonal distance versus involvement.

## Interpersonal distance versus involvement

The very fact that a relationship exists between a patient and a nurse implies a degree of interpersonal involvement, which includes the process of 'knowing the patient' (see Ch 1). Yet nurses are often warned of the dangers of becoming 'emotionally involved' with patients. The warning is based on the notion that a 'professional' demeanour requires emotional detachment in order to maintain objectivity in decision making.

The reasons usually given for warnings about involvement are brought into question by Benner's (1984) seminal research into expert clinical nursing practice. The experts in this study involved themselves with patients by identifying with them and imagining that they or someone they loved was in a similar predicament. Identification invokes involvement in the situation, not as a passive observer but as an active participant. Through identifying with patients, nurses involve themselves in a personal way in patients' experiences. This involvement, of being close to the heart of the situation, enables nurses to notice what is significant and to notice subtle changes in patients. Rather than hampering nurses' clinical judgment, involvement enhances it.

In addition to the need for objective decision making, nurses are also advised of the dangers of involvement with patients because it is perceived that such involvement will result in an emotional draining, leaving nurses unable to cope with the sometimes harsh reality of nursing. Nurses may believe they can protect themselves from hurt, from the emotional aspects of illness and from depletion of their own internal resources through distancing strategies that remove them from the situation emotionally and numb them to the reality of pain and suffering. For many years, interpersonal distancing and lack of involvement has been recognised as a defensive strategy used by nurses in an effort to cope with the distress of nursing (Jourard 1964; Menzies 1961).

When the defensive strategy is removed and efforts to relate are made, nurses do need to be capable of managing their emotional responses to patients' vulnerability and suffering. In remaining focused on the patient, they cannot allow their own emotional responses to dominate a clinical situation. Such management, termed 'emotional' labour, is starting to be recognised as an aspect of nursing work and is reviewed in Chapter 3.

Interestingly, the expert nurses in Benner's study did *not* become drained or depleted by their involvement with patients, but they also had the experience of feeling affirmed and stronger for it (Benner 1984). This is consistent with the clinicians in Graber and Mitcham's (2004) investigation in that interpersonal involvement with patients sustained and supported these clinicians and also helped with treatment efforts. Committed and involved patient–nurse relationships enable nurses to feel professional satisfaction, while patients report feeling confident, secure and satisfied when they form a bond with nurses (Tejero 2012; Turpin et al 2012).

In forming a bond with patients, nurses need to retain a sense of their 'otherness' that keeps their focus on their patients' needs but not at the expense of their own welfare. This requires a determination of the right level of emotional engagement and detachment in their relationships with patients. They must be involved enough to participate – emotionally, spiritually and intellectually – in their relationships with patients, yet remain distanced enough to maintain control and use their involvement to assist patients. In doing so, they set appropriate boundaries in their professional relationships with patients.

## Professional boundaries

There are various types of boundaries in nursing practice that provide a safe space in which nurses can function. First, there are legal boundaries, which specify the scope of nursing practice. For example, unless authorised to do so as a nurse practitioner, prescribing medications is outside the scope of most nursing practice. In addition, there are ethical boundaries of nursing practice that are specified in codes of practice (Nursing and Midwifery Board of Australia 2008; Nursing Council of New Zealand 2009). Boundary violations can carry professional repercussions such as loss of nursing registration.

While codes provide a framework, they may not provide clear answers to dilemmas that might pertain to interpersonal relationships between nurses and

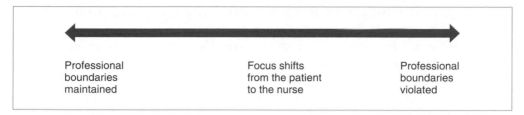

**Figure 2.1** Continuum of professional boundaries

patients. These dilemmas occur when there is a conflict between professional and personal interests. Such dilemmas can result in a boundary violation when left unresolved.

The boundaries that surround the patient–nurse relationship cannot be rule-governed at all times, as their negotiation requires professional judgment. For example, a nurse may choose to disclose a personal experience in the interest of offering the patient hope or reassurance. The judgments are made on the basis of the guiding principle for establishing the relationship – to be of benefit to the patient. Therefore, the standard by which actions should be judged is whether they are in the best interest of the patient. Boundary crossings occur when the focus of concern shifts from the patient to the nurse and are considered along a continuum (Fig. 2.1).

Actions that are obviously harmful to the patient, such as having sexual relationships with nurses while in their care, are clear boundary violations. Actions such as this are considered exploitative because the nurse is satisfying personal needs through the relationship. Boundary crossings, unlike boundary violations, are more difficult to judge. They may not result in any long-term harm to either the patient or the nurse (Holder & Schenthal 2007). There are subtle ways in which nurses may not act in the best interest of the patient, and boundaries are crossed when the needs of the nurse take precedence over the needs of the patient (Hartlage 2012). For example, nurses may disclose their own personal problems to patients in an effort to unburden their own anxieties. Complaining about work conditions to patients can be a boundary crossing if done for the purpose of sparking patient sympathy for nurses' overwork. That is, the motivation is not on benefiting the patient but rather on meeting the nurse's need. When boundaries are violated there is a risk of 'overinvolvement'.

## Overinvolvement

When nurses are overinvolved, they can no longer retain a sense of 'otherness' that enables them to maintain a sense of control. Overinvolved relationships become close personal friendships in which the nurse relinquishes the professional role and the patient relinquishes the patient role. The nurse functions as omnipotent rescuer and leaps in and takes over, assuming the patient's burdens and problems, and failing to perceive the resourcefulness of the patient. In overinvolved relationships, nurses overextend themselves – often to their own personal and professional detriment (Morse 1991). When nurses sacrifice some professional control for the bonds of friendship, they feel less satisfied and less helpful to the patient (Ramos 1992).

It is important for nurses to recognise when they are at risk of overinvolving themselves with patients. Nurses are at risk of overinvolvement when they believe they are the only ones who can help a patient, when they try to 'rescue' patients, when they cannot imagine a relationship with a patient ending and when they feel overextended or overwhelmed by a relationship with a patient.

If overinvolvement does occur, it is equally important to reflect on the situation and learn from the experience (see Ch 3), as most nurses do (Morse 1991). Talking it over with a trusted colleague (Ch 11) not only provides support but also enhances and accelerates learning from the experience.

It does happen that patients and nurses develop into lifelong friends even though their initial meeting was not social in nature. However, if this becomes an everyday occurrence in a nurse's life, it does signal a need for self-reflection (Ch 3). It could indicate that the nurse is unable to focus energy on patients. Nurses who 'make friends' with the majority of patients they meet may be treating their own needs as more important than their patients' needs.

There is an art to knowing what can be offered without an overextension of personal resources. Through reflective practice (Ch 3) and building resilience (Ch 11) nurses learn how to offer what they can without dictating results and with a clear recognition that they are not the only ones who contribute to patients' wellbeing. The key to avoiding overinvolved relationships is not to avoid involvement altogether but rather to find the right kind of involvement. The degree of involvement varies with the type of relationship that is formed between nurses and patients, and these types of relationship are covered later in this chapter.

Issues of social versus professional relationships and distance versus involvement help in bringing forward the next facet of patient–nurse relationships: superficiality versus therapeutic intimacy.

## Superficiality versus therapeutic intimacy

All relationships between patients and nurses begin at a level of superficiality. Relationships at this level are characterised by minimal self-disclosure and focus primarily on 'safe' (non-personal) content areas because there is minimal knowledge and understanding of each other, and trust has yet to be established. Social exchanges and friendly chitchat are common at this level. Having ordinary, everyday-type conversations helps to build the relationship (Wiechula et al 2016).

It is important for nurses to recognise the value of such interactions. Because deep and meaningful interaction is not occurring, they may fail to perceive the relevance of these superficial exchanges. Social interactions are valuable because they are a way for nurses and patients to get to know each other. In fact, patients use social conversation as a way of connecting with nurses and building a relationship (Henderson et al 2007; Turpin et al 2012). Being friendly and informal helps to break down authoritarian barriers sometimes associated with professional roles.

In addition, patients appreciate nurses who are friendly and lighthearted, and act like themselves, rather than enacting a 'role'.

Therapeutically intimate relationships are characterised by a high degree of mutual involvement, trust, acceptance and self-disclosure of a personal nature. Reciprocal self-disclosure is a hallmark of therapeutic intimacy (Graber & Mitcham 2004; Stavropoulou et al 2012). Patients and nurses feel free to share their thoughts, feelings and perceptions when involved in such a relationship. Topics are of a personal nature, feelings are expressed openly and freely, and both nurse and patient are committed to the relationship. However, the extent of self-disclosure is greater for the patient than for the nurse. This is in keeping with the notion that the relationship is formed not for its own purpose but for the aid of the patient. The focus of a therapeutic relationship remains on the patient.

Closely related to the concept of therapeutic intimacy is the concept of trust. Trust implies a willingness to place oneself in a relationship that may increase vulnerability; a trusting person takes a risk in self-disclosure on the understanding that the other person will behave in certain ways. In the nursing context, patients expect that they can rely on nurses; that is, they have confidence that nurses will be there to help them. Patients expect that nurses will not only care for them with technical competence but will also care *about* them, as demonstrated by concern and commitment (Lasiter & McLennon 2015).

Some relationships remain at a superficial level, with nurses providing technical care and patients being satisfied with that care. This is described by Morse (1991) as a 'clinical relationship'. Dierckx de Casterlé (2015) and Ramos (1992) described this level as 'instrumental', while Graber and Mitcham (2004) term it 'practical'. Whatever term is used, this level of involvement is characterised by the nurse focusing on the task at hand. For example, a patient visiting an outpatient clinic for a routine pap smear would not expect, or probably desire, any more than a nurse who listened, explained the procedure in understandable language and provided privacy and comfort during the procedure. Therapeutic intimacy is not warranted.

Other relationships develop beyond this level and become profoundly moving experiences for both the patient and the nurse. For example, a situation in which a nurse connects with and enables a patient to face dying with dignity, meaning, peace and comfort involves a deeply meaningful, often intimate, relationship between them.

The main differentiation between the two types of relationships is the content of the interactions and the level of trust and self-disclosure. At a superficial level, very little is known beyond the formal roles of patient and nurse. At the intimate level of involvement, the formalised roles fade into the background and the patient and nurse become known to each other as unique beings. There is a feeling of unity with the patient (Dierckx de Casterlé 2015; Graber & Mitcham 2004).

An awareness that different levels of interpersonal involvement exist between themselves and patients enables nurses to feel confident in maintaining a relationship at a superficial level and, at times, in choosing to engage in a relationship that progresses to a more intimate level. Descriptions such as 'therapeutic intimacy' imply an expectation that all relationships between nurses and patients should reach this level of involvement, or that nurses should at least attempt to have their relationships with patients reach this level. Not only is such an expectation unrealistic, and often inappropriate, it also fails to acknowledge the central characteristics of mutuality and reciprocity in the relationship.

# Mutuality and reciprocity

The level of interpersonal involvement between nurses and patients cannot be mandated. It needs to be mutually agreed upon by both the nurse and the patient (the negotiation process in which this happens is discussed later in this chapter). There must be freedom to determine how they will relate; their involvement cannot be preordained and outcomes cannot be predetermined because these remain unpredictable at the outset of the relationship. While nurses aim to understand patients' experiences, they also need to appreciate patients' desire for the relationship and felt need to connect with the nurse.

Establishing the right level of involvement is not simply a matter for nurses, because relationships are mutual endeavours between patients and nurses. Mutuality is the sharing of commonalities, including mutual goal setting. Each participant – nurse and patient – influences the level of involvement. This is referred to as 'mutuality'. Mutuality is the midpoint between nursing care that is determined by the nurse without reference to the patient and care that is determined by the patient independent of the nurse. The former is paternalistic, while the latter is autonomous.

Although it is more common for nurses to initiate the relationship, either participant may make the initial overtures. The other participant must respond in some way to this initiative. For example, the nurse solicits the patient's participation in the relationship by exploring the patient's experience, and the patient responds by disclosing information. Or, the patient solicits the nurse's help and the nurse responds by providing assistance. This call-and-response exchange is referred to as 'reciprocity'.

Reciprocity and mutuality are essential in order to establish the human connection needed for a therapeutic patient–nurse relationship (Brown 2016; Tejero 2012). Therapeutic reciprocity, the mutual exchange of meaningful thoughts and feelings, involves nurse self-disclosure in an effort to assist the patient. At times, the mutuality needed to sustain the relationship is not present; in these situations, there is a unilateral relationship.

## Mutual versus unilateral relationships

A unilateral relationship is one in which one participant is unwilling or unable to develop the relationship to the level desired by the other participant; mutuality is compromised. When patients' conditions warrant a quick response, nurses engage in unilateral decision making without making time to take the patient's understanding into account. Nurses may continue their efforts to relate at a deeper level, despite the patient's unwillingness or inability to be engaged in the relationship. Likewise, patients may try to engage a nurse in a relationship even when the nurse is unwilling or unable to make an investment in the relationship.

When relationships between patients and nurses are mutual, there is a shared sense of responsibility and commitment to maintain the relationship. Mutual relationships between patients and nurses vary in their degree of intensity and involvement, and this raises questions about how and why some relationships remain on a superficial level while others progress to the level of therapeutic intimacy. The process used in determining the level of involvement is one of negotiation between patients and nurses.

## The negotiation of mutual relationships

Through negotiation, both the nurse and the patient make a choice to move the relationship to deeper levels of involvement and commitment. The negotiation is based on patients' and nurses' perceptions of the situation and of each other.

From patients' perspectives, it is the seriousness of the situation (as they perceive it), their feelings of vulnerability (perceived absence of personal resources) and their degree of dependence that affect whether they seek interpersonal connection and involvement with nurses. When patients perceive their situation as serious, rendering them dependent on nurses for care, they are likely to make overtures and efforts to find a nurse who they feel they can trust, and on whom they can rely. In addition, when patients interpret that the demands of the situation outweigh their perceived capabilities for meeting these demands (i e, they are vulnerable), they are likely to seek involved relationships with nurses. When patients perceive their situation as minor or routine, that it does not require them to become dependent on the nurses and they feel they can cope, they expect no more than routine, technical nursing care.

Nurses base their decision about entering into a more-than-superficial relationship on their evaluation of the patient's needs and available support systems (i.e. their evaluation of the patient's situation). Because this evaluation may be different from the patient's interpretation, the importance of understanding (see Ch 6) is reinforced.

In addition to their evaluation of the patient's situation, nurses also base their choice about becoming involved with a particular patient on whether or not they sense a personality 'click', as well as their estimation of the patient as a person (Ramos 1992). Nurses choose to become involved with patients who touch or appeal to them on a personal or emotional level (Morse 1991). As such, there is often a 'perceived fit' between nurses and patients who develop relationships beyond a superficial level.

## The process of negotiation

Patients seek active connections with nurses by being friendly, likeable, cooperative and an easy patient who cooperates and complies with care and therefore does not 'rock the boat' (Stoddart 2012; Vandecasteele et al 2015). Unfortunately, they also express reluctance to make such a connection when nurses seem too busy and patients do not want to bother them (Stein-Parbury et al 2015). Nonetheless, patients do want genuine encounters with nurses who are interested in them as a person and who are available and willing to interact with them (Dierckx de Casterlé 2015).

Patients make connections with nurses by engaging in everyday chitchat that helps them to get to know each other (Turpin et al 2012). They may ask the nurse personal questions aimed at having the nurse self-disclose. Self-disclosure is associated with trust, and patients look for nurses they like and on whom they feel they can depend. Likewise, patients determine if the nurse is a 'good person' by looking for indications of kindness, empathy, enjoyment of nursing and nursing competence. They test the nurse's ability to keep a confidence by sharing a minor secret. If a nurse passes the test of dependability and trustworthiness, the patient makes friendly overtures to build the relationship (Morse 1991).

It can be seen from this description of the negotiation process that, although patients may not be able to choose the nurses assigned to their care, they do have a choice about nurses with whom they become involved. Depending on the healthcare setting, nurses may or may not be able to influence which patients are assigned to their care, but the preceding description of the negotiation process indicates that nurses choose those patients with whom they become involved.

The depth of the relationship is determined by many factors, and nurses who realise which factors are operating in a relationship are in a position to establish appropriate interactions. The goal is not to form as deep a relationship as possible but to create conditions that keep possibilities open. Unaware nurses may inadvertently hinder the development of a relationship or try to deepen relationships under circumstances where this is not warranted.

## Dislike between a patient and a nurse

Just as it is unrealistic for nurses to expect that each relationship with a patient will be deeply meaningful, it is equally unrealistic to expect that they will like every patient with whom they come into contact. The reverse side of the coin of mutually satisfying relationships is revealed whenever nurses and patients are unable to form *any* level of relationship because they dislike each other. This feeling may be unilateral or mutual.

When it is the nurse who feels antipathy towards a patient, there is often a sense of accompanying guilt. Nurses may feel they are remiss in their professional responsibility when they dislike patients. This feeling can be offset by a realisation that a nurse's responsibility is to provide adequate care for patients, irrespective of whether they actually like an individual patient. If nurses allow their dislike of a particular patient to interfere with actually caring for that patient, they are failing in their duty of care. More often, however, it is the relationship between the nurse and the patient that falters, and not the nursing care that is provided.

It is more than likely that a nurse who senses disaffection towards a patient will either try to ignore it or, worse, blame the patient for the difficulty. Either response has the potential to have a negative effect on the relationship between this patient and this nurse.

Nurses who sense dislike for a particular patient first need to admit the feeling to themselves and learn to accept it as a natural part of being a person. Through reflecting on their reactions and motivations (see Ch 3), nurses may be able to unravel their reasons for feeling negative about a patient. Even if they are unable to discover why they are reacting this way, nurses who engage in self-reflection are able to separate what may be 'their' problem from what is an aspect of the patient.

Talking to colleagues is another useful way to learn more about these reactions to patients. Most experienced nurses have probably encountered unpleasant feelings towards patients, and those who have may be able to offer valuable insights into how to manage the situation effectively. In seeking such insights, nurses are demonstrating self-awareness and willingness to learn and grow (Ch 3). In time, it may happen that a nurse develops ways of coping with situations that engender dislike of patients. Unless there is recognition and acknowledgment of the difficulty, such growth is unlikely to occur.

Admitting negative feelings about particular patients to colleagues serves another potentially useful purpose. Usually, there are other nurses working in the same area (with the same patients) who do not react negatively to that particular patient. What rubs against one nurse's grain may roll easily off another nurse. Often an agreement can be reached so that those nurses who do not feel disdain towards a particular patient can care for that patient.

Sometimes, however, all nurses working in a particular locality dislike the *same* patient, often referred as a 'difficult patient' (see Ch 10 for a full discussion). When this happens, it is useful for all nurses caring for this particular patient to discuss the situation with each other in an effort to develop a workable way of relating to that patient. Neither nurses nor patients should be blamed when they do not get along because of what may be a 'personality clash'. Reflecting on the situation, talking it over with colleagues and developing ways of working with and around the potential problem are the best approaches.

# TYPES OF RELATIONSHIPS

Through the process of negotiation, different types of patient–nurse relationships develop that are characterised by their intensity of involvement and commitment. These different types of relationships have been reported by various authors over a number of years. Dierckx de Casterlé (2015) identified three levels of relationships: instrumental, professional and skilled companionship. Ramos (1992) identified similar levels as: instrumental, protective and reciprocal. Graber and Mitcham (2004) refer to levels of interactive involvement as practical, social, personal and transcendent. These descriptors bear remarkable resemblance to three types of helpful patient–nurse relationships referred to by Morse (1991) in her seminal work: the clinical relationship, the therapeutic relationship and the connected relationship. These terms are used in this chapter.

Each type is characterised by the level of involvement and the extent to which patient *and* nurse become known to each other. In this respect, each type of relationship is associated with the different sources of knowledge that nurses use in clinical practice. These sources, identified by Liaschenko and Fisher (1999) as case knowledge, patient knowledge and person knowledge, are described in Chapter 1. The level of involvement determines the degree to which the patient is known as a person. The types of relationship outlined by Morse (1991), Ramos (1992), Graber and Mitcham (2004) and Dierckx de Casterlé (2015) are discussed here in terms of the type of knowledge that is used. In addition, the types of relationship are described in relation to the skills that are the subject of subsequent chapters (listening, understanding, exploring and intervening).

# Relevance of skill focus and type of relationship

Each set of skills – listening, understanding, exploring and intervening – is used in each type of relationship. It is not simply a matter of the type of skill used but the focus of its use. In specifying a focus for skill use, there is a danger that these specifications will be used as prescriptions (i.e. hard-and-fast rules that require rigid adherence), but they should be used as guidelines that are fluid and open to change. These guidelines are presented in an effort to fit the skills into the particular context of the type of relationship negotiated between a patient and a nurse. The focus of skill use in each type of relationship is summarised in Table 2.2.

# The clinical relationship

In clinical relationships, nurses and patients interact in a routine or standard manner. Nurses perform technical care that is usual or standard for the circumstances. These relationships are characteristically short in duration and involve a health situation that is perceived by a nurse and a patient to be minor and routine. The patient's vulnerability and dependence is almost non-existent, and the nurse follows clinical protocols in a technically competent manner. There is little negotiation involved in this relationship, although there is implicit agreement to keep the relationship at this level (Dierckx de Casterlé 2015; Morse 1991; Ramos 1992).

## Focus of skill use in clinical relationships

A clinical relationship is not cold and distant, as the words technical, routine and standard might imply. Because the care is routine, that does not mean that the patient is treated as a 'number' or a 'case', or reduced to an object. The nurse is concerned and interested, conveying this by being friendly and cordial. Social exchanges and chitchat are often part of the interactions in these types of relationships.

During interactions in a clinical relationship, attending and listening skills are present, but the focus of listening remains primarily on content (see Ch 5). Unless directly stated by patients, feelings are usually not discussed or explored. Understanding is external (Ch 6), based on the nurse's clinical knowledge rather

**TABLE 2.2** Types of knowledge and focus of skill use in various levels of involvement

| | LEVEL OF INVOLVEMENT | | |
|---|---|---|---|
| Dierckx de Casterlé (2015) | Instrumental | Professional | Skilled companionship |
| Graber & Mitcham (2004) | Practical | Social | Personal/transcendent |
| Morse (1991) | Clinical | Therapeutic | Connected |
| Ramos (1992) | Instrumental | Protective | Reciprocal |
| Types of knowledge | Case knowledge | Case knowledge and patient knowledge | Case knowledge, patient knowledge and person knowledge |
| Listening | Content | Content and obvious feelings | Content and underlying feelings |
| Understanding | External view of the clinical situation | External and some internal patient response | Primarily internal, from the patient's experience |
| Exploring | Factual data, not feelings | Factual data and patient perceptions of the immediate situation | Personal meanings of both the situation and the effects on the patient's life |
| Intervening: comforting, supporting and enabling | Explanations and factual information | Sharing information | Sharing own interpretations |
| | Reassuring presence and manner | Mobilising resources | Providing support |
| | | | Concrete and specific feedback |

than internal, subjectively-based understanding. Exploration (Ch 7) is focused on factual data, although strict adherence to a prescribed form or format is potentially alienating to the patient. Intervening skills are of the stabilising type (Ch 8), reassurance is provided through the nurse's manner and presence and explanations and factual information are shared. The nurse's self-awareness (Ch 3) during clinical relationships is focused primarily on clinical knowledge of the patient's situation, although personal biases and values may impinge on the relationship. For example, nurses may believe that patients should not complain about minor, routine procedures; they may become judgmental of patients as a result.

# The therapeutic relationship

Therapeutic relationships between patients and nurses – those in which there is recognition of the individual needs of patients – are formed in the majority of situations (Dierckx de Casterlé 2015; Morse 1991; Ramos 1992). This type of relationship is usually of short or average duration, often with the patient facing a situation that is perceived by the patient as neither life-threatening nor serious. The patient's internal and external resources for meeting the demands of the situation are adequate. Although the nurse's perspective is primarily that the patient *is* a patient, there is also recognition and understanding of the patient as a person. This type of relationship can happen in a short period of time (Mottram 2009).

### Focus of skill use in therapeutic relationships

In attending, listening and exploring, nurses focus on both content and feelings when these emotions relate directly to the patient's health situation. For example, when patients are anxious prior to surgery, nurses perceive the anxiety and explore further in order to determine the patient's need for information or reassurance. Understanding skills (see Ch 6) enable nurses to focus on the patient's subjective experience of the health event, and exploration (Ch 7) is therefore focused on both factual data and the patient's perception of the situation. Interventions are aimed primarily at maintaining and stabilising the patient's resources; nevertheless, there is the possibility that information shared by the nurse will alter the patient's perception of the situation (see types of interventions in Ch 8). Because the therapeutic relationship is more involved than the clinical relationship, nurses' self-awareness is focused on how they are affecting the patient.

## Connected relationships

A connected relationship is one in which the nurse and the patient become involved to the degree that they perceive each other as people first, and their roles as patient and nurse become secondary. At this level of involvement, nurses understand the meaning of the clinical situation for the patient as a person. These types of relationships usually take time to develop, but a degree of connection may happen in a short time when patients' situations are extreme in terms of seriousness, vulnerability or dependence (the factors affecting negotiation). Both nurse and patient choose to enter connected relationships, and trust and commitment are deep and complete. In a connected relationship, nurses often choose to 'go the extra mile' for patients, acting 'above and beyond' the call of duty (Morse 1991; Ramos 1992). These types of relationships are ones in which nurses act as 'skilled companions'; they use both their scientific knowledge and their professional obligation to treat the patient as a person (Dierckx de Casterlé 2015).

A major difference between therapeutic and connected relationships is that the nurse functions as a source of support in a connected relationship, whereas in a therapeutic relationship nurses are support mobilisers and enhancers. This is because, in a therapeutic relationship, patients' supportive resources are present, even if not immediately available. In a connected relationship, the nurse is involved and committed, although the relationship does not necessarily extend beyond the patient's contact with the healthcare setting. These relationships are memorable for both the patient and the nurse, and nurses in connected relationships feel they have made a significant difference to the patient (Morse 1991). Although they require a great deal of energy, nurses leave these relationships feeling energised by the strong bond (Ramos 1992).

The following nurse's story is an example of a connected relationship.

## A Nurse's Story

When I heard Pat's story of how she received a gunshot wound to her spine at close range from her husband during a domestic argument, I felt anger towards her husband and a deep sense of sympathy for Pat. There was virtually no hope that she would ever walk again, as the bullet had severed her spine. She was out of intensive care, out of immediate life-threatening danger, when we met. I was working as a consultation-liaison mental health nurse and the nurses had referred Pat to me for supportive counselling. I liked her the moment I met her and felt an affinity towards her. She was a physically beautiful woman of 35 who sustained a charm and graciousness that would be difficult for most people under the circumstances. We instantly 'hit it off' and over the next three months of her hospitalisation became quite close.

The fact that I often thought about her when I was off duty did not seem remarkable to me; I often thought about patients when I was at home. But there was something different about our relationship. We came to know each other on a deeply personal basis, and I no longer thought of her as a patient. I also got to know her family very well and was treated like part of their network. Her parents, three sisters, brother-in-law and three nieces were an extremely close-knit family. They maintained a continual presence at Pat's side, supporting and caring for her in every possible way. They sensed my deep commitment to Pat and expressed appreciation for it.

Neither Pat nor her family ever spoke of Pat's husband – the person I held responsible for putting her in a wheelchair. Not surprisingly, he had not been in to see her. My anger towards him grew as I became closer to Pat. How could anyone have done this to her? My sense of injustice and my firm belief in the senselessness of firearms in the home kept my anger strong. But Pat never demonstrated any anger; in fact, she never talked about 'what happened'. She accepted her situation, the complex physical problems that accompany a spinal injury, her life in a wheelchair and her altered future with equanimity and remarkable resilience. I admired her strength and supported it, for it was keeping her going against enormous odds.

When her nightmares began, and the events of the shooting were vividly replayed in them, her fear and anguish started to seep through. She shared her nightmares and her feelings with me. I encouraged her to talk about what happened only to the extent that she could make meaning and begin to build her life again. Although she expressed anger and sadness, she never dwelled on these emotions. Perhaps she knew I felt the same way; perhaps it was that I always listened – quietly encouraging her to 'get it out' while containing my own emotions. She told no one else of the emotional pain because she knew the others who were closest to her – her family – were bearing their own anguish. She never wanted to be a burden, and this internal resource saw her through the long rehabilitation process.

> When Pat was discharged from hospital to a rehabilitation centre, I stayed in touch with her and her entire family, as there were ongoing health issues with a number of them. Her sister in particular would always stop by to see me when she was at the health centre. When my own personal circumstances necessitated a relocation from the area, I drove to the rehabilitation centre to say goodbye in person to Pat and her sister. She told me of the plans that were underway to have her home converted for a wheelchair. Divorce proceedings were underway, and she was making plans to return to work.
>
> We sat in the garden of the centre and relived our relationship. She thanked me for all that I had done to help her to adjust to her new life. I thanked her for sharing so much of herself with me. I told her that my own life was enriched by seeing her strength and resilience. We knew we had touched each other in a 'special' way. I knew that Pat would continue to live a full, although dramatically altered, life. That I may have had something to contribute to this outcome filled me with great professional satisfaction.

This story illustrates the reciprocity that can exist in therapeutically intimate relationships. Not all relationships reach this level of involvement. In fact, most do not. This story also illustrates the essence of this book: the significance and value of taking the time to understand patients as people, of taking the time to notice, of being concerned enough to explore and understand their world as they experience it. Interpersonal skills enable nurses to make contact with the private, subjective experiences of patients.

### Focus of skill use in connected relationships

In connected relationships, nurses attend and listen to the entirety of the patient's story and are able to perceive themes by relating content to underlying feelings (see Ch 5). Understanding is primarily internal (Ch 6), with the nurse developing awareness of the deeply personal, subjective experience of the patient. Exploration is focused on meanings, and exploration that is based on cue recognition and perception (Ch 7) is frequent. Interventions are aimed at the nurse as being the source of support (Ch 8), and the nurse's interpretation of the situation is shared with the patient in order to assist the patient in making sense of what is happening. Self-disclosure is high, characteristic of therapeutic intimacy, and the nurse is free to share concrete and specific feedback (Ch 8) about the relationship. There is 'you–me' talk because the nurse and patient feel safe in sharing their immediate reactions about how they are experiencing each other. Self-awareness skills (Ch 3) focus on the nurse as a participant in the relationship, and both the nurse and the patient experience change as a result of their relationship.

## Summary of skill use in various types of relationships

Each type of patient–nurse relationship is qualitatively different from the other. In each, nurses use the same skills, but the focus of skill use alters as relationships become more involved and intense. A high degree of self-disclosure on the nurse's part is inappropriate in a clinical relationship, yet significantly helpful in a connected relationship. The focus of listening extends from content only in clinical relationships to themes and meanings in connected/reciprocal relationships. Understanding is primarily external in clinical relationships and primarily internal in connected/reciprocal relationships. Exploration moves from the safe areas of content in clinical relationships to the intimate area of feelings and meanings in connected relationships. Interventions in clinical relationships are of the stabilising type, while mobilising interventions characterise connected relationships.

# THE PROGRESS OF THE RELATIONSHIP

It is important that nurses understand not only the various types of relationships that are formed with patients but also how these relationships develop and progress. An ability to track the progress of development of relationships enables nurses to time their responses accordingly. For example, without trust – the major issue in beginning relationships – challenging (see Ch 8) may alienate patients, and reflecting feelings (Ch 6) could be perceived by patients as intrusive. Tracking the progress of relationships means paying careful attention to the major issues of relationship development and to how patients are responding to the efforts of nurses.

The progress of relationships is described in terms of phases of development: prior to interacting, establishing the relationship, building the relationship and ending the relationship. The major themes and issues that are characteristic of each phase serve as signals and signposts in the progress of relationships. These are indicators for nurses to notice, to be concerned about and to respond to with an awareness of their significance to developing relationships.

Not all relationships pass through each phase, and not all issues will be relevant. The phases and their central themes and issues are presented as a guide to tracking the progress of the relationship. They are not definitive but present a probable scenario. For this reason they should be treated with caution. Using the concept of phases of development runs the risk that they will be perceived as rigid, adhered to as dogma or, worse, applied in a procedural, step-by-step manner. Relationships between patients and nurses are fluid, flexible and dynamic. No one picture could ever capture the complexity and variety of these relationships. The phases presented here should be viewed with these qualifications in mind.

## Prior to interacting

The primary issue prior to interacting with patients is nurses' awareness of their own thoughts, feelings and attitudes that may affect how they approach patients. Hearing about patients in a handover report or reading about them in their healthcare records sets up certain expectations, thoughts and feelings.

When there is knowledge of a particular patient, the nurse examines what, if any, thoughts, feelings and attitudes are engendered by such knowledge. For example, there may be fear and anxiety associated with caring for a patient with a known history of mental illness. These preliminary thoughts and feelings need not be negative (e.g. a nurse may enjoy caring for patients of a particular age group, gender or clinical condition).

Self-awareness skills (see Ch 3) are especially critical during this phase of relationship development. Any or all of a nurse's thoughts, feelings and attitudes prior to interacting with a patient may affect the relationship, for better or worse. For this reason self-awareness is where the relationship begins.

# Establishing the relationship

In the initial phase of interacting, the major issue between patients and nurses revolves around trust. Both a patient and the nurse will evaluate each other at this time with questions such as:

- Can I be myself with this person?
- Will I be accepted?
- How trustworthy is this person?
- Will they like me?

The initial phase of the relationship is therefore characterised by uncertainty and mutual exploration to decrease this uncertainty, as both the patient and the nurse assess each other. Nurses assess patients in terms of their current health status and their needs for nursing care (most often accomplished by a formal nursing assessment) *and* in terms of whether or not they feel they can work with the patient (Morse 1991). Similarly, patients assess nurses in terms of deciding if they can trust the nurse and whether they can work with them. This mutual assessment provides the avenue for negotiating the relationship.

## Trust

The formation of trust is essential if the relationship is to progress beyond a superficial level because trust enables a patient and a nurse to place confidence in each other. Interpersonal trust means that one person in the relationship believes that the other person can be relied and depended upon. In the nursing context, trust can be specific to the patient's health problem and not encompass all areas of their lives as would be more likely with friendships. Unlike trust in friendships, trust in healthcare relationships is strongly connected to confidence in the healthcare provider's competence and knowledge, in addition to expressive caring behaviours such as listening and being sincerely interested in the patient as a person (Murray & McCrone 2015). In the context of nursing care trust has been defined as 'the optimistic acceptance of a vulnerable situation, following careful assessment, in which the truster believes that the trustee has his best interests as paramount' (Bell & Duffy 2009, p. 50) (*see Research highlight*).

Building trust is not simply a matter of the patient trusting the nurse; nurses must also be able to trust patients. It is a mutual process; it must be reciprocated. Trust is fostered when nurses believe in patients' competence and skill in knowing what is best for them in managing their health. Nurses demonstrate their trust

## RESEARCH HIGHLIGHT Why patients trust nurses

*Lasiter, S., McLennon, S.M., 2015. Nursing professional capital: a qualitative analysis. J. Nurs. Adm. 45 (2), 107–112.*

### Background

Numerous surveys indicate that the general public regard nursing as one of the most trusted professions because nurses are viewed as honest and ethical. As such, they possess what is termed 'professional capital'. The term 'capital' originated in the economic sense as the value assigned to material possessions. In nursing, professional capital refers how nurses use their knowledge, skills and attitudes (their capital) to promote quality and safety in healthcare. That the public perceives nurses as people who can be trusted is an example of their professional capital.

### Purpose of the study

The aim of this study was to provide qualitative evidence to support the results of quantitative surveys that indicate that nurses have professional capital because they are trusted.

### Method

This study was a secondary analysis of data that were collected in a grounded theory study that explored (through interviews) why patients felt safe in an intensive care setting, when they are critically ill and vulnerable. In the original study, the researchers were impressed with how the patients spontaneously shared their perceptions of the nature and actions of the nurses during their time in intensive care. Therefore, they conducted a secondary analysis on the interview transcripts to investigate these perceptions.

### Key findings

There were three major themes that were identified. The first was 'Taking their word for it', meaning that they knew nothing of the nurses' level of knowledge and skills, yet they placed trust in them. This trust had no real foundation; the patients just felt that the nurses had their best interests at heart. The second theme was 'They know just what to do', thus placing their trust in the nurses' capabilities. The third theme was 'I know they watch me', which referred to the nurses' constant vigilance and the monitoring of patients' health status. They felt safe because they trusted the nurses.

### Implications for nursing practice

This study provided evidence of why and how nurses are viewed as trustworthy – a perception that is borne out in public surveys of professionals. This is nurses' social capital. They do not necessarily have to earn this trust. This places nurses in a privileged position; the trust placed in them is a gift. Nurses should be mindful to not betray this trust, for example, by not engaging meaningfully with patients or not attending to their perceived needs.

in patients by treating them with respect and regard (see Ch 3) and accepting and supporting them as capable human beings.

From a patient's perspective, nurses must be perceived as trustworthy. Trustworthiness involves having goodwill and acting on behalf of the patient's wellbeing (Bell & Duffy 2009; Dinc & Gastmans 2012). Nurses are fortunate because their professional role is viewed as trustworthy by most patients. Patients expect that nurses will care for them, meet their physical needs and provide comfort. In fact, when nurses 'don't seem to care', patients will often express shock and dismay, feeling betrayed by an apparent failure of the nurses to fulfil their role.

In this respect, trust is associated with meeting patients' expectations that they will be respected, listened to and treated as individuals. However, nurses can rely on patients' inherent trust in their role only to a limited extent. They must live up to patients' expectations that they are trustworthy through consistent actions, behaviours and attitudes. Providing individualised care meets patients' expectations and helps to promote trust (Dinc & Gastmans 2012).

Another important aspect in developing trust is for nurses to share their thoughts and reactions to patients' self-disclosure. Without feedback from nurses, patients who are sharing information about themselves may feel vulnerable. Have you ever shared something of yourself – your thoughts, feelings or reactions – with another person only to be met with a silent, stone-faced response? Under such circumstances, it is unlikely that you felt trust in this person. Likewise, patients rely on responses from nurses, and understanding responses (Ch 6) are the most trust-enhancing. Moralising, evaluative and judgmental responses early in the relationship lead to patients feeling rejected.

## Mutual assessment

In this initial phase of the relationship, nurses and patients assess each other in an effort to determine if they will get along – if there is any commonality or shared interest between them (e.g. whether they are both lovers of opera) – and if they feel they can work together. Patients may question the nurse's motivation to nurse, ask how much nursing experience the nurse has and generally observe the nurse to determine what kind of person they are.

Patients test nurses as to their dependability and their ability to keep a confidence (Morse 1991). All of these are strategies used to determine how far the involvement between patient and nurse will proceed. The patient bases the decision about whether to trust the nurse on what is determined during this phase. Nurses also assess patients during this initial phase in order to consciously choose whether to make an emotional investment in the patient (Morse 1991). This personal assessment is not the same as a formal clinical assessment, which is designed to elicit information that has a direct bearing on patients' nursing care.

## The initial interview

Most frequently, the relationship between a patient and a nurse begins with an interview, during which the nurse collects pertinent data about the patient.

Depending on the setting, the data that are to be collected are often specified on a formal nursing history/assessment form. Patients are usually the source of information, although if they are unable to interact (e.g. if they are unconscious), family and friends are used as the source of information. The initial information received by the nurse forms the basis for nursing care planning.

Because this interview is also the time during which a patient and nurse begin to get to know each other, the process of how the interview is conducted is as significant as the content. The climate established during this initial contact is crucial to the subsequent formation of the relationship. This interview sets the tone and establishes some of the ground rules on which the relationship will operate.

A rapid series of questions, asked in succession, may leave patients feeling intruded upon and bombarded by the nurse. Patients may form the impression that their role is to be obedient in providing answers. Lack of an explanation by a nurse about why the information is being collected may create confusion and uncertainty about the nurse's intentions. An initial interview conducted in an automatic, routine manner may create the impression that a nurse does not care about patients as people.

While this section cannot describe all the aspects of an initial nursing assessment (e.g. observation of physical signs), it does describe ways of conducting the initial interview with the recognition that it serves to establish the relationship between nurses and patients, as much as it serves to establish an adequate nursing database. These general guidelines for conducting the initial interview relate to its process and how it is conducted rather than to its content.

Exploration skills (see Ch 7) will predominate during this interview; however, the skills of attending and listening (Ch 5), as well as responding with understanding (Ch 6), will also feature in the interview.

## Process aspects of the initial interview

It is essential that nurses establish the interview within the context. This is done by proper introductions and explanations of the meaning of the interview. Nurses who introduce themselves and clearly describe their role in the particular healthcare setting help to establish this context. A clear description of the nurse's role in the setting includes more than a simple statement of name and title. It includes a description of how often the patient is likely to interact with and see this particular nurse. Is the interview being conducted by a student of nursing who is present in the setting for that day only? In this case, the patient will not see this nurse again and should be informed of this fact without having to wonder or ask. Is the interview being conducted by a permanent member of the hospital nursing staff who is about to go on days off? Again, this should be explained clearly. It is disconcerting for the patient to share information with a relative stranger who is then not seen again, without an explanation of why this occurred.

An explanation of why the information is being sought, provided in a manner that the patient is likely to understand, also helps to set the interview within a particular context. Saying 'I need some information about you so the nurses can care for you while you are here' is hardly adequate for a patient who is unfamiliar with the particular setting. A better way would be to explain to the patient that nurses need to know 'how a particular health situation concerns you personally, how it is affecting your day-to-day functioning and how it is likely to affect you in the future', followed by an explanation that the information is used to make nursing care specific to the particular patient.

If nurses are unsure or unclear about why they are collecting the information, other than to meet a requirement of the particular healthcare agency, it is not likely that the explanation will be adequate. For this reason, nurses are encouraged to think through what they need to know about patients and why they need to know this in order to provide nursing care.

Lastly, in establishing a context for the interview, it is important to explain to patients what will be done with the information they share. The information that relates directly to the patient's nursing care will be recorded and shared with other nurses and other healthcare professionals, and this practice of sharing information should be explained to patients. Not every detail of patients' stories needs to be shared, and it is best if patients are reassured that information that will be shared will be reviewed with them at the end of the interview.

This raises an interesting point about confidentiality in the patient–nurse relationship. How can patients come to trust nurses if they believe there is little information that will be kept in confidence? In fact, as mentioned earlier in this chapter, one of the ways that patients test nurses' trustworthiness is by sharing a minor secret to see if it will be held in confidence (Morse 1991). For this reason, nurses are encouraged to question the sometimes established norm of 'telling all' to other nurses.

Confidentiality is not merely keeping patient information inside the confines of a particular setting but also considering what should be shared, through reporting and recording, with other nurses and other healthcare professionals. Information that has no direct bearing on the nursing or other healthcare of the patient should be considered confidential and treated as such.

Each of these aspects – introducing themselves, explaining the purpose of the interview and informing patients how the information will be handled – helps to set the context and climate of the interview. Once the 'stage is set' in this manner, the specific data collection – the exploration phase – can begin.

## The exploration phase

In beginning the exploration phase of the initial interview, it is best to start with 'safe' topics that allow some rapport to be established, before moving into more sensitive areas. Delving into deeply subjective experiences is inappropriate as a beginning focus when the relationship is new and possibly fragile. It is unlikely that patients will share highly personal information before trust has been established – the sharing of such information is a sign that the patient is beginning to trust the nurse, or at least wants to know if the nurse is trustworthy.

During the interview, it is important that nurses bear in mind that patients are the experts on how their health situation is affecting their lives, although the nurse may have a clinical understanding of what is most pertinent. For example, patients may not perceive the significance of a question relating to how many stairs must be negotiated in their living quarters, but for some health situations this factor is very important. Nurses rely on their clinical knowledge in directing the interview but need to mix nurse-led with patient-led exploration (see Ch 7). It has been shown that these initial interviews with patients are driven by the nurse's agenda and clinical protocols rather than what the patient knows or wants to know (Macdonald et al 2013).

The initial interview provides an opportunity for nurses to share information with patients. This is done by asking patients what questions are on their minds, as well as correcting any misinformation or misunderstandings they may have about their current health situation. Sharing information at this time also balances the interview, establishing a climate of reciprocity.

## Building the relationship

Once the relationship is established, both the nurse and the patient know where the other stands and have an idea of what to expect from the relationship. The uncertainty that characterises the beginning of the relationship is reduced. It is at this point that nurses often experience a different type of uncertainty – an uneasiness and sense of pressure about 'doing something' for the patient. Because they have encouraged patients to disclose and share their experiences, nurses may feel that they now must take action and do something about what the patient has shared. When nurses experience their sense of responsibility in this manner, this may lead to taking on and assuming patients' burdens. Under such circumstances, nurses run the risk of feeling helpless, powerless and out of control. Taking on patients' burdens is also one of the warning signals of overinvolvement. These highlight the two central issues that prove challenging when building the relationship: control and power.

### Control

An attitude that it is a nurse's responsibility to solve a patient's problems reflects issues of control. Indicators that nurses may be too controlling in their interactions include:

- talking more than listening
- evaluating more than understanding
- leading more than following
- advising more than informing.

In order to manage the issue of control effectively, nurses must remind themselves that their role in the relationship is not that of rescuer but of facilitator – one who eases burdens by enabling patients to increase their access to their own resources. Through facilitating, nurses focus less on having the answers and more on enabling patients to maintain control and develop their own answers. Helping patients to feel in control reduces their sense of vulnerability and increases their comfort. In believing their role is a facilitating one, nurses do not relinquish their responsibility to patients but assume their responsibility in a collaborative manner. In doing so, nurses operate from a position of partner in care, as distinct from the position of a provider of care.

This is not to say that every patient will want or need to be in control, or will be able to develop their own resources. Some patients prefer nurses to provide answers and offer solutions. In some clinical situations, it is appropriate for nurses to assume control because of the patient's clinical condition, desire and orientation, or a combination of these.

In building the relationship, the major focus is to develop a congruence between what the patient wants in the way of help and assistance and what the nurse offers. There could be difficulties experienced in the relationship if the nurse and patient are operating from incongruent perspectives. For this reason, nurses are encouraged to reflect on how the patient is approaching the relationship compared with how they are approaching it. It is pointless to force patients into collaboration if they believe that nurses are experts with the solutions to their problems. Likewise, to take over and exclude patients from decision making when they want this level of influence is equally pointless.

## Power

Another issue in building the relationship is power, which refers to the power that is developed through meaningful connection with patients. Simply put, power is the ability to do or act to secure desired outcomes. Nurses who are trusted and regarded favourably by patients have power to influence these patients, and its appropriate use will *enable* rather than *control* patients. This type of enabling is often referred to as 'patient empowerment' and is discussed in Chapter 8 in relation to providing information and support.

Nurses should remain conscious of the fact that they have legitimate authority by virtue of their position. It is important that they recognise the power differential between themselves and patients (Brown 2016; Delmar 2012). This is true not only because of position power but also because patients are often dependent and vulnerable, therefore decreasing their own sense of power. Nurses can exert power over patients in ways that further disempower patients such as acting as if they know best, not consulting patients with changes to care delivery and controlling and dominating interactions (Barrere 2007; Griscti et al 2016; Oudshoorn et al 2007).

Appropriate use of nurses' influencing power in their relationships with patients is an empowering process. Empowerment means relating to patients in such a way that they feel capable and competent, therefore facilitating them to exert influence and control. Benner (1984) refers to the concept of 'caring power', which is used to empower patients rather than dominate, control or coerce them. Nurses have the potential power to:

- transform patients' views of their situations
- reintegrate patients with their social world
- remove obstacles or stand alongside and support and enable patients
- mobilise patients' resources
- bring hope, confidence and trust
- affirm the human capacity to cope.

All of these processes are powerful in their own right. Nurses engaged in these processes are not operating from a traditional view of 'power over' but rather the empowerment that comes from belief in, regard for and strengthening of patients. In this sense, empowerment is similar to the characteristic of respect (see Ch 3).

# Ending the relationship

One of the major factors differentiating social relationships from professional ones is that professional relationships between patients and nurses are usually time-limited. Most patients and nurses are aware that, at some point in time, each will disengage from the relationship. Relationships between patients and nurses end for a variety of reasons: patients recover and are discharged from the healthcare setting; patients are referred to another setting for follow-up care; nurses may depart from the clinical setting; and sometimes relationships end with the death of the patient. Whatever the reason for ending the relationship, there is a need to disengage and bring a sense of closure to it. The central issues involved in ending the relationship are emotionality and review.

## Emotionality

Frequently, emotions are aroused during the disengagement process, and it is at this stage that patients and nurses are most likely to express emotions about each other and the relationship. Emotions may range from sadness and frustration to satisfaction and happiness. Most often, there is a mixture of emotions. Nurses experience satisfaction when patients recover, especially if they have played a role in that recovery. While there may be a degree of sadness in saying goodbye, this is frequently offset by the feeling of satisfaction and happiness for the patient.

Depending on the type of relationship that has developed and the degree of connection and commitment between a patient and a nurse, the emotionality that often accompanies saying goodbye may or may not be present. In clinical relationships, there may be no emotions involved, except perhaps feelings of gratitude expressed by the patient. In connected relationships, emotions may run high as both the patient and the nurse have come to know each other intimately.

Handling these emotions is a matter of bringing them into awareness (see Ch 3) and expressing them openly. Nurses who are able to express their feelings about the relationship that has developed are behaving in an authentic, congruent manner (Ch 3). In an effort to encourage the patient to reciprocate in expressing emotions, nurses may choose to reflect feelings (Ch 6).

## Review

Regardless of whether there is any emotionality in saying goodbye, the ending of the relationship is most satisfying when there is a review of what happened during the relationship. Various scenes may be relived and shared, or it may be a simple matter of reassuring the patient that all is now well. Reviewing what happened during their relationship does not mean that nurses and patients should relive every interaction but rather briefly recount significant events. Such a review brings a sense of closure to the relationship.

At times, there is no opportunity to say goodbye to patients. If nurses feel unsettled when this happens, it is often helpful to share this experience with a colleague who also knew the patient (see Ch 11). Vicariously reliving the relationship with colleagues may help to bring a sense of closure to the relationship.

# SUMMARY

The essential nature of relationships between patients and nurses is that of mutual understanding. In developing relationships with patients, nurses not only focus on understanding patients' experiences but also on understanding the level of involvement desired by patients. Relationships that develop between patients and nurses differ in their level of involvement, and nurses are encouraged to establish a level of involvement that is appropriate to the circumstances.

Negotiating the 'right' level of involvement is based on the patient's needs, level of vulnerability and degree of dependency. Regardless of the level of involvement, all the skills presented in the following chapters are used in patient–nurse relationships, but the focus of their use alters depending on the type of relationship formed. With an appropriate focus, skills are employed within the context of the relationships between patients and nurses.

Critical issues emerge at various phases of relationship development, and awareness of these issues enables nurses to address them. The issues of self-awareness, trust, mutual assessment, control, power, emotionality and review have been presented with an emphasis on the need for collaborative efforts between patients and nurses. All skills included in this book are presented from this point of view.

# REFERENCES

Barrere, C.C., 2007. Discourse analysis of nurse–patient communication in a hospital setting: implications for staff development. J. Nurses Staff Dev. 23 (3), 114–122.

Bell, L., Duffy, A., 2009. A concept analysis of nurse–patient trust. Br. J. Nurs. 18 (1), 46–51.

Benner, P., 1984. From Novice to Expert: Excellence and Power in Clinical Nursing Practice. Addison-Wesley, Menlo Park, CA.

Brown, B.J., 2016. Mutuality in health care: review, concept analysis and ways forward. J. Clin. Nurs. 25, 1464–1475.

Charalambous, A., Radwin, L., Berg, A., et al., 2016. An international study of hospitalized cancer patients' health status, nursing care quality, perceived individuality in care and trust in nurses: a path analysis. Int. J. Nurs. Stud. 61, 176–186.

Delmar, C., 2012. The excesses of care: a matter of understanding the asymmetry of power. Nurs. Philos. 13, 236–243.

Dierckx de Casterlé, B., 2015. Realising skilled companionship in nursing: a utopian idea or difficult challenge? J. Clin. Nurs. 24, 3327–3335.

Dinc, L., Gastmans, C., 2012. Trust and trustworthiness in nursing: an argument-based literature review. Nurs. Inq. 19 (3), 223–237.

Evans, E.C., 2016. Exploring the nuances of nurse–patient interaction through concept analysis: impact on patient satisfaction. Nurs. Sci. Q. 29 (1), 62–70.

Fleischer, S., Berg, A., Zimmermann, M., et al., 2009. Nurse–patient interaction and communication: a systematic literature review. J. Public Health (Bangkok) 17, 339–353.

Gadow, S., 1980. Existential advocacy: philosophical foundation of nursing. In: Spiker, S.F., Gadow, S. (Eds.), Nursing: Images and Ideals. Springer, New York, pp. 79–101.

Graber, D.R., Mitcham, M.D., 2004. Compassionate clinicians: taking patient care beyond the ordinary. Holist. Nurs. Pract. 18 (2), 87–94.

Griscti, O., Aston, M., Martin-Misener, R., et al., 2016. The experiences of chronically ill patients and registered nurses when they negotiate patient care in hospital settings: a feminist poststructural approach. J. Clin. Nurs. 25, 2028–2039.

Hartlage, H.N., 2012. Exploring boundaries in pediatric oncology nursing. J. Pediatr. Oncol. Nurs. 29 (2), 109–112.

Henderson, A., Van Eps, M.A., Pearson, K., et al., 2007. 'Caring for' behaviours that indicate to patients that nurses 'care about' them. J. Adv. Nurs. 60 (2), 146–153.

Holder, K.V., Schenthal, S.J., 2007. Watch your step: nursing and professional boundaries. Nurs. Manage. 38 (2), 24–29.

Jourard, S.M., 1964. The Transparent Self. Van Nostrand, Princeton, NJ.

Lasiter, S., McLennon, S.M., 2015. Nursing professional capital: a qualitative analysis. J. Nurs. Adm. 45 (2), 107–112.

Liaschenko, J., Fisher, A., 1999. Theorizing the knowledge that nurses use in the conduct of their work. Sch. Inq. Nurs. Pract. 13 (1), 29–41.

Macdonald, L., Stubbe, M., Tester, R., et al., 2013. Nurse–patient communication in primary care diabetes management: an exploratory study. BMC Nurs. 12 (1), Article number 20. Open access. http://www.biomedcentral.com/1472-6955/12/20.

Menzies, I., 1961. A case study of the functioning of social systems as a defence against anxiety. Hum. Relat. 13 (2), 95–123.

Morse, J.M., 1991. Negotiating commitment and involvement in the nurse–patient relationship. J. Adv. Nurs. 16, 455–468.

Mottram, A., 2009. Therapeutic relationships in day surgery: a grounded theory study. J. Clin. Nurs. 18, 2830–2837.

Murray, B., McCrone, S., 2015. An integrative review of promoting trust in the patient–primary care provider relationship. J. Adv. Nurs. 71 (1), 3–23.

Noddings, N., 1984. Caring: A Feminine Approach to Ethics and Moral Education. University of California Press, Berkeley, CA.

Nursing and Midwifery Board of Australia, 2008. Code of Professional Conduct for Nurses in Australia. ANMC, Melbourne. Online. Available at: www.nursingmidwiferyboard.gov.au/Codes-Guidelines-Statements/Codes-Guidelines.aspx#competencystandards. (Accessed 24 July 2016).

Nursing Council of New Zealand, 2009. Code of Conduct for Registered Nurses. NCNZ, Wellington. Online. Available at: http://www.nursingcouncil.org.nz/Publications/Standards-and-guidelines-for-nurses. (Accessed 24 July 2016).

Oudshoorn, A., Ward-Griffin, C., McWilliam, C., 2007. Client–nurse relationships in home-based palliative care: a critical analysis of power relations. J. Clin. Nurs. 16, 1435–1443.

Ramos, M.C., 1992. The nurse–patient relationship: theme and variations. J. Adv. Nurs. 17, 496–506.

Stavropoulou, A., Kaba, E., Obamwonyi, V.A., et al., 2012. Defining nursing intimacy: nurses' perceptions of intimacy. Health Sci. J. 6 (3), 479–495.

Stein-Parbury, J., Gallagher, R., Chenoweth, L., et al., 2015. Expectations and experiences of older people and their carers in relation to emergency department arrival and care: a qualitative study in Australia. Nurs. Health Sci. 17 (4), 476–482.

Stoddart, K.M., 2012. Social meanings and understandings in patient–nurse interaction in the community practice setting: a grounded theory study. BMC Nurs. 11, Article number 14. Online. Available at: http://www.biomedcentral.com/1472-6955/11/14. (Accessed 24 July 2016).

Tejero, L.M.S., 2012. The mediating role of the nurse–patient dyad bonding in bringing about patient satisfaction. J. Adv. Nurs. 68 (5), 994–1002.

Turpin, L.J., McWilliam, C.L., Ward-Griffin, C., 2012. The meaning of a positive client–nurse relationship for senior home care clients with chronic disease. Can. J. Aging 31 (4), 457–469.

Vandecasteele, T., Debyser, B., van Hecke, A., et al., 2015. Patients' perceptions of transgressive behaviour in care relationships with nurses: a qualitative study. J. Adv. Nurs. 71 (12), 2822–2833.

Wiechula, R., Conroy, T., Kitson, A.L., et al., 2016. Umbrella review of the evidence: what factors influence the caring relationship between a nurse and patient? J. Adv. Nurs. 72 (4), 723–734.

# CHAPTER
# 3

# Nurse as therapeutic agent

## CHAPTER OVERVIEW

- Therapeutic agency is realised through a nurse's use of self as an art.
- Interpersonal communication competence is essential in developing therapeutic agency.
- Competent communicators are responsive to what others are thinking and feeling and assertive in expressing what they are thinking and feeling.
- In nursing, emotional intelligence and emotional labour are required in order to develop interpersonal communication competence.
- Reflection on actions and intentions, as well as on personal values and beliefs, helps to develop emotional intelligence.
- Emotionally intelligent nurses are able to form meaningful interpersonal connections with the people they call patients.
- Meaningful interpersonal connections are characterised by authenticity, respect and warmth.

Visit the Evolve site for video content to support the themes and skills explored in this chapter: http://evolve.elsevier.com/AU/Stein-Parbury/patient/

# INTRODUCTION

That nurses have a sense of agency is the basis on which they form relationships with patients. A sense of agency means that nurses understand and appreciate that they can make a difference to patients' lives and that they know how to use their professional influence and knowledge to benefit patients. While such power could be used to harm a patient, a nurse's professional agency is employed in service to the patient (i.e. for therapeutic benefits).

In developing therapeutic agency, nurses need a wide and varied repertoire of interpersonal skills and an understanding of their use, as well as practical know-how. In employing their agency, nurses need an awareness of how effectively they are using their skills because such awareness enables them to evaluate their own performance. Nurses who are able to reflect upon and evaluate their own performance are in a position to learn, grow and become more skilled and effective in their interactions with patients, thus increasing their potential for therapeutic agency.

The previous chapters have outlined a moral imperative for nurses to focus their attention on patients during their interactions. This may be interpreted to mean that nurses should disregard or forget themselves whenever they engage in nursing care. By focusing on patients, at the exclusion of themselves, nurses run the risk of failing to recognise the significance of how *they* are affecting patients and how patients are affecting *them*. In the process, nurses may fail to attend to their own reactions and responses, erroneously perceiving their subjectivity to be superfluous or irrelevant to patient care.

The skills presented in the following chapters of this book can be learnt, developed and refined. Nevertheless, the skills are only as effective as the person using them. Each nurse employs the skills in a unique way. Effectively relating to patients involves more than simply using the right skill, at the right time, with the right patient. *What matters and makes a difference are not the skills themselves but the nurse who is using the skills*. Each nurse develops a style of relating to patients that is 'right' for that particular nurse. Nurses who focus solely on the skills without awareness of their own personality run the risk of contrived performance that lacks spontaneity and a personal touch. For these reasons, the initial focus of interpersonal skill development is placed on communication competence, emotional intelligence, self-awareness and reflective practice.

# THERAPEUTIC USE OF SELF

Therapeutic use of self, a term coined by Travelbee (1971), is the direct expression of the art of nursing. Use of self requires creative thinking in response to the uniqueness of each individual patient. For example, nurses who are natural comedians can effectively use humour by finding a funny side to their circumstances for patients who are distressed. Other nurses will find that their strength lies in the area of providing explanations to patients who want more information. As such there is no one description or definition that captures the use of self as an art, as each nurse's enactment of agency will be as unique as the nurse.

Developing the art of using oneself will be a career-long process for nurses whose therapeutic agency is realised. Nonetheless, there are basic requisites for developing therapeutic agency. These are communication competence, emotional intelligence and skill in labouring the emotions, as much of what makes people unique is how they feel and respond emotionally. Because nursing care situations often involve strong emotions, nurses must be skilled in effectively managing their own feelings (emotional labour) if they are going to be of value to patients.

# COMMUNICATION COMPETENCE

Nurses must be competent communicators if they are going to develop their own personal sense of agency and use their interactions with patients to be of assistance and to provide help. More importantly they must be competent in order to develop therapeutic communication skills. Therapeutic communication is employed with the intention of benefitting the patient's sense of wellbeing and comfort, and to gather information that is relevant to the patient's care. In order to be therapeutic in their communication, nurses must be competent communicators.

Competent communicators negotiate meaning and build mutual understanding in their interactions with others. They possess a wide repertoire of skills, along with the know-how of when to use them. This involves self-awareness, along with an understanding of the situation at hand. Being competent does not mean that communication will be perfect; rather, it involves adjustment and correction if the communication is not effective in achieving mutual understanding. Therefore, ongoing and continuous reflection are required; it is a lifelong process.

Communication competence involves two types of skills: those of being responsive, able to listen to and understand what others are saying; and those of being assertive, able to state their point of view and express their needs. People who are competent communicators are able to express their own ideas, opinions and feelings while also having the ability to understand the expressed ideas, opinions and feelings of other people. That is, they are skilled at balancing both assertive and responsive skills in their interpersonal interactions with others. Fig. 3.1 depicts communication competence along two axes: assertiveness and responsiveness. A competent communicator will have a balance of both types of interpersonal skills and will lie in the upper outer quadrant of the matrix.

Overly assertive people who are not able to listen to and understand others' opinions and ideas are usually considered aggressive or domineering in their communication, as they often do not listen to others while continuing to emphasise their viewpoint. As such, they are prone to override others' views. Highly responsive people – those people who are adept at understanding others yet are unable to state their own ideas – are often considered passive or accommodating in their interpersonal interactions. As such, they often miss opportunities to be heard. Neither type of person is competent in communication, as they lack a balance between the skills of responding and the skills of asserting.

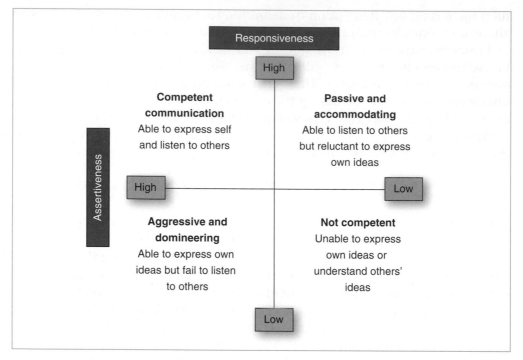

**Figure 3.1** Communication competence

Nurses need to be competent communicators because they need to be both responsive and assertive as they enact their therapeutic agency. For example, they are often in a position to advocate on behalf of a patient, thus needing to use the skills of assertion. Likewise, empathic expression, developed through using responsive skills, is necessary to understanding the experience of patients. Responding skills are covered primarily in Chapters 5 and 6, and the skills of assertion are reviewed fully in Chapters 10 and 11.

# Emotional intelligence

Competent communicators possess what is termed 'emotional intelligence'. This term was first coined by Salovey and Mayer in 1990 but was popularised in a best-selling book by Goleman in 1995. Emotional intelligence involves the ability to: recognise and manage emotional responses in oneself, as well as others; understand emotions and their meaning; assess and monitor emotions in situations; and use emotions for reasoning and problem solving (Shanta & Gargiulo 2014). People who are emotionally intelligent possess internal qualities of resilience, initiative, optimism and adaptability (Goleman 1998). In their interactions with others, they acknowledge the significance of human feelings and are able to use their hearts as well as their heads when deciding how to act.

According to Goleman (1998), there are five dimensions of emotional intelligence: self-awareness, self-regulation, motivation, empathy and social skills. These are hierarchical and interdependent, with self-awareness as the basis on which other dimensions are developed. Self-awareness includes an accurate assessment of self, along with self-confidence. Self-regulation involves control over one's emotions and being trustworthy. Motivation includes commitment, initiative and optimism. Empathy (see Ch 6), a central dimension in emotional intelligence, includes not only understanding other people but also maintaining a service orientation towards others. Finally, the social skills necessary for emotional intelligence include conflict management, cooperation and collaboration (Ch 10).

In nursing, emotional intelligence is considered to be essential because care is provided through interpersonal relationships, and emotions are vital to these relationships; nurses have a moral obligation to make emotional connections with patients in their care. Nurses need to have the capacity to understand the emotional realities of patients, and to respond empathically. However, their thinking and performance can be negatively affected if they are overcome by their own emotions. Therefore, emotional intelligence is considered to be necessary for developing both interpersonal and professional competence (Powell et al 2015). It is one mechanism for improving nursing practice through integrating nursing science and reflective, ethical care of patients (Shanta & Gargiulo 2014).

In the nursing literature there is mounting evidence that emotional intelligence improves nurses' wellbeing and patient care. It has been shown to be correlated with: reduced stress and anxiety; lower rates of burnout; improved cognitive performance; improved attitudes and caring behaviour; increased job satisfaction; and patient satisfaction (Adams & Iseler 2014; Gørgens-Ekerman & Brand 2012; Powell et al 2015; Shanta & Gargiulo 2014). Emotional intelligence is evident in stories told by nurses that reveal how they use their knowledge (Codier et al 2010). More importantly, emotional intelligence has been found to be positively associated with quality of patient care (Adams & Iseler 2014).

## Emotional labour

One aspect of being emotionally intelligent is the ability to self-regulate and manage emotional responses, especially in relation to the context in which they occur. There is a link between this dimension of emotional intelligence and the concept of 'emotional labour', as both involve the management of feelings. Emotional labour involves keeping natural emotional responses concealed in order to demonstrate an emotional response that is in keeping with the context of service provision and considered to be professionally desirable. In nursing, this involves an expectation to maintain a concerned, empathic attitude towards the patient, despite how a nurse may be feeling inside. This requires effort and is therefore part of the work of nurses.

The concept of emotional labour came to attention through the work of Hochschild in 1983 and continues to attract interest (Hochschild 2012). It has been explored as a way of understanding the work of nurses, as nurses do learn to appropriately manage their emotional responses to patients, especially when there is a perceived gap between what they feel and what they believe they should feel (Smith 2012). For example, if nurses respond to physical deformity of a patient with disgust, they must hide these feelings from the patient because they serve little useful purpose in trying to be of help. In this sense, emotional labour is considered to be necessary to therapeutic relationships.

Emotional labour involves regulating one's emotions, along with employing what is called 'surface acting' and 'deep acting' (Hochschild 2012). Surface acting is the overt expression of an emotion not felt by the person, yet thought to be needed in the situation. For example, if a nurse is feeling overtaxed by a heavy workload and a patient apologetically asks for help, stating *'So sorry to bother you ...'*, a nurse may conceal their stress and say *'No bother at all'* in a calm, pleasant manner. Deep acting involves a shift in emotional response within the nurse. For example, trying to understand a situation from the patient's perspective may result in the nurse changing their views about the situation. In nursing, deep acting is positively related to job satisfaction, while surface acting is related to emotional exhaustion and poorer job satisfaction (Chou et al 2012).

This may be because the workers in the original study on emotional labour (Hochschild 1983) suppressed their emotions in service to their company so money was not lost through poor customer service. In contrast, nurses are called to manage their emotions and respond to the complex emotional needs of patients; they act in service to the patient. The work satisfaction that is felt when enacting a professionally compassionate role, in keeping with the ideals of a caring profession, is the reward nurses often receive when they manage emotions in service to the patient. A study by Mauno et al (2016) confirmed that nurses who perceive that they can work to their ethical standards experienced fulfilment even when emotional labour was intense.

Like emotional intelligence, the concept of emotional labour is also receiving attention in the nursing and healthcare literature. In a recent review of research into emotional labour in healthcare settings, Riley and Weiss (2016) reported that half of the reviewed articles were related to nursing. They assert that the focus of emotional labour research on the nursing profession is likely to be a result of emotional work being considered women's business, as the majority of nurses are female.

Like much female-gendered work, emotional labour is frequently unrecognised, hidden and undervalued (Riley & Weiss 2016; Williams 2013). Little attention has been paid to this type of nursing work, as task-orientation and the biomedical model of healthcare dominate most work settings. Williams (2013) asserts that the emotional demands on nurses are likely to increase in contemporary healthcare as increased patient acuity, diminished resources and increasing workload place stress on nurses.

# THE IMPORTANCE OF SELF-UNDERSTANDING

An understanding of self in relation to patients, termed 'personal knowing' (Carper 1978), is considered fundamental to forming therapeutic relationships in nursing. Personal knowing assists nurses in attending to the mutual relationship, not simply the patient in the relationship. A failure to take into account the effects nurses themselves have on patients, and their relationships with them, can lead to mistaken assumptions and judgments about what patients are experiencing.

Personal knowing, referred to here as 'self-understanding', is developed for the purpose of becoming authentic, congruent and open with patients. If nurses are authentic with patients, they are sincere and genuine, not only as people who care what happens to patients but also as people who are unafraid to show they are human. The more nurses are aware of themselves, the more likely it is that their interpersonal skills will be used in an authentic and natural way. Self-understanding enables nurses to act in ways that are in harmony with who they are and congruent with and true to their unique nature and style. Openness with patients is the ability to accept patients as they are, rather than how nurses may want them to be.

Consider the following nurse's story.

## A Nurse's Story

Sylvia is an experienced registered nurse who prides herself on her ability to care for seriously injured and impaired victims of brain damage. Peter had become one of those patients who all the nurses on Sylvia's ward had come to dislike. He was labelled as uncooperative and difficult. Because some alleged his injuries had been self-inflicted, he engendered little sympathy from the nursing staff. They did not like caring for Peter and often complained bitterly to each other about their negative feelings towards him.

One day during change-of-shift report, Sylvia began to listen to her colleagues' complaints and negative judgments about Peter. After reading a journal article on the topic, she had been thinking about how some patients are labelled as difficult. She came to realise that Peter had fallen into this unfortunate category. To her colleagues' relief and surprise, she asked to be assigned to care for Peter. Little did they realise that Sylvia was challenging herself to try to understand Peter as a person rather than a label.

That day when she entered his room she noticed, for the first time, the frightened and uncomfortable look on this young man's face. His primary manner of communication was through blinking his eyes because he had sustained an unstable neck injury. His hands were restrained because he was in the habit of pulling at tubes and equipment. Sylvia stood there for a moment, noticing and absorbing his situation.

Without even thinking, she suddenly realised the cool temperature of the room and noticed that Peter had nothing more than a light sheet draped over his naked body. She looked at him and said, 'I bet you're cold'. His eyes blinked furiously in the affirmative. She immediately went to get him a warm blanket. The look of relief on his face was incredible. Throughout the entire time, no one had noticed that Peter was cold. They did not notice because they had failed to perceive him as a person.

Sylvia no longer could say 'no' to the 'personhood' of Peter by thinking of him as a label. She began to question the dynamics that had led the nursing staff to label Peter and dismiss him as troublesome and difficult. Through reflection Sylvia had become more self-aware. Her awareness allowed her to put aside the labels used about Peter and to attend to his comfort needs.

This story highlights the importance of self-understanding; through active reflection and open acknowledgment Sylvia was able to take corrective action. Sometimes nurses try to deny the existence of negative patient labels, claiming that such evaluations are unprofessional and therefore unacceptable. They do so in the erroneous belief that nurses, by virtue of being professional people, can rise above their natural human tendency to judge, or that at least nurses can put such judgments aside so they do not interfere with their nursing care. Such denial is unfortunate because it diminishes self-understanding.

A more useful strategy is to encourage nurses to actively reflect on their evaluative perceptions of patients rather than deny or ignore that their judgments can and do affect patient care. Once negative evaluations are brought into conscious awareness, nurses can explore their meaning and, like Sylvia, take corrective action if necessary. Reflection will not prevent negative evaluations, but it will assist nurses in challenging or altering them.

The more nurses know about themselves, the more likely they will come to accept themselves. The more nurses understand about themselves, the easier it becomes for them to understand patients. The more tolerant nurses are of themselves, the more tolerant they can be of patients. The more comfortable nurses are with themselves, the more comfortable they can be with patients. It is through coming to accept and understand their own perspective that nurses can come to accept and understand patients' perspectives. As nurses come to know their own experiences as human beings, they are better able to relate to the person who is the patient.

Self-understanding helps nurses to build emotional intelligence and a healthy self-concept. Self-understanding can lead to comfort with the self and genuine liking of the self. This is no easy task to achieve. It often takes a long time, as a person's relationship with the self is dynamic, not static.

Liking oneself is not the same as thinking one is without faults or failings. Liking oneself is about knowing one's strengths and areas for improvement, putting these together and concluding that what exists is acceptable, along with a continuous desire to grow and learn. When nurses know, understand and like themselves, they are less likely to hide behind their professional role and more likely to make contact with patients on a genuinely human level.

# SELF-AWARENESS VERSUS SELF-CONSCIOUSNESS

Completing Activity 3.1 often engenders feelings of self-consciousness and discomfort in people. This is because focusing on the self, especially the positive aspects, is usually a private affair and 'seeing yourself on paper', even when it is not shared with anyone else, brings the private into the open and often creates a sense of self-exposure and vulnerability.

In bringing the self into awareness, even through an activity such as this, there is a danger of becoming preoccupied with the self and uncomfortably

**ACTIVITY 3.1** What do I have to offer patients?  332

**Process**

1. Divide a blank piece of paper into two columns. In the first column, record a description of those aspects of yourself that you think are positive – ones you like about yourself. In the second column, describe those aspects of yourself that you would prefer to change – ones you do not always like about yourself. You don't need to share this list with anybody else. Be as honest as possible with yourself.

2. From your list of positive aspects (in the first column of your paper), reflect on how you could put these aspects to use in caring for and relating to patients.

3. From your list of negative aspects (in the second column of your paper), reflect on how these may affect your relationships with patients, for better or for worse.

4. Write a brief summary of how you could use your personal self in developing your professional self.

**Discussion**

1. Which was easier: describing positive aspects of yourself or negative ones?

2. Which column contains more information?

   • Frequently, when completing activities such as this, it is difficult to separate the 'you' that you want to be (ideal self) from the 'you' that exists (real self). How true was this for you in completing the activity?

   • Ask someone who knows you well and who you trust to describe what they see as positive and negative aspects about you. Compare what they say with your list and reflect on similarities and differences.

self-conscious. Self-awareness can result in self-consciousness. There needs to be a balance between the self-consciousness that is experienced through focusing too much on the self and the lack of self-understanding that leads to alienation from the self. Achieving this balance is important for nurses because the risks of focusing too much on themselves are as great as the dangers of failing to take themselves into account at all.

Egan (2014) refers to the need to be 'productively self-conscious' when engaged in helping relationships. Productive self-consciousness has positive effects because it is the ability to be absorbed in an interaction while simultaneously being aware of internal reactions and perceptions. It is the ability to raise self-understanding to a level that enhances reflection on the self while not becoming so preoccupied with the self that there is a lack of ability to focus on the person being helped.

# THE RELATIONSHIP BETWEEN SELF-UNDERSTANDING AND PROFESSIONAL GROWTH

Nurses need to be able to evaluate how effectively they are relating to patients, and self-understanding is essential in this assessment. Evaluating performance in using the skills presented in the following chapters is best achieved through the process of self-assessment. In assessing their performance, nurses begin with an awareness of how they are interacting with patients. By considering their *intentions*, *actions*, *responses* and *reactions*, nurses are able to evaluate their own performance in the interest of learning how to be more effective. Self-understanding is not simply a matter of perceiving the self as is; it is also a process of encouraging self-growth to become more effective in relating to patients. It would be irresponsible for nurses simply to accept themselves and not challenge themselves to change and grow through their nursing experiences. Through challenge comes change, and nurses willing to challenge themselves are open to personal and professional growth.

# DEVELOPING THE SELF AS A THERAPEUTIC AGENT

When relating to patients therapeutically, nurses are deliberately using their interactions for the benefit of patients. This is the conscious 'use of self' as a therapeutic agent as nurses make choices and decisions in their interactions. Benner et al (1996) define a nurse's clinical agency as an understanding of one's impact on what happens to the patient. A sense of agency is needed to influence and guide patients (see Ch 8). Most importantly, this sense of agency develops through continual learning as a result of clinical experience.

In developing this sense of agency, nurses need to become aware of what they have to offer patients (e.g. they need to know their personal strengths and their personal areas for improvement). Self-understanding enables nurses to view themselves as human beings with failures, faults, successes and strengths, as people who have something to offer patients.

Self-understanding is an essential ingredient in a nurse becoming a therapeutic agent. It is unlikely that nurses, or anyone else for that matter, will ever fully know and appreciate all facets of themselves. Nevertheless, nurses can develop their capabilities to engage in self-reflection, to perceive and accept input from others and to openly disclose themselves to others to increase their self-understanding. In fact, engaging in these processes and being motivated to keep improving are essential to becoming emotionally intelligent.

When considering how to increase self-understanding, the process of introspection, or self-reflection, often comes to mind. This often begins with noticing what elicits a personal response. 'Why did I react negatively when that patient told me he wanted to die? Why did I want to leave the room? Was it that

I felt helpless, or unsure about how to respond? Do I believe that self-destructive thoughts are unacceptable? Have *I* ever felt this way before? Why did I find it so hard to listen to what he was saying?' Often when something or somebody elicits a response, the tendency is to look to that person or thing, rather than to reflect on the self. Noticing and reflecting on thoughts about oneself involves introspection, which is one of the principal ways that self-understanding develops.

Paying attention to such thoughts and feelings (i.e. allowing them to enter into rather than forcing them out of awareness) encourages nurses to discover more about themselves. Introspection and listening to oneself mean trusting oneself, being honest with oneself, accepting oneself and sometimes challenging oneself. Nevertheless, introspection is only effective in increasing self-understanding when personal thoughts and feelings are used for the purpose of discovering more about oneself.

Many nurses interpret the need to maintain control over their emotions, as in the self-management of emotional labour, to mean that they should be void of emotions. Rather than deny their emotional responses, although they may be concealed from patients, it is better for nurses to be aware of and reflect on such reactions. Without awareness, it is likely that these emotions will be expressed inadvertently to patients. Nurses who keep in tune with their emotional responses have a greater chance of maintaining true control than those who try to control emotions by ignoring them.

More importantly, nurses' feelings and reactions to patients serve a purpose because they provide useful information in measuring how the relationship with a patient is progressing. For example, anger and frustration towards a patient, when left unexamined, may lead to labelling that patient. It could be that the feelings of anger and frustration are a result of the nurse's inability to understand what the patient is experiencing. Perhaps the patient is not conforming to the nurse's expectations of a 'good patient'. A host of other possibilities exist. Self-reflection enables nurses to discover what their emotional reactions might be revealing about *their* relationships with patients. Reflecting on personal thoughts and feelings triggered through interaction with patients provides useful sources of information about oneself.

# REFLECTION AND REFLECTIVE PRACTICE

Reflection is an active exploration of personal experiences, consciously employed for the purpose of making sense of those experiences. Ongoing reflection is essential to becoming a skilled and competent communicator. Some people naturally engage in reflective processes, thinking deeply on life and their experiences of it. Other people may need guidance and assistance to be reflective.

Reflection and reflecting practice are built into professional competency standards and codes of conduct for nurses in many countries (Goulet 2016; Nursing and Midwifery Board of Australia 2008, 2016; Nursing Council of New Zealand 2007, 2009). This is because nursing knowledge is embedded in practical experience, and reflection is required as a means to promote continuous learning.

A spirit of enquiry sparks reflective nurses to think about their actions while they are engaged in clinical practice (Goulet et al 2016). In this sense, reflection is a way of functioning. It involves a here-and-now pursuit to make sense of the everyday world of nursing practice as it unfolds; this is reflection that 'looks on', referred to as 'reflection-in-action'. Reflection also involves thinking about experiences after they have occurred, which involves a 'there-and-then' thinking process in order to use experience for the purpose of considering new ways to practice. This is reflection that 'looks back', referred to as 'reflection-on-action'. Finally, reflection can occur prior to action, as nurses consider their intentions and plans for patient care. This is reflection that 'looks forward', referred to as 'reflection-for-action' (Asselin et al 2013). Regardless of whether it occurs before, during or after clinical practice, reflection is a process for understanding and appreciating experiences.

Schön (1983) is credited with coining the term 'reflective practice' and the processes of reflection-in-action and reflection-on-action. The potential of reflection was recognised by nurses as a valuable process because the profession is practice-based, with knowledge embedded in practice. Reflection became considered as central to the advancement of nursing knowledge and professional practice because thinking about clinical situations leads to insights for change (Asselin et al 2013; Bulman et al 2012; Goulet et al 2016; Miraglia & Asselin 2015), the purpose of which is to improve practice, especially when experiences are novel or formidable. Such improvements are aided and enhanced by linking reflections to theory. In this sense, reflective processes accompany learning, encouraging nurses to develop theoretical understandings that will serve as guides for future action. They promote continuous professional development and the courage to try different approaches.

While many students of nursing are taught to reflect on action (after the fact), Rolfe (2014) argues that Schön's original contention was that reflection-in-action was the process in which professionals engaged. In this sense, reflection is a form of experimentation through 'on-the-spot' thinking. Schön (1983, 1991) makes reference to the 'swamp' to indicate that professionals face problems and challenges that are messy and uncertain. In the 'swamp' there are rules or a set techniques to follow; solutions to problems are not straightforward.

This point is of particular relevance in relation to the use of interpersonal skills in nursing. Because each patient is unique and their response to their circumstances is specific to them, there are no set techniques or rules to follow. This is in contrast to the technical rationality that underpins evidence-based practice. When interacting with patients, nurses need to continuously assess how the patient is responding, and adjust their approach accordingly.

Nonetheless, beginning practitioners of nursing may struggle to simultaneously reflect while they are in the process of interacting with patients. Therefore, students of nursing will need to begin the process of reflection by first leaning how to reflect-on-action. Continuous reflection of this type then has the potential to develop into the art of reflection-in-action.

In a study that explored whether experienced nurses did engage in the process of reflection, it was found that they do engage with reflection-on-action (Asselin et al 2013). The clinical situations that the nurses described were ones that required immediate intervention. Their reflection about this situation occurred in four distinct phases. The first phase involved 'framing the situation' in light of their professional role and emotional responses. Next was pausing to consider what to do, which was followed by engaging in active reflection in order to gain insight into the situation. The final phase was moving to an intention to change practice in light of the insight gained (*see Research highlight*).

## RESEARCH HIGHLIGHT Problems encountered by experienced nurses in reflective practice

*Asselin, M.E., Schwartz-Barcott, D., 2015. Exploring problems encountered among experienced nurses using critical reflective inquiry, J. Nurses Prof. Dev. 31 (3), 138–144.*

### Background

Reflection is viewed as a critical process for professional development and advancement of nursing practice. There is an assumption that reflection is a deliberate process that develops over time. While the process of reflection is used extensively in nursing education, there is little evidence for what actually happens in practice. Previous research focused on the situations and problems that triggered reflection.

### Purpose of the study

The aim of this study was to describe the difficulties that experienced nurses in acute care perceived when employing reflective practice.

### Method

This was a secondary analysis of qualitative data that was obtained during a study (Asselin et al 2013) exploring how 12 experienced acute care nurses used reflective processes in a structured group setting.

### Key findings

There was a considerable stall in the nurses' reflection; they kept reliving the situation (sometimes for months and years) but could not move forward in the process of reflection. They became stuck in the process of reflection, replaying a situation over again but not moving forward in their thinking. They questioned themselves as to whether they had 'done the right thing' but could not consider what else could have been done. The group discussion did facilitate reflection and assisted the nurses in moving forward.

*cont.*

> *Research Highlight continued*
>
> ### Implications for nursing practice
>
> Nurses can become delayed in their reflections and ruminate for a long time without moving forward. Discussion with other nurses helps in moving forward and developing new insights. Reflective practice needs to be supported at the organisational level to assist nurses to use the reflective process to its full potential. Structured, facilitated reflection has the potential to enable nurses to move their *intentions* to change to *actual* changes in practice.

# Processes for reflection

The conditions that are essential to the reflective practice include: a desire to learn, openness in sharing, honesty, the belief that change is possible and the courage to act (Goulet et al 2016). Reflection needs to be practised regularly, and active strategies support the process. This means that the most successful reflection is accompanied by structured activities such as keeping a professional diary or completing the activities in this book. Unless there is some means of tracking an individual nurse's reflections over a period of time, sustainable professional growth through reflection may be difficult to attain.

With increasing frequency, clinical supervision (see Ch 11) is considered by many as an ideal method to encourage and support reflective practice. Clinical supervision, whether conducted individually or in groups of nurses, is aimed at using reflective processes for the purpose of improving the quality of nursing care. The process is useful in developing interpersonal skills and in increasing self-understanding.

# Pitfalls in reflection

Despite its obvious benefits, reflection does have its potential pitfalls. It is important to remember that effective reflection will inevitably lead to anxiety because the process of reflecting involves change and challenge. It requires nurses to show a willingness to be challenged to view experiences in different lights and to reconsider what may be long-held and cherished beliefs. The anxiety and discomfort that accompanies effective reflection points to the need for support systems to be in place (e.g. colleagues who serve as skilled facilitators and mentors).

Another pitfall in using reflection is perhaps the most challenging of all in relation to beginning practitioners and students of nursing. It is that a nurse needs to be clinically experienced in order to benefit from reflection (Goulet et al 2016). This implies that the nurses who most need to learn in terms of clinical experience may be least able to benefit from the process of reflection. Nevertheless, structured reflection, especially under the guidance of a more experienced nurse, is a useful way for beginning nurses to assess their own interpersonal skills and to improve self-understanding through raised awareness of the impact of self on nursing practice.

## Input from others / interactive reflection

There are limits to how far self-understanding can progress and develop through introspection alone. Natural 'blind spots', the ease with which self-reflective thoughts can be ignored, dismissed and defended, along with the tendency to protect the self through self-deception, pose barriers to the introspective process.

Other people provide useful information through the way they react and respond. For this reason, another effective way to complement, not replace, self-reflection occurs when nurses attend to feedback from others, be it solicited or unsolicited. Feedback from good friends is useful and can be solicited. Feedback from patients is another useful source of information, although nurses usually do not solicit it.

## Input from patients

Patients are not only expressing information about themselves when they interact with nurses, they also are expressing information about how they perceive the nurse. Patients reveal how they feel and what they think about the nurses who are interacting with them by the manner in which they behave. What they choose to discuss, how freely they disclose information and how comfortable they seem during an interaction are examples of input that patients provide about how they see the nurse. The cues that indicate the effect nurses are having on them automatically surface throughout interactions. Nurses need to be receptive to such input from patients because this feedback informs them about themselves. In this regard, nurses need not actively solicit patient feedback.

Perceiving such input from patients begins with an awareness and understanding of its relevance. Next, nurses need to be open to receiving the information. Asking themselves questions such as 'What is it about me that enables patients to openly express their feelings?', 'Why is this patient telling *me* this?' and 'Have I inadvertently communicated that I don't want to hear what this patient is saying?' enables nurses to become open to input from patients.

It is natural for nurses to ignore or reject input and feedback about themselves when this information lacks congruence with personal images (what nurses believe they are or want to be). Nurses who are feeling inept may not notice when patients reveal that they *are* quite effective. For this reason, feedback and input from others, especially patients, may challenge nurses to reconsider their current perspectives.

# SELF-SHARING

Another process that is effective in increasing self-understanding arises out of a combination of self-reflection (introspection) and interactive reflection (input and feedback from others). It is the process of self-sharing – the disclosure of personal thoughts, feelings, perceptions and interpretations by openly expressing them to others.

## How self-sharing increases self-understanding

Self-sharing enhances self-understanding because it triggers (and therefore solicits) feedback from others and also because it intensifies self-reflection. When internal thoughts, feelings and attitudes are made external through open discussion, they are often internally clarified, expanded and accepted. Sometimes self-sharing persuades nurses to internally challenge and alter their thoughts, feelings and attitudes. In this sense, self-sharing often transforms into a process of 'thinking aloud' and then having a dialogue with the self while using the other person as a sounding board.

At other times, self-sharing enables nurses to test the validity of their current thoughts, feelings and attitudes. In 'testing' their internal responses, nurses are asking others what they think or feel about these responses. This often leads nurses to reconsider their responses in light of what others think and feel.

The relationship between self-sharing and self-understanding is a circular one (see Fig. 3.2). While a certain degree of self-understanding is helpful to begin self-sharing, it is not vital. Through self-sharing, further input is received, both from others and from the self, which is then useful in increasing self-understanding.

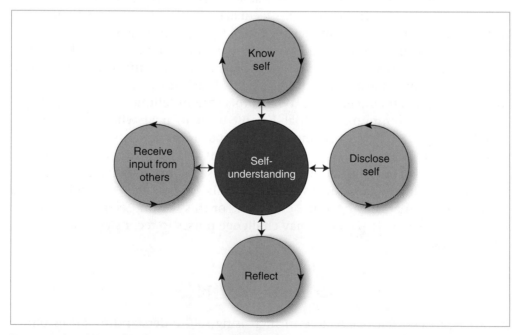

**Figure 3.2** Relationship between self-sharing and self-understanding

# Risks of self-sharing

Despite its potential value for increasing self-understanding, disclosing oneself to others is not always easy to do. There are many reasons for keeping to oneself and choosing not to disclose. Activity 3.2 is designed to uncover some of the reasons why self-sharing may be difficult.

---

## ACTIVITY 3.2 Difficulties in self-sharing

### Process

1. Working on your own, rank each of the following topics from 1 to 12, according to what is easiest for you to disclose about yourself (1) to what is hardest to disclose (12). Place these topics in the context of interacting with someone you do not know very well.

   **a.** Talking about my fears

   **b.** Sharing my hopes and dreams

   **c.** Discussing my family life

   **d.** Describing my previous health problems

   **e.** Stating what I dislike about other people

   **f.** Complaining about a mark on an assignment

   **g.** Expressing my political views

   **h.** Stating what I want or need

   **i.** Expressing confusion or uncertainty

   **j.** Describing how I like to be treated by others

   **k.** Complaining about being treated unfairly

   **l.** Telling others that I am not pleased about something they have done

2. Review your answers and reflect on those items that you determined as easy to discuss (those ranked 1–5). Record your reasons for evaluating these items as easy to disclose.

3. Review your answers again, this time reflecting on those items that you determined as difficult to disclose (those ranked 8–12). Record your reasons for evaluating these items as difficult to disclose.

4. Compare your responses with two other participants. Discuss your responses to steps 2 and 3. Summarise what is easy to disclose and what is hard to disclose, focusing on your reasons.

5. This step lists some of the reasons for lack of self-disclosure. Working individually, rate each of these reasons in terms of how often it is true for you. Use the following descriptions:

*cont.*

*Activity 3.2 continued*

- often
- sometimes
- rarely.

If I tell others what I think and feel ...

**a.** I may hurt them

**b.** They may take advantage of me

**c.** I may appear weak

**d.** I may become emotional

**e.** They may hurt me

**f.** They may talk to others about me

**g.** I may discover something about myself that I'd rather not know

**h.** They may use what I've said against me

**i.** I may discover problems I never knew I had

**6.** Working in the same groups of three as for step 4, discuss those items that you rated as 'often' and 'sometimes'. What similarities are there in your responses? What differences are there?

### Discussion

**1.** What are the major reasons for reluctance to self-disclose?

**2.** What are the major disadvantages of self-disclosure? What are the major advantages?

**3.** How does self-disclosure promote self-awareness?

The major difficulty in disclosing self is the exposure that it brings. Once people are exposed, they often feel vulnerable, especially if the disclosure has been about problem areas or negative thoughts, feelings and perceptions. There are risks of being rejected, being hurt and being challenged by others. This sense of vulnerability is not necessarily destructive to nurses because of its potential to increase feelings of empathy with patients, who often feel exposed and vulnerable when they disclose themselves to nurses. While there are obvious risks in exposing oneself, these are offset by its potential benefits.

## The climate conducive to self-sharing

Because of the exposure and vulnerability that self-sharing can bring, it needs to take place in an atmosphere of trust and respect – trust in the sense that the disclosure will not be met with rejection and respect in the sense that disclosed information will be considered, and not dismissed or ridiculed.

As a general rule, there is ease and comfort with disclosure when it is likely that personal thoughts, feelings and attitudes will be understood and appreciated by the other person. This is more likely to happen when the other person shares similar experiences. For this reason, nurses often benefit by disclosing themselves to other nurses (see Ch 11). Through the process of self-sharing, nurses can be supported by other nurses. They may also be challenged at times to reconsider their perceptions, thoughts and feelings.

# SELF-DISCLOSURE WITH PATIENTS

Self-disclosure with patients (see Chs 5, 6 and 7) is different from self-sharing. Self-disclosure with patients is employed as a therapeutic skill and is therefore for the benefit of the patient, not the nurse. Although self-disclosure with patients may result in increased self-understanding for the nurse, this is not its primary focus. The intent of self-disclosing with patients is to promote interaction and increase interpersonal involvement with patients. The primary intent of self-sharing with people other than patients is increased self-understanding in the nurse.

## Areas of self-exploration

It is important that nurses not only understand the processes for promoting greater self-understanding but also that they recognise those areas of themselves that are most relevant to the nursing-care context. There are many facets of each nurse's personal self that are woven together to create the essence of the person who is the nurse. While many aspects of the self can be considered, those addressed in Activity 3.3 have a potential to affect the way nurses approach helping patients.

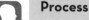

**ACTIVITY 3.3  Beliefs about helping in nursing practice**  ↻ 333

### Process

For each of the following statements, record on a separate sheet of paper the response that most closely identifies your personal beliefs and attitudes. Use the following scale:

3   For the most part, I *agree* with this statement.

2   I am *undecided* in my opinion about this statement.

1   For the most part, I *disagree* with this statement.

   **a.**  Patients should be encouraged to accept that they have contributed to their own health problems.

   **b.**  What happens in patient–nurse relationships is more the nurse's responsibility than the patient's.

   **c.**  People are masters of their own destinies; solutions to whatever problems they have are in their own hands.

*cont.*

*Activity 3.3 continued*

**d.** There are many social factors contributing to health problems that are beyond individual control.

**e.** Whether they realise it or not, people engage in behaviours that cause health problems.

**f.** Effective health education could prevent major health problems.

**g.** Patients should be encouraged to find solutions and take action on their own behalf when dealing with health problems.

**h.** It irritates me when I hear somebody say that a patient caused their own health problems; most of the time people can't help it.

**i.** Providing advice to patients is an essential aspect of effective healthcare.

**j.** People should be presented with options for healthcare so they can choose what suits them best.

**k.** In recovering from an illness, it is essential that patients heed the advice of healthcare professionals.

**l.** Most people could change their problematic health habits if they really wanted to.

**m.** Patients should determine their own goals when working with healthcare professionals.

**n.** I don't have much time for patients who won't follow the advice of knowledgeable healthcare experts.

**o.** Diseases and illnesses are largely a result of biological and genetic factors, which are usually beyond individual control.

**p.** Patients should place themselves in the hands of qualified healthcare professionals who know best what to do about health problems.

## Discussion

1. Reflect on your responses and consider whether you tend to hold people responsible for their health problems.

2. Consider your responses in light of whether you tend to think that people should take responsibility for their own healthcare.

3. In general, what do your responses reflect about your beliefs about health and healthcare?

# PERSONAL PHILOSOPHY ABOUT HEALTH

Personal value systems, the 'shoulds' and 'oughts' that direct individual behaviour, are part of all people's lives. These values and beliefs, which are personal and unique to the individual, assist a person in making choices and decisions about living. They provide direction about what is important, what matters, what is seen as significant and what is worthwhile. These values and beliefs are not static; they are altered, revised and adapted through life experiences. Nurses often find that their beliefs and values alter throughout their professional lives.

One aspect of personal value systems that is particularly relevant for nurses is their beliefs about health and helping. For example, nurses may feel less inclined to care for patients who they believe are responsible for their own health problems.

Activity 3.3 is designed to make participants think about how they would approach helping other people on the basis of two central issues: *blame* and *control* (Brickman et al 1982). Blame is the degree to which people are held responsible for causing their problems, and control is the degree to which they are held responsible for solutions to their problems. Both involve questions of personal responsibility, and assumptions about personal responsibility have direct effects on the type of help offered. Brickman et al (1982) conceptualised four models of helping based on the issues of blame and control (see Fig. 3.3).

Although developed many years ago, this conceptualisation remains evident in current literature, especially in relation to how people are 'blamed' for their health problems (e.g. Beames et al 2016; Koski-Jännes et al 2016). In the nursing literature, it has been shown that nurses blame patients who they judge as being responsible for their problems (Karman et al 2015; Michaelsen 2012).

The view from within the 'medical model' is that people are neither responsible for creating their problems nor responsible for solutions to their problems. The

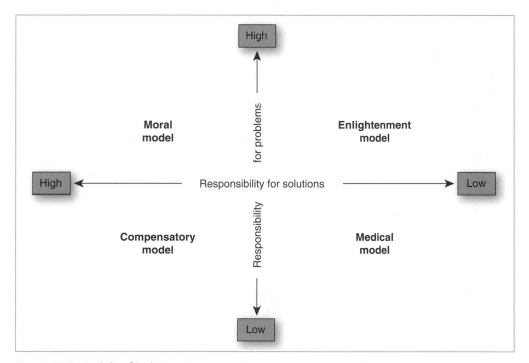

**Figure 3.3** Models of helping
*Based on Brickman et al (1982). Models of helping and Coping. Am Psych 37 (4), 368–384*

'compensatory model' operates from beliefs that people cannot be blamed for their problems but are held responsible for doing something about them. Beliefs within the 'enlightenment model' are that people are responsible for creating their problems but need to rely on others in solving these problems. The 'moral model' holds people responsible for both creating their problems and developing their own solutions.

Each stance results in an orientation to how to be of help to patients. The 'medical model' relies on expert advice and treats patients as passive recipients of assistance. Patients are expected to seek and heed such advice and assistance. While people are not blamed for their problems, they may be blamed if they fail to cooperate with the solutions offered. Helping in the 'compensatory model' centres on the mobilisation of needed resources and providing opportunities to compensate for what are seen as failures and weaknesses that are outside individual control. Acceptance of personal blame and reliance on an external authority is the helping approach used in the 'enlightenment model'. The 'moral model' focuses helping on motivating people to change through persuasion, appeal, reprimand and reproach.

In nursing practice, there is likely to be a mixed application of these models, as illustrated in the following examples. Nurses might hold active smokers responsible for problems such as lung cancer, while lung cancer acquired from passive smoking usually does not bring such blame. In both of these situations, people would not be held responsible for the possible solutions/treatment for the lung cancer. Nursing care would be provided to the active smokers ('enlightenment model'), although some nurses may question the use of healthcare resources on this population ('moral model'). The victims of passive smoking might be approached using the 'medical model', in which case they would not be held responsible for the cause or the solutions. A person with diabetes mellitus may not be held responsible for acquiring the disease but will be expected to be actively involved in its control ('compensatory model'). A suicidal person may be blamed for the problem and expected to find solutions through effort and willpower ('moral model').

Help may not be effective if the person desiring help and the person offering help are operating from a different set of assumptions about personal responsibility (Brickman et al 1982). For this reason, it is important not only that nurses realise their own orientation to helping and its underlying assumptions but also that they are aware of and understand patients' orientations to helping.

# PERSONAL VALUES AND BELIEFS

Nurses' personal values and beliefs directly affect their interactions with patients. They have the potential to restrict effective relationships with patients; however, they can also enhance these relationships.

One way that nurses' values and personal beliefs may hinder effective relationships with patients stems from the fact that these values and beliefs often function as perceptual filters. Perceptual filters allow some aspects of patients' stories to be accepted, while others are rejected. When values and personal beliefs function as filters, the skills of listening (see Ch 5) are most affected. Cultural stereotypes (Ch 4), another possible hindrance in relating effectively with patients, often stem from values and personal beliefs.

Another way that personal values create interference occurs when nurses impose or project them onto patients, rather than keeping them in abeyance. When values and beliefs are imposed on patients, they are used as yardsticks for measuring them. Whenever nurses make judgments about what patients 'should' or 'should not' be, there is a chance that they are evaluating patients in terms of their own value system. For this reason, nurses are encouraged to reflect on these types of judgments.

On the other hand, certain values and personal beliefs enhance and strengthen nurses' ability to relate to patients. For example, a personal belief that people are capable, worthwhile and dependable works in favour of establishing effective relationships with patients. Such beliefs help to create a climate of respect and regard for patients.

When relating to patients, nurses cannot be expected to abandon their values and personal beliefs; however, they need to be able to distinguish their own philosophical stance from that of a patient. The more aware nurses are of their own values and personal beliefs, the less likely it is that interference will occur, and the more likely it is that the values that enhance effective relationships will be strengthened.

Most nurses enter nursing with some goal in mind. It might be to secure a job with the promise of sustained demand. It could be that part-time work is appealing. An advertisement in the local newspaper might have sparked interest in nursing in a 'Why not? I'm not doing anything else with my life …' fashion. Assuming there were options available, nursing is usually chosen because of an interest in people. In all likelihood, this interest in people is directly related to a desire to help.

Activity 3.4 probably highlights a common myth about nursing: the belief that all benefits in nursing are for the patient, never the nurse. By focusing solely on their desire to help and to assist others, nurses fail to acknowledge the potential benefits of nursing for themselves. The 'ideal' nurse is often perceived as self-sacrificing – so 'others-oriented' that there is a denial of self. Such an ideal does not exist in reality.

# PERSONAL NEEDS

Forming meaningful relationships with patients and assisting them with health issues and problems often has benefits for nurses as well as patients. For example, nurses derive satisfaction in seeing patients recover from illnesses, especially when they know they made a difference to the recovery. Does this mean that nurses meet their own needs through their nursing relationships? A recognition and acknowledgment of the personal benefits of nursing results in an affirmative answer to such a question.

## ACTIVITY 3.4 Expectations of nursing

### Process

1. Think of all the reasons why you chose nursing as a career. Record these on a sheet of paper. Do not place any identifying information about yourself on the paper.

2. Now complete the following sentences, recording your answers on the same sheet of paper:

   **a.** If I could do anything as a nurse it would be to …

   **b.** In my role as a nurse I see myself as …

   **c.** Nurses help others because they …

   **d.** My greatest disappointment as a nurse would be if I …

3. Collect all the sheets of paper and distribute them among all participants.

4. Record, on a sheet of paper visible to all participants, all the reasons identified by the participants for choosing nursing. If a reason is given by more than one participant, record how many times it is stated.

### Discussion

1. Discuss the responses to each of the items in step 2 of the process. Remember, you are not discussing your own responses but the ones of the anonymous participant who authored the paper you received.

2. Do motivations for becoming a nurse and expectations of nursing focus exclusively on helping others, or are there references to personal gains and benefits?

Nevertheless, there are obvious risks involved because nurses' personal needs may interfere whenever relationships with patients are used as the *primary* source of meeting these needs. For example, relying on patients to satisfy the nurse's need for personal recognition, appreciation and validation is fraught with danger. For this reason, nurses need to develop awareness of potential trouble spots – those personal needs that may interfere in their relationships with patients.

## ACTIVITY 3.5 Needs that may interfere

### Process

1. Use one of the following descriptions to rate questions a–j:

   • hardly ever

   • sometimes

   • most of the time.

How often do I ...

**a.** Let people take advantage of me because I am afraid to say no to their requests?

**b.** Focus on problems and negative aspects of a situation, so I fail to take into account the positive side of people and their strengths?

**c.** Feel as if I must 'do something' to make other people feel better – to rescue them?

**d.** Think I need to have all the answers when other people discuss problems with me?

**e.** Worry about whether or not other people like me?

**f.** Feel the need to be needed?

**g.** Need to be in control of situations?

**h.** Want other people to take care of me?

**i.** Feel controlled by other people?

**j.** Act as openly with other people as I want them to act with me?

2. Review your answers. If the majority of your answers are 'sometimes', go back and change them to either 'hardly ever' or 'most of the time'. All of the items will be true for most people some of the time!

3. Identify the items that are 'hardly ever' and 'most of the time'. Reflect on these in terms of how these aspects of yourself may affect your relationships with patients.

**Discussion**

1. The items included in this self-assessment relate to three general areas of basic human needs: the need to feel attached to other people (included); the need to be in control; and the need for affection and affirmation from other people. Which one of these general areas of personal needs is predominant for you?

2. Discuss each of the three basic human needs and how, if they are predominant in a nurse, interactions and relationships with patients may be affected, for better or worse.

# CHARACTERISTICS THAT HELP INTERPERSONAL CONNECTEDNESS

The focus of the preceding sections of this chapter has been on increasing self-awareness because such reflection leads to self-understanding, self-challenge and eventual acceptance of aspects that characterise each nurse. Other than considering how these aspects of the self potentially affect relationships with patients, no effort has been made to evaluate them (or the nurse they characterise) in terms of right/wrong, good/bad or desirable/undesirable. No evaluation has been attempted because nurses must first develop awareness of 'what is' before considering 'what should be'. Understanding 'what is' provides a starting point – a reference from which to work towards 'what should be'.

There are certain characteristics, personal beliefs, values and orientations towards helping that enhance nurses' abilities to relate effectively to patients. In this regard, they are in the 'what should be' category. When they are present in the nurse, these characteristics help to facilitate interpersonal connections with patients because they help to create the necessary interpersonal climate for developing patient–nurse relationships. The presence of this climate enables nurses to effectively use the skills and processes described in this book. If the facilitative climate is absent, the use of the skills may become hollow, mechanical and artificial.

## ACTIVITY 3.6  Characteristics of effective helpers

**Process**

1. Think of someone in your life who is helpful to you (i.e. the person you go to for understanding, assistance and guidance).

2. Think about what this person is like. What personal characteristics do they possess? Focus on specific characteristics that are helpful to you. Describe these on a sheet of paper.

3. Now think about what this person does that you find helpful. What specific things does this person do? Describe these on your sheet of paper. Do not be concerned if there are similarities between answers to steps 2 and 3. In some instances, your answers may be exactly the same.

4. Review what you have written. Briefly summarise what, in your opinion, enables this person to be effective in helping you.

5. Compare your descriptions with those of all other participants by compiling an overall description of a person who is helpful. Record this in a place visible to all participants.

6. Select key words from the description and record them.

**Discussion**

1. What are the similarities in participants' individual descriptions? What are the differences?

2. Focusing on the key words identified in step 6 of the process, describe personal characteristics that are essential for being a helpful person.

3. Is there anything you would add to this list of personal characteristics?

From Activity 3.6, you may discover that people perceived to be helpful embody certain characteristics (what they are), demonstrate certain skills (what they do) and possess a degree of understanding about people (what they know). It is the personal characteristics associated with helpful people that are discussed here.

Characteristics that enhance the ability to be helpful include:

- authenticity and congruence
- respect and warmth
- confidence and assertiveness.

The characteristics are described in Table 3.1.

| TABLE 3.1 Characteristics of a helpful person | | |
|---|---|---|
| **CHARACTERISTIC** | **DESCRIPTION** | **BENEFIT** |
| Authenticity | Being true to oneself<br>Not 'hiding' behind the role of nurse | Patient will know that the nurse is human |
| Congruence | Consistency in beliefs, feelings and action | Patient will come to trust the nurse |
| Respect | Acceptance of the patient's reality and experiences, and inherent belief in the patient's capabilities | Patient will feel free to express their concerns and feelings |
| Warmth | Friendly, non-verbal demonstration of concern and interest | Patient will feel at ease because the nurse is approachable |
| Confidence | Belief in self and secure in the knowledge that can be helpful | Patient will be reassured that the nurse can be of assistance |
| Assertiveness | Ability to express own ideas and feelings and to explore difficult subjects | Patient will come to know that the nurse is actively interested |

# Authenticity and congruence

Frequently, when nurses try to use the skills described in this book, feelings of awkwardness and lack of authenticity accompany their first attempts. This is especially true if the skill being tried is unfamiliar and foreign to the nurse's current repertoire of skills. While a skill may be unfamiliar, the personal values from which it emerges may not be. For example, a nurse may be unaccustomed to reflecting feelings (see Ch 6) because of being raised in an environment where feelings were hardly ever expressed and never discussed openly. Unless this nurse believes that patients' feelings are important to understand and comes to realise that, for some patients, feelings are the most significant facet of their experience, the nurse may fail to try to use feeling reflections with patients. This nurse must tap into the authentic desire to help patients in order to overcome feelings of reluctance and awkwardness.

Congruence is related to authenticity because with congruence comes consistency between what nurses believe, how they feel and what they do. The skills described in this book are only effective if they are used in conjunction with an attitude that matches their intent. There is little point in pretending to listen through appropriate attending behaviour (Ch 5) if a nurse is not currently interested in what a patient is expressing. A listening posture without an attitude of genuine interest lacks congruence. A congruent manner is one in which the nurse's intent and related action are in harmony.

# Respect and warmth

Respect operates from an attitude of 'being for' patients. To be respectful is to assume the patient's goodwill (Egan 2014) and to believe that patients are doing their best to cope, to adapt and to change. With respect comes a deep concern for a patient's individual experiences – an acceptance of their perspective and feelings. Respect emerges from the value that each human being has inherent worth and dignity. When they are respected, patients are free to be themselves; they need not fear that they will be placed against a standard of what they 'should' be experiencing.

Holding personal judgments in abeyance (see Ch 5) is one of the most striking ways nurses convey respect to patients. This highlights and reinforces the need for self-understanding. Unless nurses are cognisant of their personal values and beliefs, they may inadvertently judge patients against a personal value system. An attitude that is suspicious of patients' motives and behaviours lacks respect if suspicion is the nurse's first reaction.

Warmth is a feeling primarily conveyed through non-verbal behaviour that demonstrates an active interest in and regard for patients. Warmth is an active demonstration of respect because it conveys active concern. Warmth is not emotionally effusive or overly friendly behaviour. Too much warmth creates a sense of false solicitude, lacking genuineness. Patients might become frightened at the prospect of a nurse whose concern seems extreme, especially if this occurs early in the course of the relationship. Too little warmth distances patients because this gives an impression of lack of concern and regard.

# Confidence and assertiveness

Even when nurses are congruent and authentic, and able to convey respect and warmth, unless they also have an ability to express themselves confidently and assertively they may not be able to make interpersonal contact with patients. Knowing what to say and how to say it becomes inconsequential if nurses fail to use interpersonal skills because they are apprehensive and hesitant.

Assertiveness is most often presented as a means of resolving conflict (see Ch 11) and defending individual rights if they have been violated. However, conflict is not the specific focus here. In the general context of patient–nurse relationships, being assertive means that nurses are able to take advantage of opportunities to make interpersonal contact with patients.

While nurses often recognise the need to be assertive when advocating *for* patients (e.g. when another healthcare professional is disregarding a patient's request), they often express concerns about being assertive *with* patients. Whenever nurses think 'I can't say *that* to a patient', they are experiencing concerns about what will happen. These concerns include a fear of upsetting patients, a discomfort with the expression of feelings, a perception that it is intrusive to ask personal questions and a reticence about delving into the subjective experiences of patients. Apprehensions such as these often inhibit nurses and may even restrict them from meeting their professional responsibilities to patients. For example, if a nurse is reluctant to explore a patient's apparent distress (out of fear of compounding that distress), vital information about the patient's experience may be missed or overlooked.

The concerns that inhibit nurses are often based on faulty assumptions such as 'patients will become *more* upset if asked to discuss their distress', 'nurses should be passive and obedient' and 'it is impolite to discuss sensitive and personal matters with a relative stranger'. In becoming assertive with patients, nurses need to overcome these concerns by challenging these assumptions.

First, nurses do not have the 'power' to 'make' patients more upset simply on the basis of bringing a patient's distress into the open (although this is different from abuse of power, which is discussed in Ch 10). When patients are distressed, they are often relieved to share their emotional pain with an interested and understanding nurse. Rather than compounding their tension, open discussion can actually provide comfort. Second, while it would be impolite to discuss highly personal matters with a stranger in a social situation, patient–nurse interactions are different from usual social interactions. In caring for patients, nurses need to discuss personal matters with them because this is part of their professional responsibility.

At times, being assertive translates into making the decision 'not' to discuss something. For example, when a patient is coping by maintaining their emotions within manageable limits, a nurse can make an active decision *not* to explore or focus on feelings. As long as the decision not to say something is based on an assessment of the situation, rather than the nurse's internal fear, assertiveness is present. Being assertive in relating to patients means that nurses have both the courage to say something and the wisdom to remain silent.

# DEVELOPING A PERSONAL STYLE

Authenticity, congruence, respect, warmth and assertiveness are desirable characteristics that each nurse demonstrates in a unique way. Although these characteristics help to create an interpersonal climate that enhances meaningful connections, they should not be construed as personality prescriptions for nurses. Each nurse develops personal capabilities for relating to patients.

Skills that are useful in establishing these relationships can be learnt and developed. There are certain conditions, such as respect and warmth, that enable nurses to use the skills most effectively. These conditions can be enhanced and developed. There are approaches to helping patients that can be employed (e.g. challenging patients to reframe their experiences) (see Ch 8). These approaches can be understood and developed.

Each nurse finds a way to use the skills to express the necessary characteristics and to integrate a variety of approaches in a unique expression of that nurse's personality. Some nurses are good at challenging patients and do so quite effectively and naturally, while other nurses find this approach difficult and are frustrated when they attempt to use it.

In developing a personal style, nurses must learn how to blend the skills and characteristics with their own personalities and to discover how their personal selves merge into their professional selves. A concerted effort to understand, practise and employ the skills results in this blending. Engaging in the processes of self-understanding accelerates the development of a personal style in relating to patients. Nevertheless, some unique challenges arise when nurses attempt to learn and develop the skills of interacting in a manner that is unique to them.

Developing a personal style of relating to patients poses certain learning challenges because beginning nurses have developed a characteristic style of communicating and relating to other people prior to entering nursing practice. Although these familiar patterns of interacting may be comfortable for the individual nurse as a person, they may not be suitable within the nursing context. In learning the skills and developing them for the nursing context, nurses are often challenged to alter or change their customary and usual patterns of interaction. In meeting this challenge, a total transformation of a nurse's particular manner is not necessary because such transformation may not reflect the nurse's personality. Nevertheless, alterations to existing patterns of interacting are often necessary in order to develop a personal style that is both authentic to an individual nurse and appropriate to the context of nursing care. While the person who is the nurse has not changed, the nursing care context signals the need for a change in approach.

# LEARNING THE SKILLS

The following chapters contain descriptions of a range of skills that enable nurses to interact effectively with patients. While theoretical understanding of the skills is a vital aspect of learning, understanding not accompanied by technical know-how in the use of the skills is insufficient. For this reason, learning the skills of interacting with patients is achieved most effectively through performing the skills.

Every nurse is encouraged to attempt each of the skills to see how they fit the particular nursing context and determine what alterations can be made to help them fit better. Some of the skills will be familiar, and using them will come naturally because they already exist in the nurse's repertoire. Other skills will be foreign, and nurses may feel awkward and unnatural when initially attempting to use these skills. Selecting some of the skills because they are comfortable to use and ignoring others because 'they don't feel right' limits practical learning opportunities and potential.

## The need to 'unlearn'

It is more than likely that the skills presented in the following chapters will be recognisable as everyday activities. For example, listening (see Ch 5) is a process that people engage in daily, whether it be effective or ineffective. This familiarity with some skills, however, presents a specific dilemma to nurses as they approach learning how to fit skills into a nursing care context as well as blending the skills with their personality.

Because nurses have been interacting with other people all of their lives, they may believe they already know how to talk to patients, and they may be disconcerted to find out there is more to learn. But these familiar patterns of interacting may not be effective within the nursing care context. As a result, some nurses may fail to recognise and appreciate the alterations that may be needed to make their interactions with patients more effective.

Learning how to use interpersonal skills within the nursing care context is often a matter of 'letting go' of habitual and automatic ways of interacting – ways that have become comfortable. For example, offering advice and giving solutions is a common response to someone who presents a problem. In Chapter 6, this way of responding is shown to be less effective than a response that demonstrates understanding. If offering advice and giving solutions is their customary way of responding to those in need, nurses are challenged to refrain from their usual way of responding. The necessity of letting go of familiar patterns and 'unlearning' ways that may have become entrenched presents a major hurdle in learning and developing effective interactive skills with patients.

Departing from the comfort zone of usual and customary patterns of interacting and attempting new and unfamiliar ways initially results in feelings of being untrue to oneself. Nurses may become confused by this apparent lack of authenticity, which has been discussed as a core condition for effective interactions. Nurses may feel inept, clumsy and overly self-conscious as they struggle to let go of the familiar and to meet the demands of learning new ways of interacting.

Such feelings are often unavoidable during initial attempts to use any new skill, and this highlights the need for continuous self-assessment, which raises awareness and understanding of self. Through self-assessment, nurses come to appreciate what they are attempting in their interactions with patients, why they are attempting this and how it is affecting patients. Nurses are encouraged to promote their own growth as people and as nurses and to challenge growth within themselves by trying various ways of interacting with patients, even when these ways initially feel awkward. With continuing practice, self-understanding and acceptance (as well as patience with the learning process), the skills will eventually become natural. At this point a personal style will emerge.

## Reactions to learning the skills

Some nurses fail to perceive and appreciate the significance of learning interpersonal skills simply because they *have* been interacting with other people all their lives. These nurses view the skills of interacting with patients as little more than commonsense and 'doing what comes naturally'. Because the skills used when interacting with patients are not exclusive to nursing, these nurses fail to perceive the importance of spending time learning them or recognising how the nursing care context necessitates an alteration in interaction patterns.

Such reactions fail to take into account the fact that commonsense is not innate but learnt behaviour. Toddlers do not have the commonsense to recognise the dangers of running onto a street full of moving vehicles. While the commonsense that nurses have developed throughout their lives could assist them in learning the skills, there is also a danger that this commonsense approach may inhibit learning. For example, commonsense may dictate that patients should not be worried or alarmed by what the nurse perceives to be a minor situation. Under such circumstances, the commonsense approach may be to try to talk patients out of their 'needless' worrying with platitudes and clichés. While such an approach seems to have a rational, objective basis, it fails to acknowledge the reality of patients' experiences and is therefore less effective than approaching patients by trying to understand their experiences.

In believing that interacting with patients is nothing more than commonsense, nurses may fail to develop the self-understanding necessary to recognise when their approach is not effective. They may fail to reconsider habitual and automatic responses and attitudes and to realise that the context indicates a need for a change in these usual approaches. In simply 'doing what comes naturally', nurses fail to learn how to develop skills specific to the nursing context.

At the opposite end of the spectrum are those nurses who accept the importance of learning how to interact with patients and immerse themselves in learning the skills. For these nurses, a different type of learning challenge may present itself. In attempting to learn the skills, these nurses may become reticent about saying anything to a patient out of fear of making a mistake and saying the wrong thing. If they do attempt to employ the skills, these nurses may have a stilted manner.

Most often this reaction is a result of a common misconception that talking to patients is somehow dramatically different from talking to people who are not patients. The nurses who become almost paralysed when trying to use the skills, or who use the skills in a stilted way, are often stifled by a belief that 'being therapeutic' means being completely different from usual. The major consequence of this belief is that it retards development of a personal style.

The nurses who are resistant to learning new ways of interacting because they believe that interacting with patients is nothing more than commonsense assume that relationships with patients have no special features. The nurses who are reticent to interact with patients out of fear of making a mistake assume that relationships with patients are entirely different from other types of human interactions and that a common ground cannot be established. Both groups are misguided and are acting on false assumptions. The first response reflects a rejection of the professional self ('I'll just be myself'), while the second response fails to recognise the use of personal self ('I no longer *can* be myself').

While relationships with patients have characteristics that are different from social relationships such as friendship (see Ch 2), the person who is the nurse remains the same. Nurses must come to realise that their professional self emerges from their personal self; neither is a separate entity.

These reactions to learning the skills of interacting within the nursing context highlight the need for continuous self-appraisal and self-challenge. By focusing their efforts on becoming more aware, nurses who react to learning the skills in the ways described in the preceding paragraphs are able to meet the challenges posed by these reactions. By reflecting on their responses, nurses not only become aware of their faulty perspectives (if any exist) on interactions with patients but are challenged to review and revise these perspectives. The essential aim in developing such an awareness when interacting with patients is to be able to assess and evaluate how current perspectives and interpretations could be affecting the development of effective interpersonal skills.

# SELF-ASSESSMENT OF INTERPERSONAL SKILLS

Active and ongoing self-assessment is a dynamic strategy for reflection and is one of the most effective ways to increase interpersonal effectiveness as a nurse. Self-assessment draws on all of the processes for developing self-understanding that are described in this chapter. Nurses need to develop the ability to observe themselves as they participate in interactions with patients. This requires nurses to develop abilities to stand apart from themselves temporarily and to tune their senses to recognise effective and ineffective interaction patterns. Observing feedback and input from patients, which indicates how patients are responding to the nurse's attempts to interact, adds to this self-evaluation. Discussion with other nurses about relationships with patients offers opportunities to be both reassured and challenged. Finally, sharing motives, intentions, thoughts and feelings, both with oneself and with other nurses, offers further opportunities for growth in interpersonal effectiveness with patients.

## Advantages of self-assessment

Self-assessment is a useful way to approach the development of skills for a variety of reasons. First, focusing on self-assessing, especially when initially attempting to use the skills, helps to release nurses from the fear of saying the wrong thing. Through the process of self-assessment, 'mistakes', when made, are viewed as indicators for further growth and development rather than outright failures. Nurses who can recognise when they either miss the point or could be handling an interaction more effectively have an opportunity to recover and move the interaction back on track. When awareness is lacking, errors and omissions go unrecognised and future learning opportunities are missed.

Second, self-assessment has the advantage of using the nurse's firsthand experience in the interaction. Nurses who have participated in an interaction know best what happened. In this sense, 'being there' provides essential input. Nurses who 'were there' understand their own intentions during the interaction and can therefore evaluate an interaction in light of these intentions. In this regard, evaluation of performance is placed within the context of actual interactions, as opposed to employing rules that are context-free. This approach takes into account the specific factors relevant to a given interaction and places evaluation within the light of these factors.

Finally, and perhaps most importantly, developing the ability to self-assess enables nurses to engage in continual learning. Through awareness and self-assessment, nurses come to understand their personal strengths and areas for improvement, and performance is evaluated in terms of these personal aspects. When every interaction is viewed as an opportunity for learning, nurses engage in continuous professional growth. In this respect, self-assessment (the evaluation of one's own performance) is considered an essential ability, even a skill in its own right.

Self-assessment is useful in evaluating interpersonal effectiveness after an interaction has occurred, and this is the most common way in which it is initially developed. When developed to its fullest, self-assessment also enables nurses to determine how best to approach a given situation *during* an interaction.

During interactions with patients, nurses have a range of skill options to employ, assuming their repertoire of skills is extensive. For example, the choice to encourage a patient through attending and listening (see Ch 5), through the use of exploration (Ch 7) or through the use of empathy expression (Ch 6) depends on a nurse's ability to evaluate their own performance in the immediate situation and to track the progress of the relationship (Ch 2). Through maintaining an orientation towards self-assessment, the choices that are made have a sounder basis than those made by using either a trial-and-error approach or a standard textbook description.

## Approaches to self-assessment

Beginning and experienced nurses are encouraged to begin their self-evaluation with an assessment of how they are currently functioning with their interpersonal skills. Activity 3.7 is designed to increase awareness of current interaction patterns. It relies on the process of introspection, discussed earlier in this chapter, and is therefore an activity that should be completed in solitude.

In addition to reflecting on 'everyday' interactions, it is essential that nurses reflect on their interactions with patients. Interactions with patients are different from everyday interactions in the sense that nurses are often focused on being helpful to patients. While helping others does occur during everyday interactions, this is not always the primary intent of such interactions.

In order to determine how best to approach situations with patients, nurses must be able to observe and reflect on the interaction while simultaneously participating in the interaction. The complexity of self-assessment is often overwhelming as a result of these demands. Because the ability to become a participant–observer during interactions can be quite cumbersome to manage all at once, it is often useful to break up the process of self-assessment into manageable units. Although the ultimate aim is to combine all units, mastering smaller units first helps

## ACTIVITY 3.7 Assessment of current skills

### Process

1. Observe your interactions for approximately 10 days. Focus on situations in which you are aware of how you are interacting. These situations should contain interactions during which you felt you were effectively interacting with the others, and those that you felt were not as effective. These should be situations that illustrate how you typically communicate and interact with other people. Some examples of the type of situations you may observe include:

   - introducing yourself to a stranger
   - needing to clarify something you have not understood
   - asking another person about themselves
   - speaking in a group
   - asking someone for a favour
   - wanting to say 'no' to a request
   - giving or seeking information
   - receiving negative feedback about yourself
   - explaining why you did or said something
   - disagreeing with someone
   - seeking assistance from someone
   - expressing concern for someone else
   - wanting to help someone else
   - demonstrating to someone that you care about them.

2. Record these situations as soon as possible after they occur. Include a description of what happened, what you thought about what happened and how you felt about what happened.

3. After you have recorded these situations for about 10 days, review them in order to determine your major strengths when interacting with other people and those areas in which you think you could improve.

### Discussion

1. Write a brief summary of your interactions, using the following as a guide:

   - what you observed about your interpersonal interactions (e.g. 'I notice that I don't always listen when I am worried about what I am going to say')
   - your strengths and areas for improvement (e.g. 'I'm good at starting conversations with people I don't know')
   - your personal goals for improving your ability to interact and relate to others (e.g. 'I would like to be able to seek clarification so that I'm sure I understand').

develop the art of self-assessment. The following approaches and activities focus on these smaller units: observing, perceiving, reflecting, evaluating and making alterations on the basis of the evaluation.

# Reflection after interactions with patients

An effective approach to assessing performance, and one of the most commonly used approaches, is a reflective evaluation of an interaction after it has occurred. This approach to self-assessment is used after nurses have spontaneously participated in an interaction with a patient. Through reflection, nurses are able to identify skills that were used, assess the effects of these skills and, using patient responses and theoretical concepts as a guide, construct a probable explanation of why the skills were effective or ineffective.

Activity 3.8 is presented as a way for nurses to reflect personally on interactions with patients, be they positive or negative experiences.

Nurses may fall into the trap of being overly critical of themselves whenever they reflect on their interactions with patients because they place pressure on themselves to 'do it right'. Rather than viewing interactions as opportunities for growth, nurses who want to 'do it right' perceive interactions as tests of effective performance. This view often stifles personal and professional development.

Whenever nurses are asked to reflect on their interactions, there is a danger that they will recall only those interactions during which they felt ineffective. For this reason, it is important that nurses focus on positive, fulfilling and beneficial

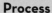

## ACTIVITY 3.8  Guide to self-reflection

**Process**

1. Describe (either through speaking or writing) an interaction in terms of what happened. Do not think about why it happened. Just think about what happened between you and the patient.

2. Answer the following questions:

   **a.** What did you say that was helpful to the patient?

   **b.** What was your intent in saying this?

   **c.** How did you know it was helpful?

   **d.** What did you say/do that was not helpful to the patient?

   **e.** What was your intent in saying this?

   **f.** How did you know it was not helpful?

   **g.** What could you have said that would have been more helpful?

   **h.** What were you feeling during this interaction?

   **i.** What do you think the patient was feeling during the interaction?

   **j.** How would you change this interaction if you could do it again?

interactions, as well as on those interactions that could have been more effective. Satisfying and successful interactions are as informative as those that are not.

## Focus on specific skills during an interaction

At times, nurses will want to develop a specific skill or related set of skills because they perceive these skills as difficult, uncomfortable to use or hard to understand. Under these circumstances, an effective way to self-assess is to focus on these skills during an interaction.

## Maintaining an ongoing record

The previously described self-assessment methods are most effective whenever nurses keep track of a number of patient interactions. Such a record is sometimes referred to as a 'journal' or 'diary'. In maintaining such a record, nurses are able to develop their understanding and use of interpersonal skills by referring to a variety of situations and circumstances. When a variety of situations are evaluated, comparisons and contrasts can be made and patterns begin to emerge. Keeping track of various patient situations, and various ways of interacting in these situations, enables nurses to formulate a more complete understanding than simply focusing on isolated events or isolated skills.

## Soliciting help from other nurses

In addition to the introspection that the previous approaches encourage, it is useful for nurses to solicit feedback from other nurses about how they are interacting with patients. The questions in Activity 3.8 can be used to prompt information from other nurses. The questions are exploratory. They refrain from passing judgment and encourage other nurses to reflect and determine how they are interacting.

This approach to helping other nurses is preferable to providing solutions and offering advice. When solutions and advice are given, nurses are not encouraged to generate their own solutions. Also, it is only the nurse who 'was there' during a given interaction who knows exactly what happened. Nurses who were not present, yet receive a second-hand account of what happened, are relying on the nurse giving the account and are processing the information through their own filters. It is preferable for the nurse who 'was there' to process the interaction through their own perceptual filters because this approach has the greatest possibility for promoting self-understanding. Other nurses may offer alternative perspectives, thus encouraging a reappraisal of the situation, but it is best to begin with attempting to understand.

## Pitfalls in self-assessment

The tendency to judge or evaluate one's own performance is often automatic, even natural, for nurses. Nevertheless, a negative evaluation can be quite troublesome when the perceived stakes are high. In evaluating their interactions with patients, the stakes are often high for nurses because of a need to maintain a positive professional image. Most nurses will want to be effective in their interactions with patients, and a performance judged as ineffective may threaten a nurse's professional image and professional esteem. For example, when nurses recognise that they have blocked or inhibited an interaction with a patient, they may find this behaviour unacceptable in a professional sense. In order to preserve and maintain an image as effective professionals, they may overlook, diminish, justify or even reject flaws and mistakes in their performance.

Overcoming this potential pitfall is best achieved through recognition and continuous awareness that self-assessment is done for the purpose of professional growth and development. Continual reflection and evaluation of performance enables nurses to build on their experiences and learn from them. Through self-assessment, nurses determine what was right or wrong, and effective or ineffective, about their interaction skills and patterns. Nevertheless, this evaluation is not the endpoint of self-assessment. Self-assessment is employed primarily for the purpose of seeking ways to improve. It is not simply an evaluative process but a learning process. A commitment to continual learning is an essential aspect of professionalism.

Another potential pitfall in using self-assessment is a tendency to gloss over performance, perceiving it globally as either all good or all bad. Focusing exclusively on positive aspects is as much a pitfall as focusing exclusively on negative aspects of performance. Nurses who can focus only on mistakes or flaws in their interactions with patients are being too harsh in their self-evaluation. Nurses who can focus only on positive aspects of their performance are failing to recognise areas for improvement and learning, which exist in the majority of situations.

The tendency to view performance globally as either all good or all bad is kept in check through the realisation that most interactions will contain a mixture of positive and negative aspects. Whenever nurses can perceive only one type or the other, their self-assessment lacks accuracy and completeness. If this happens, nurses are encouraged to reflect further in order to develop a balanced view of evaluation.

A final potential pitfall in using one's self as the assessor of performance emerges whenever nurses lack understanding of the criteria on which to base their evaluations. A lack of understanding of how and why interpersonal skills are used is addressed through further reading and discussion about the theory of effective interactions in nursing. Additionally, nurses may need to solicit assistance from an external authority (e.g. an experienced nurse or an educator) in developing appropriate criteria on which to base their self-assessment.

## SUMMARY

Nurses need to become competent communicators who display emotional intelligence in their practice environment. In order to do so, they need to develop acute self-understanding whenever they engage in interactions and relationships with patients because the primary tool they are using in these circumstances is themselves. Without self-understanding, nurses run the risk of imposing their values and views onto patients. *Values that serve the nurse may be detrimental or useless to patients.* There is a danger that without self-understanding nurses may confuse their own values with those of their patients. Although connected through the relationship, nurses need to maintain an identity that remains separate from those of their patients.

More than any other parts of nursing, interpersonal relationships with patients are likely to engender feelings within nurses. The processes of self-reflection provide assistance in handling such reactions to patients.

This chapter has reviewed three processes for developing self-understanding:

- introspection
- input from others
- self-sharing.

Nurses are encouraged to use these processes in their day-to-day encounters with patients. Reflection, both in solitude and through interaction with others, as well as self-sharing, enables nurses to meet the challenges of self-growth.

Self-understanding is the primary means through which nurses are able to evaluate their effectiveness in relating to patients. Through self-understanding, nurses remain in touch with what they are doing, and how this is affecting patients for whom they care.

# REFERENCES

Adams, K.L., Iseler, J.I., 2014. The relationship of bedside nurses' emotional intelligence with quality of care. J. Nurs. Care Qual. 29 (2), 174–181.

Asselin, M.E., Schwartz-Barcott, D., 2015. Exploring problems encountered among experienced nurses using critical reflective inquiry. J. Nurses Prof. Dev. 31 (3), 138–144.

Asselin, M.E., Schwartz-Barcott, D., Osterman, P.A., 2013. Exploring reflection as a process embedded in experienced nurses' practice: a qualitative study. J. Adv. Nurs. 69 (4), 905–914.

Beames, J.R., Black, M.J., Vartanian, L.R., 2016. Prejudice toward individuals with obesity: evidence for a pro-effort bias. J. Exp. Psychol. Appl. 22 (2), 184–195.

Benner, P., Tanner, C., Chelsea, C., 1996. Expertise in Nursing Practice: Caring, Clinical Judgment and Ethics. Springer, New York.

Brickman, P., Rabinowitz, V.C., Karuza, J., et al., 1982. Models of helping and coping. Am. Psychol. 37 (4), 368–384.

Bulman, C., Lathlean, J., Gobbi, M., 2012. The concept of reflection in nursing: qualitative findings on student and teacher perspectives. Nurse Educ. Today 32, e8–e13.

Carper, B.A., 1978. Fundamental patterns of knowing in nursing. Adv. Nurs. Sci. 1 (1), 13–23.

Chou, H.Y., Hecker, R., Martin, A., 2012. Predicting nurses' well-being from job demands and resources: a cross-sectional study of emotional labour. J. Nurs. Manag. 20, 502–511.

Codier, E., Muneno, L., Franey, K., et al., 2010. Is emotional intelligence an important concept for nursing practice? J. Psychiatr. Ment. Health Nurs. 17, 940–948.

Egan, G., 2014. The Skilled Helper, tenth ed. Brooks/Cole, Belmont CA.

Goleman, D., 1995. Emotional Intelligence. Bantam, New York, NY.

Goleman, D., 1998. Working With Emotional Intelligence. Bloomsbury, London.

Gørgens-Ekerman, G., Brand, T., 2012. Emotional intelligence as a moderator in the stress-burnout relationship: a questionnaire study on nurses. J. Clin. Nurs. 21, 2275–2285.

Goulet, M., Larue, C., Alderson, M., 2016. Reflective practice: a comparative dimensional analysis of the concept in nursing and education studies. Nurs. Forum 51 (2), 139–150.

Hochschild, A.R., 1983. The Managed Heart: Commercialisation of Human Feeling. University of California Press, Berkeley, CA.

Hochschild, A.R., 2012. The Managed Heart: Commercialization of Human Feeling (Updated). University of California Press, Berkeley, CA.

Karman, P., Kool, N., Poslawsky, I.E., et al., 2015. Nurses' attitudes towards self-harm: a literature review. J. Psychiatr. Ment. Health Nurs. 22, 65–75.

Koski-Jännes, A., Pennonen, M., Simmat-Durand, L., 2016. Treatment professionals' basic beliefs about alcohol use disorders: the impact of different cultural contexts. Subst. Use Misuse 51 (4), 479–488.

Mauno, S., Ruokolainen, M., Kinnunen, U., et al., 2016. Emotional labour and work engagement among nurses: examining perceived compassion, leadership and work ethic as stress buffers. J. Adv. Nurs. 72 (5), 1169–1181.

Michaelsen, J.J., 2012. Emotional distance to so-called difficult patients. Scand. J. Caring Sci. 26, 90–97.

Miraglia, R., Asselin, M.E., 2015. Reflection as an educational strategy in nursing professional development: an integrative review. J. Nurses Prof. Dev. 31 (2), 62–72.

Nursing and Midwifery Board of Australia, 2008. Code of Professional Conduct for Nurses in Australia. NMBA, Melbourne. Online. Available at: www.nursingmidwiferyboard.gov.au/Codes-Guidelines-Statements/Codes-Guidelines.aspx#competencystandards. (Accessed 24 July 2016).

Nursing and Midwifery Board of Australia, 2016. Registered Nurse Standards for Practice. NMBA, Melbourne. Online. Available at: http://www.nursingmidwiferyboard.gov.au/Codes-Guidelines-Statements/Professional-standards.aspx. (Accessed 24 July 2016).

Nursing Council of New Zealand, 2007. Competencies for Registered Nurses. NCNZ, Wellington. Online. Available at: http://www.nursingcouncil.org.nz/Publications/Standards-and-guidelines-for-nurses. (Accessed 24 July 2016).

Nursing Council of New Zealand, 2009. Code of Conduct for Registered Nurses. NCNZ, Wellington. Online. Available at: http://www.nursingcouncil.org.nz/Publications/Standards-and-guidelines-for-nurses. (Accessed 24 July 2016).

Powell, K.R., Mabry, J.L., Mixer, S.J., 2015. Emotional intelligence: a critical evaluation of the literature with implications for mental health nursing leadership. Issues Ment. Health Nurs. 36, 346–356.

Riley, R., Weiss, M.C., 2016. A qualitative thematic review: emotional labour in healthcare settings. J. Adv. Nurs. 72 (1), 6–17.

Rolfe, G., 2014. Rethinking reflective education: what would Dewey have done? Nurse Educ. Today 34, 1179–1183.

Salovey, P., Mayer, J.D., 1990. Emotional intelligence. Imagin. Cogn. Pers. 9 (3), 185–211.

Schön, D., 1983. The Reflective Practitioner: How Professionals Think in Action. Basic Books, New York.

Schön, D., 1991. The Reflective Practitioner, second ed. Jossey-Bass, San Francisco.

Shanta, L., Gargiulo, L., 2014. A study of the influence of nursing education on the development of emotional intelligence. J. Prof. Nurs. 30, 511–520.

Smith, P., 2012. The Emotional Labour of Nursing Revisited, second ed. Palgrave Macmillan, Basingstoke.

Travelbee, J., 1971. Interpersonal Aspects of Nursing, second ed. FA Davis, Philadelphia.

Williams, A., 2013. Hochschild (2003) – The managed heart: recognition of emotional labour in public service work. Nurse Educ. Today 33, 5–7.

# 4

# Considering culture

## CHAPTER OVERVIEW

- Culture is a set of values, beliefs and practices, based on a worldview, that are shared by a group of people.
- Because all people have a culture, there is a danger of viewing others through one's own cultural lens.
- Cultural stereotyping is based on simplistic and narrow views.
- Healthcare systems have their own cultures that may be at odds with patients' worldviews, especially beliefs about health and illness.
- Culturally congruent care means that healthcare practices are adjusted to accommodate a patient's worldview; it is provided by culturally competent providers.
- Cultural safety includes the awareness that healthcare systems that are not culturally congruent are disempowering.
- Nurses must know how to work with interpreters when there are language differences.

Visit the Evolve site for video content to support the themes and skills explored in this chapter: http://evolve.elsevier.com/AU/Stein-Parbury/patient/

# INTRODUCTION

This book demonstrates the importance of cultural competence for all nurses in order that they provide patient-centred care. Nurses who work towards cultural competency appreciate getting to know more about their patients' cultural values, beliefs and the ways they view the world, which may be different from their view of the world. Differences in cultural understanding commonly lie outside conscious awareness. That is, cultural understandings are often taken for granted. It is for this reason that nurses need to develop conscious awareness and appreciation of cultural diversity when interacting with patients. Doing so forms the basis of culturally congruent nursing care. The development of cultural competence is an ongoing process for cultural congruence, as is the promotion of cultural safety in nursing practice.

# WHAT IS CULTURE?

When considering the influence of culture, there is a tendency to think that culture is something that pertains to *others* and not the self. Likewise, it is often viewed as something that is 'exotic' or 'foreign', such as rituals pertaining to death and burial. Of utmost importance is the recognition that culture is something that pertains to every human being. Everybody has culture.

Culture encompasses a view of the world that is shared by a group of people and learnt through social interactions within the group. This includes a wide range of behaviours, values, beliefs, attitudes and customs, and is reflected in the language, dress, foods and social institutions of a group; culture determines how people live, how they view the world and how they communicate (Bearskin 2011; Garneau & Pepin 2015; Parisa et al 2016). These values and beliefs are often taken for granted and are therefore not always in conscious awareness.

Culture provides the framework for a particular society's way of life; it influences the way social life is regulated and guides interactions between members of a social group. Cultural understandings influence the way members of a group make sense of their world. Culture shapes perceptions, decisions and relationships with others. A person's social group culture is reflected in all aspects of everyday life including customs, greetings, methods of communication, attitudes to the family, beliefs about marriage, attitudes to illness and approaches to healthcare.

Traditional views of culture are based on the assumption that culture is defined, static and unchanging for a particular group of people. This view contrasts with a more contemporary one in which culture is viewed as dynamic and evolving; shared meanings develop through an ongoing, relational process of transmitting and using knowledge (Garneau & Pepin 2015).

Nurses and other healthcare professionals come from a variety of cultures and backgrounds and they must bear in mind that their worldviews may not be understood by others. There is a danger that they may base interpretations on their own views and values, rather than considering that others may not share these. Differences between healthcare professionals and patients, as well as among them, can lead to misunderstandings and outright conflict. This is especially important as the healthcare workforce is multicultural in nature.

Healthcare organisations and healthcare professionals have their own cultures and languages, which can be foreign, confusing and alienating for patients. The care practices within an organisation reflect its cultural values and beliefs. Those new to that culture must learn the cultural ways in order to become part of that group. The importance of organisational culture is recognised as influencing patient care, satisfaction and outcomes, as well as nurse satisfaction (see Ch 11).

# CULTURAL STEREOTYPING

Culture affects many aspects of living, including choice of clothing, food and friendship affiliation. Stereotyping is categorising individuals into groups based on an oversimplified set of these characteristics. For example, a stereotypical Australian male wears thongs and stubbies and has a beer in hand. This tends to produce a narrow and biased viewpoint; people are reduced to a few characteristics. The ultimate danger, however, involves generalisation of these stereotypes in their extreme forms and an associated reluctance to recognise the extent to which individual differences do exist within all groups and breach basic human rights for respect.

---

### ACTIVITY 4.1 Cultural awareness: stereotypes

**Process**

1. Think about all the different groups to which you belong and form your identity, for example, female, family (e.g. mother), Buddhist, university student and sports club.

2. Record these on a board or paper so everybody can see them.

3. Discuss how each of these groups is similar and dissimilar.

4. Discuss whether there are any commonly held beliefs or attitudes about any of the groups listed. These are often the basis of stereotypes.

**Discussion**

1. Were there more similarities or dissimilarities in the various groups?

2. How do stereotypes develop and persist?

3. How do stereotypes affect the way people are treated?

---

When nurses rely on stereotypes and act on them, they miss an opportunity to get to know the person on any more than a superficial level. The cost of not getting close enough to patients to gain insight into their respective individualities may result in a failure to identify and meet their specific needs, thus compromising quality nursing care and causing harm to the patient by increasing their vulnerability.

The menace inherent in stereotypes is that they are intransigent, pervasive, self-fulfilling, self-perpetuating and dangerous. If a patient is viewed by nurses as 'a typical hysterical Mediterranean patient', interactions will be coloured by that perception. When nurses apply the stereotype of a 'druggie' (i.e. irresponsible, immature, needy and worthless), they avoid taking the risk of getting to know and value the patient. Nurses need to continually challenge their own use of stereotypes in order to minimise the influence they exert on patient–nurse interactions and nursing practice.

The tendency to stereotype can be lessened by recognising the influence that values have on behaviour (see Ch 3) and by appreciating the range of values that lie behind the behaviour of specific groups. To be truly culturally aware, it is important to recognise that while there are differences *between* different cultural groups, there are also as many or even greater differences *within* them.

More importantly, stereotypes can lead to stigmatising people and even racism (Cameron et al 2014; Durey et al 2011; Ferdinand et al 2015; Huria et al 2014; Kelaher et al 2014) by reducing people to simplistic categorisations that can affect their access to and experience of healthcare. Consider the following patient's story.

## A Patient's Story

Brenda has strong links to and relationships with Indigenous Australians because of her heritage and identity. People sometimes find her background confusing because she has pale skin and blonde hair. When people seem genuinely interested, she always takes the time to explain the meaning of being an Aboriginal Australian. On the afternoon that she arrived at a hospital emergency department (ED) with her seriously ill two-year-old son, she had no time to explain anything, although she ticked the box on the admission form to identify her son as an Indigenous Australian.

She attended the ED of a busy metropolitan hospital because her son was having an extreme allergic reaction to peanuts. That day her family and friends had come together for a children's birthday party for her five-year-old daughter. The party was a large gathering of toddlers and preschoolers who enjoyed an afternoon's festivities. Near the end of the party, following the cutting and eating of the cake, she noticed her two-year-old son was showing signs of a severe allergic reaction. She had seen it before and knew exactly what to do.

Not knowing for sure what had caused the reaction, she administered adrenaline and set out for the local hospital, a two-minute car trip from home. On the way, she remembered that she had decorated the cake with 'hundreds and thousands' that had been stored in a jar that previously contained peanuts. Her two-year-old son had reacted immediately after eating the cake.

On arrival she quickly explained what was happening to the triage nurse in the ED. She told him of her son's history and the events of the day, stating that she and her son needed to be seen immediately as her son has severe allergic reactions to peanuts. The nurse's response was not in keeping with the seriousness of the circumstances and he asked her to be seated. She became quite distressed, stating in a loud voice that she and her son must be seen immediately. He replied, 'Have a seat and wait like everybody else'.

Knowing she had no time and knowing of another hospital two minutes away she picked up her son, who by now was unable to walk, and went to the second hospital. There, her son was stabilised in the ED and admitted to the intensive care unit. Although he recovered physically, Brenda had difficulty recovering emotionally from her treatment in the ED of the first hospital; she felt traumatised.

She retained the services of a lawyer and obtained the ED record of her son's admission under the right to freedom of information. On the record she read: 'Aboriginal woman, dishevelled, wearing dirty clothes, with two-year-old child in her arms, loudly demanding to be seen immediately. Child appears dirty, unkempt and possibly neglected, not in keeping with developmental milestones as he is crawling. Strong smell of alcohol on mother's breath. Mother seems hysterical and believes child is having a reaction to peanuts. Not able to confirm allergy. Plan is to contact the children's services department and have the child seen by a social worker. Mother told to wait. Triaged to category 3'.

Brenda filed a formal complaint against both the hospital and the nurse. She was pleased to hear that this resulted in action being taken against the nurse, who was removed from further triage duty. Brenda was satisfied knowing that this nurse would not have further opportunity to make decisions that could have dire consequences purely on the basis of a racial stereotype.

Brenda's story is extreme, but common. It illustrates what can happen when people make decisions on the basis of stereotyping. Had the nurse asked a few pertinent questions, he would have found logical explanations for the circumstances. First, anyone who goes to a children's birthday party will often have soiled clothing at the end. Second, Brenda did have one glass of champagne at the start of the party, well over two hours before she arrived in the ED, so was unlikely to be inebriated as the nurse suggested. Third, her son was unable to walk because he was critically ill by the time he arrived at hospital. Unfortunately, the nurse made decisions not on these facts but on his image of 'an Aborigine' (i.e. a stereotype).

## CULTURE AND HEALTHCARE

There is substantial evidence that the cultural background of patients has an impact on the quality and safety of healthcare delivery and outcomes. For example,

## ACTIVITY 4.2  Feeling different

### Process

1. Think of a time when you were in a group of people and you felt different. The basis for feeling different could be based on skin colour, ethnicity, age, gender, body size or type of clothing.

2. Depict how you felt by drawing a picture or writing words on a piece of paper.

3. Record how you got the message that you were different.

4. Share your experience with another person.

### Discussion

1. What was the basis of feeling different?

2. How did it feel to be different?

3. What would have helped in the situation?

4. What conclusions can be drawn from the experience of feeling different?

Indigenous people in Australia, New Zealand and Canada experience health disadvantages, lower life expectancy and poorer access to healthcare services when compared with non-Indigenous people (Bearskin 2011; Huria et al 2014; Katterl & Bywood 2012; Khoury 2015; van Schaik & Thompson 2011). As a result, the World Health Organization (2010) has endorsed a resolution to make reducing these inequities a priority for all countries.

People from a culturally and linguistically diverse background also experience poorer health and access to healthcare than those of the mainstream society (Bhui et al 2015; Cioffi 2013; Ferdinand et al 2015). A failure to appreciate the cultural differences between patients and healthcare professionals has been shown to negatively impact on the quality of care and patient satisfaction (Cameron et al 2014). A lack of understanding of a patient's culture can result in negative patient outcomes and actual patient harm (Probast & Imhof 2016; Wain et al 2016).

There are numerous reasons for disparities and inequalities in health and healthcare such as transport problems, socioeconomic status and educational factors. However, those that are most relevant to the subject matter in this book are cultural perceptions and belief systems about health and illness, language barriers and healthcare providers' poor awareness and understanding of cultural healthcare practices. Each of these has direct bearing on the mismatch between healthcare as it is delivered and the healthcare language and cultural needs of people who are served by a healthcare delivery system.

Healthcare professionals may feel inadequate and ill-equipped in meeting the challenges of addressing cultural diversity (see *Research highlight*).

## RESEARCH HIGHLIGHT Attitudes of healthcare professionals working in Aboriginal health

*Wilson, A.M., Magarey, A.M., Jones, M., et al., 2015. Attitudes and characteristics of health professionals working in Aboriginal health. Rural and Remote Health 15 (1), Article 2739 (online).*

### Background

Reducing the gap between the health status of Aboriginal Australians and non-Aboriginal Australians needs to be addressed as a matter of priority. Because the majority of healthcare professionals in Australia are non-Aboriginal, it is essential that they have the knowledge, skills and attitudes to meet the challenges in closing this gap.

### Purpose of the study

The aim of this research was to explore the opinions and attitudes of non-Aboriginal healthcare professionals who were working in a community-based healthy eating and exercise program that was delivered to Aboriginal Australians in both rural and metropolitan settings.

### Method

Semi-structured interviews were conducted with 35 non-Aboriginal healthcare professionals who were working in the healthy eating and exercise program, or who had worked in other Australian Aboriginal health settings. The interviews were an in-depth exploration of their perceptions and experiences of participating in an Australian Aboriginal health initiative. Data from the interviews were coded into themes, using a critical social research framework.

### Key findings

The analysis revealed four attitudes expressed by the participants. The first was termed 'don't know how', which reflected a lack of practical knowledge. The next was 'too scared', which was based on the participants' fears about addressing issues related to Australian Aboriginal health issues. The third theme was termed 'too hard'. This theme reflected a perception that addressing issues in Australian Aboriginal health was too difficult to manage. The final theme, 'barrier breaker', related to those healthcare professionals who learnt how to practise within the context of Australian Aboriginal health, thus overcoming the perceived barriers that were expressed in the other three themes.

### Implications for nursing practice

In order to address the health disadvantages experienced by Indigenous Australians, non-Aboriginal healthcare professionals need to overcome their lack of practical knowledge and fears about how to address the health problems faced by Aboriginal Australians. They need to reflect on their feelings and attitudes in order to bring about needed changes in the delivery of healthcare for Aboriginal Australians. More importantly, open dialogue is needed to bring about these changes.

# The culture of healthcare

The disparities and inequalities in healthcare of culturally diverse patients are due, in part, to the actual culture of healthcare itself. Healthcare systems and institutions are themselves imbued with shared values, beliefs, practices and rituals that construct and are constructed by their culture. Nurses working in such systems may not be consciously aware of these cultural norms as culture tends to be 'taken for granted' and viewed as 'the way things are'.

In the Western world the culture of healthcare is dominated by a biomedical view of health and illness that determines how problems are recognised and what is worthy of attention (Khoury 2015; Kirmayer 2012). Healthcare is disease-oriented, based on an understanding of pathophysiology and psychopathology. This imposes a monocultural system that is alien and depersonalising for people whose cultural beliefs about health and illness are different. Healthcare systems become inaccessible because they are not culturally appropriate (Chapman et al 2014; Tranberg et al 2016).

Patients' personal, subjective experiences of illness are imbued with cultural meaning, which may or may not fit biomedical explanations of ill-health. For example, Indigenous peoples of Australia believe that disharmony and discontinuity cause ill-health, and healing seeks to reintegrate people with one another and with the environment (van Schaik & Thompson 2011). In many Indigenous cultures the development of cancer is viewed as fate or destiny, or as punishment or payback for wrongdoing (Tranberg et al 2016). Latino immigrants in the United States believe that depression is a result of personal transgressions and supernatural causes (Caplan et al 2013). Knowledge developed in the field of biomedical science does not accommodate such understandings as diseases and their cause and cures are viewed through a different lens.

Nurses from social and cultural backgrounds that are different from the patient may not understand cultural meanings of health and illness, especially if they operate from an exclusively biomedical orientation. This leads to misunderstandings and makes the process of empathic communication difficult. More importantly, patients whose health beliefs are different from those supported by the biomedical model often avoid talking to healthcare professionals because they perceive a lack of empathy and openness (Tranberg et al 2016).

In addition, the ideology of Western healthcare is based on the autonomous individual, with a high value placed on independence and self-agency. This orientation does not accommodate people from cultures in which collective identity and interdependence take precedence over individual autonomy and independence. For example, individual autonomy in Indigenous cultures means honouring the family and community rather than the individual (Stevenson 2016). Therefore, consent to healthcare treatment involves obtaining permission from the right person(s) within the family, and this can extend to a wider community. The standard process of consent to treatment does not match cultural sensibilities.

The movement in healthcare, evidence-based practice in which approaches to care are based on the 'best available evidence', can result in a 'one size fits all' attitude that can exclude cultural sensibilities (Whitley et al 2011). Importantly, nurses should recognise that the majority of the evidence is based on research that excludes people who don't speak English.

In a similar vein nurses can hold the common misconception that equity in healthcare means that 'every patient is treated exactly the same'. This misconception stems from the fact that nurses recognise their moral and professional responsibility to care for patients regardless of their ethnic background, cultural beliefs, religious practice or even how they are dressed. Equity in healthcare means that people have equal *access* to care, not that they are cared for in exactly the same way. Approaches to individual patients must be adjusted and adapted not only to meet their unique needs but also to accommodate their cultural values and beliefs.

Adjusting and adapting approaches to individual patients can be particularly challenging when patients are from a culture that is not understood or, worse, rejected. This poor understanding (or outright rejection) is not always in conscious awareness because it often stems from ethnocentrism, a tendency to see the world as having one standard – that of one's own cultural group – and to judge other cultural groups in relation to it. An ethnocentric individual is unlikely to perceive or acknowledge differences in the ways that people view the world and to fail to appreciate the advantages of living in a culturally diverse society. Ethnocentricity is also present in the healthcare system itself. To interact effectively with people from different cultural groups, nurses need to become aware of an inherent tendency to be ethnocentric.

## Perceptions of health and illness

The influence of culture is particularly evident when considering the meaning of illness because beliefs and explanations about health and illness are often culturally determined (see illness representation, Ch 9). For example, people may believe that illness is a punishment for past wrongdoings, with suffering being a means of atonement. Others may share a belief that illness is nothing more than chance. That is, there is no reason other than the 'luck of the draw' for becoming sick.

People may believe that members of their social group who are well have an obligation to pay respect to the sick and to attend to their needs. Family and friends are expected to visit the sick, provide them with food and help them to rest and regain their health. The sick, in turn, have an obligation to accept these attentions. Making brave attempts to care for oneself, and indicating that such attentions are not needed, may be regarded as ill-mannered.

The approaches of the belief systems described above contrast with those that place a high value on independence and avoidance of relying on others beyond what is absolutely necessary. For these people, attempts to get well quickly and to resume normal roles are admired and praised by others who are important to them. In cultures such as this, people who are sick have an obligation to make every effort to minimise the time that they are dependent on others. Nurses who, due to their own cultural backgrounds, value such independence may have trouble understanding the patients who do very little for themselves in relation to healthcare.

When nurses do not understand cultural sensibilities such as these, serious misunderstandings may occur. For example, traditional Vietnamese healing methods that include 'coin rubbing' to dispel poisons believed to be responsible for colds and flus may result in skin marks and breaks and could be interpreted as parental child abuse (Narayan 2010). Likewise, Chinese people may be stoical and show no emotion when experiencing pain due to a belief that suffering is a part of life (Tung & Zhizhong 2015).

Culturally-responsive nurses acknowledge that much of their world and the world of patients is socially constructed and that the way it is constructed depends largely on cultural beliefs. In becoming culturally aware, nurses develop an understanding and acceptance of the differences that exist between different groups of people and are willing to investigate the practices and belief systems that are associated with different cultural groups.

The initial step in developing cultural awareness is to increase understanding of one's own culture. This is best done through the process of reflection about the origin and nature of a personal value and belief system. For example, nurses might reflect on how illness was perceived and managed in their family of origin. Of central importance is a reflection on how members of the cultural group 'expect' people to behave when ill. For example, in some cultures people do not complain when in pain, while in others a dramatic outward expression of pain is accepted as 'normal'.

# Culturally congruent care

Although necessary, awareness of cultural diversity is not sufficient for professional nursing practice that is culturally congruent. Culturally congruent care is respectful of and responsive to the patient's culturally based values and beliefs. It is based on mutual understanding between a nurse and a patient. Culturally congruent care involves an abandonment of ethnocentric thinking in order to appreciate cultural diversity. This includes awareness of differences between and within different cultures. Developing an understanding of a patient's values and beliefs is essential. This requires skills in interacting with patients that builds mutual understanding. In providing culturally congruent care, nurses must be receptive to learning from patients, as it is the patient who can best explain their values and beliefs.

There are different approaches to conceptualising culturally congruent care (Garneau & Pepin 2015). The first is based on identifying the particular traits, values, customs and beliefs of identified cultures, which can be found on lists of cultural characteristics and traits. Learning about culture in this manner produces a cognitive understanding of cultural groups, and it is assumed that it will result in culturally congruent care. This approach is problematic and considered to be outdated (Kirmayer 2012) because it can lead to superficial understandings that are based on stereotypes and fails to take into consideration that there is as much diversity within cultural groups as between them. Learning a set of characteristics and traits of a particular culture border on stereotyping and preconceived notions (Florczak 2013). In addition this assumes that culture is stable and does not recognise the diversity that exists within cultural groups (Garneau & Pepin 2015). More importantly, this traditional view does not consider the relationship between a nurse and a patient in relation to power and privilege (Doutrich et al 2012).

## ACTIVITY 4.3  Cultural responses to illness

### Process

1. When you were a child and you felt unwell …

   a. How did others in your family expect you to behave?

   b. Were you encouraged to complain or express discomfort and pain?

   c. Were you permitted to take time off school and your other usual activities, or just expected to carry on as usual?

   d. What attempts were made to help you recover? (e.g. special food, medications, staying in bed, going to see a doctor)

2. What were you told about why you became unwell? (e.g. not enough sleep, not eating well)

3. Were you held responsible for your illness?

4. What role were you expected to play in recovering?

5. Form small groups of six to seven people and discuss your answers.

### Discussion

1. What similarities were there in the responses to the questions? What were the differences?

2. What were some of the reasons people were given for becoming ill?

3. What were some of the actions that people took to get better?

Another approach to culturally congruent care is through developing 'cultural humility'. Cultural humility means that nurses appreciate that their culture, both as an individual and as reflected by healthcare culture, is not the yardstick by which patients should be evaluated; this is the opposite of an ethnocentric view. Rather than relying on a set of cultural attributes or adhering to popular beliefs about a culture, culturally humble nurses will enquire into the individual patient's personal interpretations and beliefs. They are open, self-aware, egalitarian and self-reflective (Foronda et al 2016).

The development of cultural humility is an ongoing process of awareness and reflection (see Ch 3). Nurses who are 'culturally humble' will not impose their value system on a patient but enter the relationship with openness to different ways of seeing the world. They are ready to learn from the patient and negotiate care that is based on the patient's cultural belief systems. In doing so, they may develop cultural competence.

# Cultural competence

Cultural competence is a multidimensional concept currently used to describe the conditions necessary for appropriately delivering healthcare that is culturally congruent. Cultural competence encompasses awareness, knowledge, understanding, sensitivity, tolerance and skill (Garneau & Pepin 2015). It is directly related to the capacity to fully understand a patient's perspective and, more importantly, to provide healthcare that incorporates this perspective.

Culturally competent practitioners will have the desire and motivation to seek cultural encounters with patients whose culture is different from theirs in order to obtain further knowledge and skill. That is, cultural competence is an ongoing process in which nurses continually strive to deepen their understanding and appreciation of cultural diversity. As such, developing cultural competence involves ongoing critical self-reflection (see Ch 3). Being open, challenging one's own perspectives and integrating different realities, within the context of the relationship with the patient, are necessary for this reflection (Garneau 2016). Moreover, cultural competence extends beyond the individual nurse to include developing healthcare systems that are culturally congruent to the population being served.

Nurses who work with a specific population of people should make every effort to learn about that group's cultural beliefs, values and healthcare practices. For example, Australian Aboriginal cultures, although having much diversity within them, hold a tradition of not using a deceased person's name because doing so calls their spirit back to earth (McGrath & Phillips 2008). A nurse could inadvertently disturb this sensibility by asking for specifics of family members' names when collecting healthcare information. Culturally competent nurses would know not to do so. When nurses routinely care for a population of patients whose language is different from their own, their cultural competence will include making an effort to learn a few key words or phrases in the language that is used by that population. Doing so can not only prevent misunderstandings but also demonstrates a sincere desire to be 'for' the patient.

Each of these approaches to addressing issues of culture and healthcare, cultural congruence, awareness and competence is based on the individual nurse and fails to take into account either the relationship between a nurse and patient or the overall context of healthcare. The broader concept of cultural safety encompasses both.

# Cultural safety

Nurses are morally and professionally bound to provide care that is safe. The notion of safety extends beyond physical and psychological parameters to include care that is culturally safe. Developed in New Zealand by Ramsden (1993) and her nursing colleagues, this concept was a result of nurses who were discontented with the nature of healthcare. Cultural safety is becoming widely recognised internationally as an important cultural concept in healthcare (Bearskin 2011; Doutrich et al 2012; Downing et al 2011; Kirmayer 2012; McEldowney & Connor 2011; Parisa et al 2016).

Cultural safety is more than simply learning about cultural practices and beliefs; it is an ethical standard that recognises the position of cultural groups and how they are perceived. Culturally 'unsafe' care includes any actions in which the patient feels inferior, humiliated, alienated or deprived of care on the basis of their culture (Bearskin 2011; Parisa et al 2016). Imposing an ethnocentric biomedical perspective on illness while dismissing beliefs that do not fit a biomedical model is an example of culturally unsafe practice.

Unlike notions of 'cultural awareness' or 'cultural sensitivity', which can be evaluated by professional standards, cultural safety can only be judged by the patient or recipient of care (McEldowney & Connor 2011). Cultural safety does not mean that all recipients of care are treated the same, as is often touted as the key to cultural awareness and sensitivity. Rather, the tenets of cultural safety imply that nurses adjust their care in accordance with the cultural sensitivities of each individual patient.

Cultural safety is more than recognition of the uniqueness of cultural identity and the need for equity in healthcare. Cultural safety also includes recognition of social structures that disempower cultural groups and cause harm. It is a means by which nurses examine healthcare structures that disadvantage some people, rendering them powerless in that structure (Doutrich et al 2012; Kirmayer 2012).

Culturally safe nurses recognise social structures that account, in part, for lack of access to adequate healthcare for some cultural groups. Culturally safe nurses accommodate and respect a diverse range of views on health and healing. They are not limited to one particular pattern of thinking about illness, be it a biomedical orientation or one that derives from their own cultural background.

Reflection on and in actions (see Ch 3) is the key to becoming culturally safe (Doutrich et al 2012; Parisa et al 2016). To become culturally safe, nurses need to engage in the process of continuous contemplation as to how their own culture and the culture of healthcare is impacting on every interaction with patients.

# LANGUAGE DIFFERENCES

In certain situations, it is likely that patients will have difficulty understanding the language used by nurses. Such language barriers pose a risk to patient safety because misunderstandings and inadequate nursing assessments may result in patient harm (van Rosse et al 2016). In addition, language barriers have been shown to decrease the amount of information offered to patients and the number of questions patients ask (Probast & Imhof 2016). As a result, effective communication is impeded.

With patience and care, it is possible to convey simple information to a person who has minimal English. It is important to speak slowly and clearly.

Avoid using jargon and phrases that can be readily misunderstood such as 'that wound seems to be breaking down; we had better keep an eye on it'. It is best to use plain, correct English, avoiding ambiguities and, above all, avoiding forms of 'pidgin' English, which is used to simplify language but may actually make it more confusing. For example, a nurse may ask a patient, 'When you see doctor; what he say?' Ambiguity in tense may cause patients with little English to wonder if the interaction under discussion was in the past or is to occur in the future.

It is also important for nurses to recognise that non-verbal communication varies across cultures, especially in relation to eye contact. In some cultures it is considered rude to look directly into another person's eyes, especially if that person is in a position of authority. Staring at the floor could indicate that the patient is listening, and remaining silent demonstrates respect.

Where the difficulty is related to the non-English speaking background of the patient, a member of a medical interpreter service may be brought in to translate. If this is not possible, a member of the patient's family who does speak English is often asked to act as an interpreter, but this has potential problems.

Where the interaction difficulty is related to the age of the patient (e.g. a young child) or to specific communication problems (e.g. an intellectual disability), members of the family or individuals who are familiar with the patient are commonly used. It should always be remembered that interacting through a third person increases the likelihood of misinterpretation or reinterpretation of the content. This may be due to the filtering process associated with a third person and the interpretations and meanings attached to the content by that person. In addition, the intermediary may make a conscious decision to alter the meaning by omitting, adding or distorting the content of the message, or patients may withhold information because of the personal relationship that exists between themselves and the intermediary.

All of the alterations to the content mentioned in the previous paragraph are more likely to occur in situations where the topic under discussion creates a high level of discomfort for those involved in the interaction (e.g. if a male adolescent is asked to interpret while his mother's personal and obstetric history is taken, or an unfamiliar, middle-aged male is interpreting for a female adolescent patient who is being questioned about her sexual activity).

The following scenario illustrates problems that may occur when an untrained interpreter is used.

## SCENARIO

A Lebanese cleaner was asked to interpret for a couple who had given birth to an infant with Down syndrome or 'mongolism'. The cleaner told the parents that they had given birth to a 'Chinese baby', a literal translation. This caused a great deal of conflict between the husband and the wife and was not cleared up for many months. This situation would have been avoided if a trained healthcare interpreter had been used.

When language barriers exist, nurses need to rely on a third person to act as an intermediary. Healthcare systems have established health-interpreter programs to meet the need for interpreters with the expertise required to work within health-related areas. If it is necessary to use an untrained interpreter in an emergency situation, a professional interpreter should be employed as soon as possible to check the understanding of the patient and the family. Working effectively with an interpreter is a skilled activity, and there are enormous advantages in making the effort to acquire the skill.

Interpreters who are trained to work in the healthcare system are able to translate medical terminology accurately and have proven useful in bridging gaps between the culture of the healthcare professional and that of the patient. Misunderstandings arising both from language barriers and from differences in cultural beliefs and practices may, therefore, be prevented or minimised with the help of a trained interpreter. Whenever important or sensitive discussion is needed, or when complex information is sought or given, it is important that an interpreter, bound by the ethic of confidentiality that applies to all healthcare professionals, is involved.

While the importance of using interpreters is recognised, and embedded in healthcare policy, they are often underutilised, either because they are not available or because their use requires extra time (Ian et al 2016). When the situation at hand is urgent, and a family member or another member of the healthcare team is available, professional interpreters are often not summoned (van Rosse et al 2016). Patients often prefer a family or staff member to function as an interpreter because they do not trust that confidentiality will be maintained; likewise, family members may not want an interpreter because they fear that information may be relayed that they do not want the patient to hear (Probast & Imhof 2016).

It is important to appreciate that the role of interpreter involves dilemmas and challenges. In studies investigating the experience of interpreters, it is reported that they find it difficult to simply be a 'conduit' of spoken language (Butow et al 2012; Hsieh & Nicodemus 2015). They are challenged by the need to also act as a cultural interpreter both to the patient in explaining how the healthcare system operates and also to the clinicians in providing explanations as to the meaning of certain behaviours. In this regard they may play a role as a patient advocate. A real challenge for them is the requirement that they remain emotionally neutral; when patients became distressed they felt the patient's suffering and it was difficult for them to not try to provide comfort.

## Guidelines when using an interpreter

The guidelines for working with an interpreter are presented in Table 4.1 and follow the sequence of the interaction. Prior to the interaction, it is especially important that some rapport is established between the patient and the interpreter if there is to be a discussion of sensitive and private matters. In instances when sexual or personal details must be discussed, it may be important that the interpreter be of the same gender as the patient.

## ACTIVITY 4.4  Working with an interpreter  333

### Process

1. Form as many groups of three as possible where two members of the group are fluent in the same language, which should not be English. The remaining participants are observers.

2. Using the given situations, one foreign language speaker plays the role of a nurse and the other an interpreter. The third person plays the role of the patient. If there is more than one group, different groups can play each situation. Alternatively, the same group can play the two situations consecutively.

3. The role-play is set in an emergency department where a patient has been admitted with severe asthma. Emergency treatment has been instituted and the patient is now breathing more comfortably. The nurse has arranged for an interpreter to help collect information for a nursing history. For the purpose of this role-play, any nursing history format may be used.

   **Situation A:** The nurse and interpreter face each other and the nurse directs questions to the interpreter using the third person. For example, 'Has he/she ever been in hospital before?'; 'When did he/she have his/her last meal?'; 'Is he/she allergic to any medications?'. The role-play ends when the history is completed.

   **Situation B:** The nurse introduces the interpreter to the patient. The interpreter sits next to the patient. The nurse addresses questions directly to the patient. After the history is completed, the nurse asks the patient if they have any questions about any aspect of treatment or care. Answers are directed to the patient, not to the interpreter. After the interview, the nurse is the first to leave while the interpreter stays and chats briefly with the patient before leaving.

### Discussion

1. How did it feel to be the 'patient' in situation A? How did it feel to be the 'patient' in situation B?

2. What difficulties did the 'nurses' in situation A experience? What difficulties did the 'nurses' in situation B experience?

3. What principles should be observed when working with an interpreter? Compare your answers with the following text about using interpreters.

During the interaction, the patient needs to feel that the interpreter is an ally so the patient is less likely to feel outnumbered and disadvantaged. Speaking directly to the patient, not to the interpreter, not only enables the nurse to develop rapport with the patient but also facilitates observation of the patient's non-verbal communication.

The interaction usually works best if the interpreter is able to interpret the words simultaneously, *as they are spoken*. This is the 'trailing' method of interpreting and is most likely to promote a good rapport between the patient and the nurse. In the other type of interpreting, *consecutive interpreting*, the patient completes a

| TABLE 4.1 Guidelines for working with an interpreter | | |
|---|---|---|
| **SEQUENCE** | **GUIDELINE** | **RATIONALE** |
| Prior to the interaction | Nurse explains to the interpreter the purpose of the interaction. Interpreter explains the purpose to the patient and establishes rapport. | All parties need to understand the purpose of the interaction. |
| During the interaction | Interpreter sits next to the patient and directs interpretations directly to them. Nurse focuses attention on the patient by maintaining eye contact (within culturally accepted limits) and speaking directly to the patient. | Interpreter is aligned with the patient, acting as an ally. The nurse's relationship is with the patient, not the interpreter. |
| After the interaction | Nurse leaves the interaction first. | The interpreter can then have a chat with the patient. The nurse should not directly engage in a discussion with the interpreter in the patient's presence. |

whole sentence or phrase before it is translated. Regardless of which approach is used, it is especially important to assure mutual understanding by paraphrasing and clarifying.

After the interaction, there should be an opportunity for the patient and interpreter to have an opportunity to chat in the nurse's absence. The nurse should avoid engaging the interpreter in lengthy discussions in which the patient is not involved, as the interpreter should be seen to be aligned with the patient, not the nurse.

Although an interpreter should be used whenever there is important information to convey, it is often necessary to manage without an interpreter when interacting with a patient who has limited English. At times, there may not be an interpreter who is immediately available. Therefore, it is important for nurses to prepare for such times by learning key phrases for the population that is being served. In addition, a list of basic words in the patient's language should be compiled for use by all staff.

# SUMMARY

As societies become increasingly culturally diverse, nurses are challenged to appreciate and accommodate the multiple perspectives on health that cultural diversity brings. This chapter is a beginning step in developing such appreciation and accommodation. Material in the chapter has focused on the importance of understanding cultural diversity and developing nursing practice that is culturally safe. In addition, the chapter has enabled nurses to consider some of the impediments to such understanding (e.g. cultural stereotyping). Some of the challenges of working with interpreters and communicating non-verbally have also been reviewed. Readers should bear in mind that this chapter represents a very brief introduction to the challenges of cross-cultural communication.

# REFERENCES

Bearskin, R.L.B., 2011. A critical lens on culture in nursing practice. Nurs. Ethics 18 (4), 548–559.

Bhui, K.S., Aslam, R.W., Palinski, A., et al., 2015. Interventions to improve therapeutic communications between black and minority ethnic patients and professionals in psychiatric services: systematic review. Br. J. Psychiatry 207, 95–103.

Butow, P.N., Lobb, E., Jefford, M., et al., 2012. A bridge between cultures: interpreters' perspectives of consultations with migrant oncology patients. Support. Care Cancer 20, 235–244.

Cameron, B.L., del Pilar, M., Plazas, C., et al., 2014. Understanding inequalities in access to health care services for Aboriginal people: a call for nursing action. Adv. Nurs. Sci. 37 (3), E1–E16.

Caplan, S., Escobar, J., Manuel Paris, M., et al., 2013. Cultural influences on causal beliefs about depression among Latino immigrants. J. Transcult. Nurs. 24 (1), 68–77.

Chapman, R., Smith, T., Martin, C., 2014. Qualitative exploration of the perceived barriers and enablers to Aboriginal and Torres Strait Islander people accessing healthcare through one Victorian emergency department. Contemp. Nurse 48 (1), 48–58.

Cioffi, J., 2013. Being inclusive of diversity in nursing care: a discussion paper. Collegian 20, 249–254.

Doutrich, D., Arcus, K., Dekker, L., et al., 2012. Cultural safety in New Zealand and the United States: looking at a way forward together. J. Transcult. Nurs. 23 (2), 143–150.

Downing, R., Kowal, E., Paradies, Y., 2011. Indigenous cultural training for health workers in Australia. Int. J. Qual. Health Care 23 (3), 247–257.

Durey, A., Thompson, S.C., Wood, M., 2011. Time to bring down the twin towers in poor Aboriginal hospital care: addressing institutional racism and misunderstandings in communication. Intern. Med. J. 42 (1), 17–22.

Ferdinand, A.S., Paradies, Y., Kelaher, M., 2015. Mental health impacts of racial discrimination in Australian culturally and linguistically diverse communities: a cross-sectional survey. BMC Public Health 15, 401. doi:10.1186/s12889-015-1661-1.

Florczak, K.L., 2013. Culture: fluid and complex. Nurs. Sci. Q. 26 (1), 12–13.

Foronda, C., Baptiste, D., Reinholdt, M.M., et al., 2016. Cultural humility: a concept analysis. J. Transcult. Nurs. 27 (3), 210–217.

Garneau, A.B., 2016. Critical reflection in cultural competence development: a framework for undergraduate nursing education. J. Nurs. Educ. 55 (3), 125–132.

Garneau, A.B., Pepin, J., 2015. Cultural competence: a constructivist definition. J. Transcult. Nurs. 26 (1), 9–15.

Hsieh, E., Nicodemus, B., 2015. Conceptualizing emotion in healthcare interpreting: a normative approach to interpreters' emotion work. Patient Educ. Couns. 98, 1474–1481.

Huria, T., Cuddy, J., Lacey, C., et al., 2014. Working with racism: a qualitative study of the perspectives of Māori (indigenous peoples of Aotearoa New Zealand) registered nurses on a global phenomenon. J. Transcult. Nurs. 25 (4), 364–372.

Ian, C., Nakamura-Florez, E., Lee, Y., 2016. Registered nurses' experiences with caring for non-English speaking patients. Appl. Nurs. Res. 30, 257–260.

Katterl, R., Bywood, P., 2012. The closing the gap initiative: success and ongoing challenges for division of general practice. Aust. Fam. Physician 41 (7), 523–527.

Kelaher, M.A., Ferdinand, A.S., Paradies, Y., 2014. Experiencing racism in health care: the mental health impacts for Victorian Aboriginal communities. Med. J. Aust. 200, 1–4. doi:10.5694/mja13.10503. (online).

Khoury, P., 2015. Beyond the biomedical paradigm: the formation and development of indigenous community controlled health organizations in Australia. Int. J. Health Serv. 45 (3), 471–494.

Kirmayer, L.J., 2012. Rethinking cultural competence. Transcult. Psychiatry 49 (2), 149–164.

McEldowney, R., Connor, M.J., 2011. Cultural safety as an ethic of care: a praxiological process. J. Transcult. Nurs. 22 (4), 342–349.

McGrath, P., Phillips, E., 2008. Australian findings on Aboriginal cultural practices associated with clothing, hair, possessions and the use of name of deceased persons. Int. J. Nurs. Pract. 14 (1), 57–66.

Narayan, M.C., 2010. Culture's effects on pain assessment and management. Am. J. Nurs. 110 (4), 38–47.

Parisa, B., Reza, N., Afsaneh, R., et al., 2016. Cultural safety: an evolutionary concept analysis. Holist. Nurs. Pract. 30 (1), 33–38.

Probast, S., Imhof, L., 2016. Management of language discordance in clinical nursing practice—a critical review. Appl. Nurs. Res. 30, 158–163.

Ramsden, I., 1993. Kawa Whakaruruhau: cultural safety in nursing education in Aotearoa (New Zealand). Nurs. Prax. N. Z. 8 (3), 4–10.

Stevenson, S.A., 2016. Toward a narrative ethics: indigenous community-based research, the ethics of narrative, and the limits of conventional bioethics. Qual. Inq. 22 (5), 365–376.

Tranberg, R., Alexander, S., Hatcher, D., et al., 2016. Factors influencing cancer treatment decision-making by indigenous peoples: a systematic review. Psychooncology 25, 131–141.

Tung, W.-C., Zhizhong, L., 2015. Pain beliefs and behaviors among Chinese. Home Health Care Manag. Pract. 27 (2), 95–97.

van Rosse, F., de Bruijne, M., Suurmond, J., et al., 2016. Language barriers and patient safety risks in hospital care: a mixed methods study. Int. J. Nurs. Stud. 54, 45–53.

van Schaik, K.D., Thompson, S.C., 2011. Indigenous beliefs about biomedical and bush treatment efficacy for indigenous cancer patients: a review of the literature. Intern. Med. J. 42 (2), 184–191.

Wain, T., Sim, M., Bessarab, D., et al., 2016. Engaging Australian Aboriginal narratives to challenge attitudes and create empathy in health care: a methodological perspective. BMC Med. Educ. 16, 156. doi:10.1186/s12909-016-0677-2.

Whitley, R., Rousseau, C., Carpenter-Song, E., et al., 2011. Evidence-based medicine: opportunities and challenges in a diverse society. Can. J. Psychiatry 56 (9), 514–522.

Wilson, A.M., Magarey, A.M., Jones, M., et al., 2015. Attitudes and characteristics of health professionals working in Aboriginal health. Rural Remote Health 15 (1), Article 2739 (Online).

World Health Organization (WHO), 2010. Indigenous health – Australia, Canada, Aotearoa New Zealand and the United States – Laying claim to a future that embraces health for us all. Available online at http://www.who.int/healthsystems/topics/financing/healthreport/IHNo33.pdf, (Accessed 15 July 2016).

# PART

# 2

# THE SKILLS

This part of the book explores specific interpersonal skills that nurses must develop in order to interact with patients effectively and form therapeutic relationships. Chapters 5–7 focus on the individual skill sets of listening, understanding and exploring. In Chapter 5 listening is considered with specific reference to the patient–nurse relationship and that which is relevant and meaningful in nursing care.

The role of empathy in therapeutic relationships is highlighted in Chapter 6, as this is considered the key concept to understanding a patient as a person. The skills of exploration are reviewed in Chapter 7 and include the role of probing through the use of questions, as well as prompting through the use of statements. While there are numerous references to how each set relates to other sets, separating them by chapter enables readers to develop skills within manageable learning segments.

Chapter 8 offers insight and guidance to nurses as they move from understanding patients' situations to taking meaningful action to comfort, support and enable patients. The numerous learning activities that appear throughout these chapters serve to deepen readers' understanding of the skills and how to use them effectively.

# CHAPTER
# 5

# Encouraging interaction: listening

## CHAPTER OVERVIEW

- Listening is a complex process that involves more than hearing.
- Nurses need to listen to patients in order to gather relevant information and to understand the patient.
- Nurses need to listen to that which is most directly related to nursing care.
- Listening effectively involves being receptive and fully present.
- There are a variety of listening skills that include attending, observing, perceiving, interpreting and recalling.
- Nurses need to evaluate whether listening has been effective.
- The chapter concludes with a description of how to evaluate whether listening has been effective.

e Visit the Evolve site for video content to support the themes and skills explored in this chapter: http://evolve.elsevier.com/AU/Stein-Parbury/patient/

# INTRODUCTION

'It wasn't much; I mean, I really didn't do anything to help. All I did was to listen.' Comments such as these fail to acknowledge or demonstrate an appreciation for the complexity and power of effective listening. 'Just listening' seems so simple, as if no effort is required and no expertise is needed. In nursing, listening is powerful because it encourages patients to share their experiences; it validates patients as people with something to say; it promotes understanding between a nurse and a patient; and it provides the nurse with information on which to act.

It is not nearly as 'simple' as it sounds on the surface. Quite a lot is happening when nurses 'just' listen. When nurses listen, *just* listen, they pay careful attention to what they hear and observe, they focus on what is explicitly expressed by the patient and they try to determine what the patient is meaning. Effective listening requires receptivity, sustained concentration and astute observation. It is a planned, deliberate act, which can hardly be viewed as 'not doing anything'.

Nursing care is based on an understanding of patients' personal experiences of health and their responses to illness. In order to reach this level of understanding, nurses must first listen to patients' stories. The skills of listening are fundamental to patient–nurse relationships. Listening permeates the entire relationship; if meaningful interpersonal connections are to occur, listening must occur throughout every interaction.

Listening actively demonstrates nurses' presence with, and interest in, patients. Nursing presence, which is the foundation of listening, is the intentional act of being with the patient, both physically and psychologically (McMahon & Christopher 2011; Penque & Kearney 2015). Through listening, nurses orient themselves as being 'for' the patient. Listening encourages patients to express themselves because it provides the necessary time and space. Listening enables patients to experience being heard and accepted by nurses. Listening enables nurses to understand and appreciate patients' experiences, especially in relation to their nursing care needs. As such, it sets the stage for effective interpersonal connections and assessment of the patient. Nurses base their responses to patients on what is perceived through listening. Once the stage is set, the players can enact their roles (the one helping and the one helped), but it is vital that the stage remains set throughout the relationship.

# THE LISTENING PROCESS

Listening is a complex process that encompasses the skills of reception, perception and interpretation of input. The process begins with input. Sights, sounds, smells, tastes and tactile sensations are received through the sensory organs. The initial step in the listening process is the reception of this input, predominantly through the eyes and ears. The ability to receive the input is dependent upon the listener's state of readiness – when receivers are 'tuned in'. Next, the received input must be noticed as important; it must be actively perceived. During this stage of the process, external and internal distractions often interfere with accurate perception and create filters, which partially or completely block the input. Almost as soon as the input is perceived, the listener attaches meaning to it – an interpretation is made.

The meaning attached to a particular piece of sensory input is connected to the listener's culture, memory, previous experience, expectations, desires, wants, needs and current thoughts and feelings. For example, nurses working in a hospital unit know when they hear a particular buzz and see a light over a doorway to a patient's room (sensory input received and perceived) that the patient in that room has turned on the call light, requesting assistance (interpretation). To an outsider, the sound and sight of the call light activation may be received and noticed but no particular meaning is derived unless there is a familiarity with how hospitals are equipped. If they are busy, nurses who notice the call light may interpret the patient's request for assistance as a nuisance. Likewise, a nurse may decide that the patient requesting assistance is not in immediate need if this particular patient turns on the call light for minor reasons (interpretation based on experience and expectations).

Effective listening encompasses not only receiving sensory input but also perceiving it and interpreting its meaning. When nurses correctly interpret what patients are expressing, listening has been effective.

# HEARING AND LISTENING

Hearing and listening are not the same. Any person with the apparatus for detecting audible tones can hear but may or may not be capable of listening. People without hearing capabilities may be able to listen, while those with hearing capabilities may fail to listen. Listening involves paying active attention to what is being said; it is more than simply receiving sensory input.

## Active and passive listening

Effective listening, the active process of taking in, absorbing and eventually understanding what is being expressed, requires energy and concentration on the part of the listener. Have you ever been in a conversation with somebody who claimed to be listening to you but was attending to another matter, for example. watching television or reading? No matter how much this person may try to convince you that they are listening, it is not likely you will believe it because they are not offering their full attention.

Hearing, without fully concentrating and attending, is passive listening. Active listening is for the purpose of understanding. Not only does it require the reception of sensory input but also astute observation, undivided attention and the processing or interpretation of what is heard. While some people may be capable of listening to background music while reading or studying, this type of passive reception does not serve listeners well during engaged interpersonal interaction. Effective listening is only achieved in an active and involved manner. It cannot be done passively.

Hearing involves 'being there' for patients, while listening involves 'being with' patients. Hearing promotes interpersonal contact between a patient and a nurse, with the emphasis on task-related activities. Listening promotes interpersonal connection between a patient and a nurse at a deeper level of commitment. A patient's desire for contact or connection is important to consider, and this reinforces the negotiated aspects of the level of involvement in the relationship (see Ch 2).

# BENEFITS OF LISTENING

It is important that nurses understand the benefits of effective listening in order to more fully appreciate its power and helpfulness. Although considered essential to effective communication and relationship building, there is little empirical evidence in the nursing literature on the subject of listening (Kagan 2008b). Nonetheless, listening is recognised as a powerful agent for healing (Browning & Waite 2010). The benefits of listening are described as those for the patient, those for the nurse and those for the relationship between them.

## For the patient

Effective listening is consistent with the concept that nurses care about patients. When nurses take and make time to listen to what patients are expressing, they demonstrate genuine interest in and regard for patients. Listening is one of the clearest ways for nurses to convey respect for and acceptance of patients. By listening, nurses actively demonstrate to patients that what they have to say matters – that the patient matters. Nurses give of themselves when they listen. Patients feel worthwhile because they have been given the nurse's time, energy and attention.

Listening reinforces the inherent worth of patients and, as a result, patients feel comforted because they feel valued. Their sense of wellbeing and mental ease are enhanced when nurses are fully present and available to interact because they feel acknowledged and validated as a person (Finfgeld-Connett 2006; Kagan 2008a). Patients report that they value nurses who make an effort to be attentive through listening (Marshall et al 2012). Patients, likewise, associate nurses' caring with their capacity to be fully present and available to them, as they feel protected and calm (Kostovich & Clementi 2014). In contrast, 'not being listened to' has negative effects on their sense of wellbeing and healthcare (Courts et al 2004).

## For the nurse

Any verbal response that nurses make is based on what is perceived through listening to the patient. Listening to patients enables nurses to receive information about patients, collect data on which to base nursing care activities and reach deeper levels of understanding with patients. It is vital to the processes of patient assessment and care planning. Being fully present with a patient, as would be evidenced through listening, has been linked to effective clinical decision making in nursing (du Plessis 2016).

Theoretical understanding of a particular clinical situation offers possibilities and probabilities, but listening to an individual patient's experience offers concrete, personally unique data on which to base responsive nursing care. For example, chronic illness often affects a patient's sense of self-worth (a theoretical possibility). But by listening to an individual patient's experience of and reactions to chronic illness, the nurse comes to understand concretely and specifically how this particular patient's sense of self-worth is, or is not, affected by the experience. Listening encourages patients to open up and tell their stories and, as a result, nurses are in a better position to understand patients and become cognisant of their nursing care needs.

## For the relationship

Listening encourages further interaction between patients and nurses. It is a catalyst in promoting trust in their relationship because patients will come to know that they can rely on the nurse to 'be there'. When patients feel listened to, they feel a sense of connection with nurses, thus enabling the relationship to progress (Jonas-Simpson et al 2006; Kagan 2008a).

At times, listening with understanding is all that is needed in an interaction; it is an end in itself. For example, listening to a patient's expression of sadness in response to a loss may be just what the nurse needs to do in order to be of help. At other times, listening is a means to another end – a responsive nursing action based on understanding that is achieved through listening. For example, as a result of listening to a patient express a lack of understanding about a current medication regimen, the nurse can explain why it is important (e.g. to take medication prior to eating). Thus, nursing care is based on what the nurse has assessed through listening.

## LISTENING WITH NURSING EARS

The general benefits of listening in the nursing care context are important to appreciate; however, the benefits refer primarily to how meaningful interaction between a patient and a nurse is enhanced. What about the content of listening in the nursing care context? When nurses listen, they need to listen for aspects of the patient's experience that are significant in the context of nursing assessment and care planning. What should be the focus when listening to patients? What kinds of meanings and understandings are specific to the clinical practice of nursing? What particular aspects of patients' experiences are most relevant to nurses? Listening with 'nursing ears' is listening for specific nursing-related meanings, and an understanding of these meanings forms the basis of listening goals within the nursing context.

## ACTIVITY 5.1 Listening goals in nursing

### Process

1. Form small groups of about five participants.

2. Discuss the answers to the following questions:

   a. 'What do I need to know and understand about patients in order to care effectively for them?'

   b. 'When I am listening to patients, what is most significant for me to notice about what they are expressing?'

3. Record and compare your answers with the other groups.

### Discussion

1. Do the answers to the questions provide any focus for listening in nursing? If so, what is the focus?

2. Are there aspects of patients' experiences that are more significant to nursing than other aspects? What are these?

3. What are the major goals of listening in the nursing context? List them.

4. Listening with nursing ears means focusing on goals. Compare your list in step 3 with the following goals (presented in question form):

   a. What effects do the current health status of patients have on their daily living?

   b. How do patients interpret their health status?

   c. How are patients reacting to the healthcare they are receiving?

   d. How are patients reacting to your nursing approach in particular?

   e. How much do patients understand about their health status and healthcare? How much do they want to understand?

   f. Who or what is most important to patients? What do they value the most in life?

   g. What worries patients the most about their health status and healthcare?

Activity 5.1 poses challenges because it suggests that certain limitations can be imposed on listening. Does listening with 'nursing ears' mean that nurses should ignore, avoid or filter out aspects that are not directly related to nursing care concerns? The answer is no, as it implies partial listening. While it is important for nurses to recognise what concerns them *as nurses*, there is potential danger when listening goals are overemphasised. When this occurs, goals for listening become barriers.

Rather than perceiving these goals as limitations, it is better to think of them as focusing lenses through which to view patients. To take the analogy further, imagine looking through the lens of a camera and focusing on a particular subject within a scene. While the entire landscape is in view, the camera lens brings some aspects of the picture into sharper focus than others. Such is the case when using listening goals in the nursing context. While the entire 'picture' (i.e. the patient) is in view (received), some aspects are brought more sharply into focus (perceived) because these aspects have direct relevance to nursing care.

Another way to employ listening goals in nursing is to use them as orienting and guiding frameworks during the interpretation of received messages. Attention needs to be paid to the patient's entire message; however, the message is interpreted in light of the goals of listening. The message is perceived as is, but the meaning is interpreted using a nursing framework. This framework, or orientation to listening, is then viewed as enhancing rather than limiting because it provides direction to the nurse's listening. Consider the following nurse's story.

## A Nurse's Story

When she first met James, Maddie, an experienced cardiac nurse, was completing the usual admission procedure onto the cardiac surgical ward. She had to complete all the necessary observations of James' physical condition but, more importantly, she needed to get to know James as a person. As Maddie listened to his story of a lifelong problem with his mitral valve, she realised that James understood the implications of his scheduled valve replacement surgery. James told Maddie that he knew the surgery would need to be done someday.

Naturally, James was concerned about the surgery itself, but he reassured himself with the knowledge that he was in the capable hands of an experienced cardiac surgery team. As she listened, Maddie began to realise the potential impact of the surgery on James' life. He was employed as a night-shift supervisor of a large coal preparation plant, a position he worked hard to obtain and an achievement of which he was proud. Nevertheless, his job involved a great deal of walking around the plant and James noted his increasing inability 'to get around like I used to'. He was afraid that he might become disabled after the surgery, unable to continue in a job he obviously enjoyed. He understood the details of the surgery, recognised that it was necessary and accepted it. Yet he was worried about what it might mean for his future.

In focusing on James' concern about the potential impact of the surgery and of what it might mean in terms of his daily life, Maddie was listening with 'nursing ears'.

# READINESS TO LISTEN

Effective listening requires a certain amount of mental preparation in order to achieve a state of readiness. A nurse's 'readiness to listen' is as important as the act of perceiving actively and fully what a patient is expressing. Even before messages are received, the conditions necessary for receiving input must be realised. First, nurses must have the intent and desire to listen to patients. Positive intentions and desires alone, however, are not enough; they need to be conveyed to the patient.

Effective listeners demonstrate the readiness to listen through these attitudes and behaviours.

## ACTIVITY 5.2 Indicators of listening

### Process

1. Think of someone in your life who really listens to you. Visualise this person. Reflect on your reasons for choosing this person. Why do you think of this person as one who listens? What does this person do that leads you to believe that they listen?

2. Record your thoughts and reflections about this person.

3. Now think of someone in your life who does not seem to listen to you. Visualise this person. Reflect on your reasons for choosing this person. Why do you think of this person as one who does not listen to you? What does this person do that leads you to believe that they don't listen?

4. Record your thoughts and reflections about this person.

### Discussion

1. Compare your recordings of each person – the listener and the non-listener. What differences do you note?

2. Summarise the major differences between people who listen and people who do not.

3. If working in a group, compare your summary with the summaries of other participants.

Activity 5.2 highlights characteristics of effective listeners, namely:

- availability to interact
- having the time to listen
- not interrupting the speaker
- not judging, evaluating, advising or imposing their own ideas on the speaker
- not merely listening for what they want to hear
- openness to whatever is being expressed.

People who are inpatients in acute care hospital settings have reported that nurses often appear 'too busy' with the completion of tasks and therefore do not have the time to interact with patients (Chang et al 2005; McCabe 2004; Shattell 2005). It may be that nurses are feeling overwhelmed by their workload as they attend to the numerous tasks that occupy their workday, but this may communicate to patients that there is little time available to listen. When this happens, nurses cannot convey a readiness to listen. Focusing on tasks reflects a value that the tasks are more important than the people who are the patients. Patients are left with the feeling that the nurse's time is too precious to interrupt.

When the desire to help is present, yet there is a perception that there is no time to listen, nurses are placed in a bind. There is a fear that the demands of current healthcare systems on nurses are increasingly distracting them from interacting with patients (Penque & Kearney 2015; Papastavrou et al 2012). Lack of time and competing demands can prevent nurses from being fully present and available to listen. The focus on clinical pathways, tasks and increasing documentation has the potential to compromise care (Kuis et al 2015). When there is little time for nurses and patients to connect interpersonally, the quality of care diminishes.

# Receptivity

In order for a television set to receive a signal or transmission, the set has to be tuned into the correct frequency so the signal can be processed. This analogy is useful in understanding the readiness to listen. Nurses must 'tune into' patients' signals and adjust their receivers so the messages are not only audible but also comprehensible. This involves the mental preparation of focusing concentration on a patient's messages and developing antennae to notice what a patient is expressing.

Tuning in to a patient's message is hard work. Some signals are easier to receive than others. At times, there is so much interference that the signal cannot be received at all.

# Reducing interference

Interference stems from distractions that draw attention away from the patient and prevent clear reception of a message. Such distractions originate externally (from outside of the nurse) and internally (from within the nurse).

## External interference

It is important to pay careful attention to the external environment when attempting to listen. For example, the sights and sounds of a busy, bustling hospital setting often present many potential sources of external interference. The ringing of telephones, a variety of healthcare personnel coming and going and patients being transported from one area to another are potential distractions. When nurses visit patients in their home setting, distractions such as the playful noise of small children or a radio or television may be sources of interference. It is not always possible to eliminate external sights, sounds and other stimuli, but attempts should be made to reduce them as much as possible when listening to patients.

In a hospital setting, drawing the curtains around a patient's bed not only provides a degree of privacy but also decreases the number of external distractions and potential interferences. This simple act is effective in reducing the amount of visual distractions but may not reduce the audible ones. Also, it sends a clear message to others that a meaningful activity is occurring.

Interruptions from other staff members can be particularly distracting – even the fear of being interrupted is a potential distraction. Nurses working together in a clinical setting need to be mindful of this; they should assess the need to distract another nurse who is engaged in an interaction with a patient.

Sometimes there are aspects of patients themselves that are sources of external interference. Examples of this kind of interference include: patients who speak in accents that are distracting to a nurse; patients who express themselves in a disjointed, rambling manner; and patients whose speech is barely audible and halting. In these instances, nurses can reduce the interference by attempting to put aside the distractions and concentrating carefully on what the patient is expressing.

In general, reducing external interference occurs whenever attempts are made to exclude the outside world. This is done by placing barriers between the outside world and the patient and nurse, or by consciously tuning out external noise.

## Internal interference

When nurses are ready to listen, they are able to forget themselves for the moment. They allow themselves to be engrossed in the interaction with a patient and to notice and perceive what the patient is expressing. Internal interference – the nurse's own thoughts, feelings, preoccupations or value judgments – are often more difficult to control than external interference. A noisy television set (an external interference) can simply be switched off in order to eliminate it as a source of distraction. Internal interferences cannot simply be switched off.

### Thoughts as internal interference

One common preoccupation that interferes with listening is the worry a nurse often feels about how to respond to the patient: 'What am I going to say to this patient?'; 'What am I going to do for this patient?'. Thoughts such as these are often related to a self-expectation that nurses must 'do something' in order to help patients. As a result, nurses become so preoccupied with their own anxieties that they fail to listen and perceive what the patient is expressing. An internal reminder that something is being done – 'I am listening to what this patient is expressing' – can help to draw a nurse's focus away from their own thoughts and onto the patient. If something else can be done, it will become evident *after* the nurse listens with understanding to what the patient is expressing.

Other thoughts that potentially interfere with listening include any preoccupations that a nurse may have at any given moment. These range from 'Have I remembered to defrost something to eat for dinner tonight?' to 'There is a waiting room full of mothers and babies and I am not going to have time to see each of them' to 'Ms Holmes will need pre-op medications soon. I wonder how long this conversation is going to last. How can I bring it to a close?'. Sometimes these thoughts can be excluded from conscious awareness, while at other times they signal the need to attend to another matter, and then return to the interaction at hand. At yet other times such thoughts are impossible to exclude from conscious awareness, but nurses pretend to be listening. It is far better to cease the interaction until such time that undivided attention can be given to a patient than to feign listening.

## Value judgments as internal interference

The natural tendency to judge what is heard as right or wrong, good or bad, interesting or boring is one of the greatest sources of internal interference when attempting to listen. This tendency is considered natural because it happens automatically, often without conscious awareness: 'That's a stupid way to react'; 'I don't think he should be feeling that way'; 'What's she going on about? It's really nothing'. Such thoughts are judgmental because they channel the patient's message through the nurse's personal interpretive filter. They interfere with listening because they close off possibilities that do not match the nurse's internal frame of reference.

What is heard may be evaluated negatively and rejected outright as unacceptable. Even if what is heard is evaluated in a positive light, it interferes with a nurse's ability to fully appreciate and understand the uniqueness of a patient's experience because the nurse is still relying on a personal frame of reference.

While it is almost impossible to prevent valuative thoughts, nurses who are aware recognise them as stemming from a personal value system and are therefore able to separate their own value system from the patient's. Personal judgments, once separated, can then be held in suspense, deferred and kept peripheral to the patient. Being non-judgmental is a near impossible goal to achieve; however, keeping one's value system separate and suspended is achievable. The most critical aspect of suspending judgment is the nurse's self-understanding (see Ch 3).

## Feelings as internal interference

Sometimes, internal interference stems from a nurse's lack of ability to cope with what the patient is expressing; for example, a feeling of despondency might overwhelm a nurse listening to the sorrow of a young mother dying of cancer. Nurses may fail to listen because of their own anxieties, and they may, unwittingly or unknowingly, either change the subject or avoid interacting with the patient altogether. There are times when nurses' own circumstances create a sense of vulnerability that prevents them from being fully present with a patient. When emotional demands are high, nurses are at risk of 'switching off' in an effort to protect themselves (Barrett et al 2005).

On the majority of occasions, nurses fail to listen to distressing patients' stories out of fear of not knowing what to say or how to respond. Not listening or even avoiding a patient for these reasons potentially compounds the patient's distress because it isolates and distances a patient from the nurse, thus disabling the relationship.

Nurses must remind themselves that listening to a patient's distress, no matter how disturbing, is comforting simply because it shows they are fully present and genuinely interested in the patient. Words spoken by nurses in an attempt to comfort may actually intrude. Listening is 'being there' with these patients. Often, patients do not want or need words in these extreme situations. The caring of another human being is more than adequate and helps to make the 'unbearable bearable'.

When nurses become overwhelmed, and perhaps paralysed, by their own feelings as a result of what patients are expressing and experiencing, seeking support from other nurses is preferable to avoiding or emotionally abandoning the patient (see Ch 11).

Once the state of readiness to listen is achieved, a nurse is available to be fully present during an interaction with a patient. Attention is focused and undivided, perceptual filters are open, antennae are up and interference is reduced. This state of readiness, when maintained throughout the interaction, not only enables nurses to listen but also encourages further interaction.

# NURSING PRESENCE

All of the factors described as 'readiness to listen' are encompassed in the concept of nursing presence because this is an essential requisite for effective listening. Presence involves mindfulness, being in the moment and fully observant (see Ch 11). This ability involves 'being with', 'being there' and 'being there *for*' patients; it does not necessarily involve 'doing for' them (Kuis et al 2015). Nursing presence requires intention, dedication and openness on the part of the nurse.

Nursing presence is beneficial for the patient, the nurse and their interpersonal relationship. Patients feel protected, calm, safe and secure when nurses are fully present, and nurses achieve job satisfaction when making meaningful connections with patients. Their relationships are enriched as presence enables the nurse to know and understand the patient.

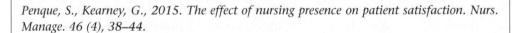

## RESEARCH HIGHLIGHT Nursing presence and patient satisfaction

*Penque, S., Kearney, G., 2015. The effect of nursing presence on patient satisfaction. Nurs. Manage. 46 (4), 38–44.*

### Background

Nurses demonstrate human presence by being in close physical proximity to patients, demonstrating that they are available and attending to patients' needs. In a similar vein they show respect by meaningfully engaging with patients. Nursing presence is beneficial to patient care and patient satisfaction. While nursing presence is a useful concept, its use as an intervention has not been systematically studied in relation to patient satisfaction.

### Purpose of the study

The purpose of this study was to determine the effects of a nursing presence intervention on nurse-sensitive indicators of patient satisfaction.

### Method

This was a quasi-experimental study comparing patient satisfaction data from two groups of patient participants – one prior to the intervention and one after. The intervention was that nurses, who were first educated about presence, spent standardised amounts of uninterrupted time with individual patients. They did not undertake any tasks during this time; they simply spent time being with the patient. During the first three weeks, they spent five minutes with each assigned patient. The time was increased to 10 minutes, then 15 minutes. The setting was an acute care hospital unit and all nurses employed there participated in the study.

### Key findings

The intervention of nursing presence improved overall patient satisfaction and three nurse-sensitive indicators: clear nurse communication; courtesy and respect of nurses; and nurse listening. Five minutes of time was enough to improve the perception of nurse listening. When the time was increased to 15 minutes, there was also improvement in perception of courtesy and respect of nurses. Of note is that the 15-minute intervention required the support of the nursing manager. There was no difference in the indicator of clear nurse communication.

### Implications for nursing practice

Patient satisfaction can be improved if nurses dedicate time to simply being with patients. As little as five minutes spent with a patient can make a difference to their perception of nurse listening. Increasing the time leads to patients feeling greater respect for nurses. Nursing presence can be useful as an intervention in and of itself.

# THE SKILLS OF LISTENING

The groundwork involved in achieving the readiness to listen is an inward process initiated by nurses as they prepare both themselves and the environment. Readiness alone, however, is not sufficient for effective listening because two-way communication with a patient has not yet begun. This section explores the interactive nature of listening because the skills of listening are enacted through interchange with another person. The skills of listening are divided into five areas: attending, observing, perceiving, interpreting and recalling.

## Attending

Attending behaviour is the outward, physical manifestation of a nurse's readiness to listen. It communicates to the patient that the nurse is available to listen and accessible to interact. The outward behaviour of attending conveys the message: 'Go ahead, you have my attention; I'm here with you now'. Patients find it valuable when nurses give their time to be available to patients and associate such attending behaviour with helpful communication (McCabe 2004).

The messages of attending are sent through non-verbal channels, predominantly body posture and eye contact. For example, a nurse checking a patient's healthcare record for recent documentation (no matter how casually) while attempting to listen is not fully communicating their intent because they are not demonstrating attending behaviour to the patient.

Attending behaviour has two key elements: the spatial position of the nurse in relation to the patient and the maintenance of eye contact. While attending, nurses physically place themselves in a manner that promotes interaction between themselves and patients. Attending behaviour demonstrates active interest in the patient. Egan (2014) presents general guidelines for attending using the acronym SOLER, which stands for:

**S**   Squarely facing the person in a front-on presentation

**O**   Open posture, conveying an acceptance and openness to the other person

**L**   Leaning forward, demonstrating active interest

**E**   Eye contact maintained, including being at the same eye level as the other person

**R**   Relaxed posture, demonstrating an ease with self, the other and the situation.

Attending promotes active engagement between nurses and patients and encourages patients to continue expressing themselves.

Attending encourages further interaction between patients and nurses, while non-attending is discouraging. In Activity 5.3, person A will probably not wish to continue the conversation after person B begins non-attending. No matter how intent a nurse may be on listening, without attending, a patient will not be encouraged to continue.

## Some words of caution about attending

The intensity of attending is not always appropriate because it is not always warranted by the topic at hand. Try assuming the posture during a conversation about the weather. You will note that intense attending feels awkward when the subject of the conversation is of little consequence. A discussion about the weather, unless there has recently been a significant event related to the weather, does not warrant such an intense listening response. This is important for nurses to bear in mind. There are times when patients discuss subjects that do not require the intensity of attending and for a nurse to assume the posture is not only awkward but inappropriate.

The attending guideline about maintaining eye contact is another area that presents some difficulty, and caution needs to be exercised when applying this guideline. Unbroken eye contact is unnatural, awkward and even threatening

## ACTIVITY 5.3 Attending and non-attending

### Process

1. Divide into pairs and designate one person as A and the other as B.

**Instructions to A**

2. Tell a story to B about something exciting or interesting that has happened to you. Talk for about five minutes on the subject.

**Instructions to B**

3. Begin the interaction by assuming the attending posture (i.e. face A, maintain eye contact, lean forward and remain relaxed and open). After about a minute or two, start to lean back, fold your arms and look away from A. Focus on something other than what A is saying (e.g. stare out the window, clean your nails, flip through a book). Do anything to violate the rules of attending. Remain silent, do not interrupt or change the subject, but do try to keep listening.

4. Stop the conversation after about five minutes.

### Discussion

1. How did A feel during the interaction? What happened to A when B began non-attending?

2. How did B feel during the interaction? What happened to B when they began non-attending?

3. How did the conversation change when B no longer appeared interested?

because of the discomfort it creates. The head-on position of attending forces eye contact that is then difficult to break. When nurses are attending, it is important to bear in mind that occasional breaks in eye contact are not only natural but also desirable in maintaining comfort and ease during the interaction.

Finally, an attending posture, which focuses on eye contact as one of its central aspects, may not be appropriate in some cultures. Maintaining eye contact can be a sign of disrespect when there are cultural norms about status. Looking directly into the eyes of a person who is of a higher status is unacceptable when these cultural norms are operating. Likewise, eye contact may vary with age and gender. Nurses need to be sensitive to how patients are responding to their attempts to encourage interaction through attending behaviour, and a large part of this sensitivity is awareness of cultural variances (see Ch 4). For example, in some cultures it is considered rude to look a person in authority (as nurses are often viewed) directly in the eye (i.e. to make eye contact with them).

## Attending within the clinical nursing context

In nursing it is sometimes difficult to assume the classic attending posture. Nurses must learn to adapt the attending posture to the realities of their particular clinical setting. For example, it is not always possible to face the patient squarely. In a hospital, when patients are lying in bed and the nurse is standing nearby, the attending mandate of squarely facing the other may be impossible to achieve. More importantly, Stickley (2011) asserts that this 'square on' posture may be interpreted as confrontational and recommends sitting at an angle. Nurses need to physically situate themselves in such a manner to establish eye contact, maintain a relaxed stance and be close enough to interact in a meaningful manner but far enough away to maintain comfort.

Standing at the side of the bed is preferable to standing at the foot of the bed. Although the foot position would allow a nurse to squarely face a patient, it may actually discourage interaction because it leaves too much distance between the patient and the nurse and places the nurse in an authoritarian stance. By placing themselves at the side of the bed, nurses are almost facing the same direction as the patient. This may be preferable to the 'squarely facing' position because it demonstrates that a nurse is attempting to view the world *with* the patient, sharing a common perspective.

While standing at the side of the bed, nurses are faced with the challenge of lowering themselves to the eye level of the patient, unless the height of the bed is at a level that places the patient at the same eye level as the nurse. Sitting down is the most logical way to meet this challenge. This also sends the message to the patient that the nurse intends to remain there – to interact. While seated, nurses are obviously accessible and available to patients.

Awareness that being seated is preferable can pose a dilemma for nurses. There may be a shortage of chairs. If they seat themselves, they may be reprimanded or frowned upon by other nurses for not working hard enough. The hard work of listening to patients is often unrecognised and unacknowledged, especially in the hospital setting where so much 'other work' needs to be accomplished. In long-term residential settings, such as nursing homes, it is vital for nurses to lower themselves to the level of the patient and establish eye contact in an effort to gain their attention.

# Silence

Obviously, when nurses are attending and listening to patients, they are silent. Silence plays a major part in effective listening, and its value is important to recognise. To be silent and not interrupt patients who are expressing themselves is a sign of respect and interest.

Silence can also go further in its helpfulness. Both the patient and the nurse may be silent for short periods of time. Silent moments are useful because they allow the patient and the nurse time to collect their thoughts and reflect on what has been expressed; they provide an opportunity for either the patient or the nurse to change the direction of the conversation; and they slow the pace of the interaction. Nevertheless, nurses frequently experience difficulty in remaining silent because of a felt need to say or do something.

There are times when silently being with a patient, fully attending and being fully present is quite helpful. Patients who are in severe physical pain may not wish to talk or be spoken to but would like to have a nurse present. Patients who are psychologically depressed may feel pressured to interact and would benefit from a nurse's silent, undemanding presence. These two situations provide examples of contexts in which the silent presence of nurses is appropriate and helpful.

During a verbal interaction, it is important to ascertain when to allow the silence to proceed and when it is better to break the silence with speech or action. Nurses can employ some general guidelines when they are faced with the decision. First and foremost, silence should not be used as a substitute or excuse for not knowing how to respond or what to say. When used in this way, silence could be interpreted by the patient as rejection or lack of interest on the part of the nurse. It is better for nurses to admit to feeling 'at a loss for words' under these circumstances. Silence is also ineffective if the patient expects or wants a verbal response from the nurse. Careful attention to the flow and direction of the interaction allows nurses to 'check its pulse' and perceive patient cues that indicate discomfort with the silence.

Silent periods also have limitations if they last longer than about 10–15 seconds. When silence progresses beyond these time limits, the flow of the interaction may be stifled, rather than enhanced. Try this experiment the next time you are interacting with another person: when a silent period ensues, unobtrusively check the time. Alternatively, sit on your own quietly for 10–15 seconds. It is surprising how long a 10–15-second period of silence actually feels.

# Observing

Effective listening includes astutely observing the patient. A large part of listening is not only paying careful attention to what is expressed but also how it is expressed. During listening, nurses have a good opportunity to observe the non-verbal aspects of the patient's expressions. Subtle and obvious cues about patients' experiences are better understood when nurses perceive patients' non-verbal behaviour. Non-verbal cues often shed light on the feeling aspects of a patient's experience. Feelings are most often expressed through facial expression, eye contact, body posture and movements and other non-verbal behaviour. Such patient cues are signals for further exploration (see Ch 7), but the nurse must first notice the cues. Noticing cues and their initial interpretation occur in the context of listening.

There is no doubt that participants in Activity 5.4 will experience a heightened awareness of the non-verbal indicators of feelings because they are asked to determine what feelings other participants are expressing. Their perceptual antennae are ready for the reception of non-verbal input. It is beneficial for nurses to develop and maintain this degree of heightened perceptual awareness when interacting with patients. Heightened perceptual awareness enables nurses to be more astute in their observations. It makes them notice the way in which a patient is relaying messages.

The inherent difficulty in accurately interpreting non-verbal messages is also demonstrated in Activity 5.4. This highlights and reinforces the need for nurses to check their perceptions through exploration (Ch 7). Noticing and observing

## ACTIVITY 5.4  Non-verbal expressions of feelings

### Process

1. Form groups of five to six participants and decide on a topic for discussion. The chosen topic can be of any nature, but it needs to be one about which participants can express emotions. Controversial topics are most effective (e.g. euthanasia, abortion, IVF, rights of smokers).

2. Participants should reflect on their feelings or emotions in relation to the selected topic. Each participant records this feeling or emotion on a slip of paper. These slips of paper are not shared with other participants.

3. Participants should reflect on how they usually express their chosen emotion non-verbally.

4. In small groups, discuss the chosen topic. Throughout the discussion, each participant expresses their chosen feeling through non-verbal means only. Participants are not to express their chosen feeling in a verbal manner (i.e. they cannot say how they feel).

5. Stop the discussion after about 10 minutes.

6. Each member of a small group should record what feeling they believe was being expressed by each of the other members, as well as the non-verbal behaviour that led to this conclusion. Participants do not consult with any other members at this point.

7. Each group member takes a turn asking other members what feeling they thought they were expressing. After each states their conclusion, the member whose feeling was being discussed shows the other members the feeling recorded during step 2. Continue around the small group until each member's feeling expression is discussed.

### Discussion

1. On what basis did participants determine what feeling was being expressed? Would this differ between cultural groups, age groups or gender groups?

2. How accurate were the guesses about what feeling was being expressed? What discrepancies existed between what others interpreted and what the participant intended to convey? Why?

3. What does this say about the valid interpretation of non-verbal messages?

non-verbal cues of patients is significant in the context of listening. The cues must then be validated by the patient as to their correct meaning because listening enables nurses to observe them but not necessarily to interpret them accurately.

## The importance of non-verbal communication

Both attending and observing rely on a nurse's awareness of the importance of non-verbal communication. It is a nurse's non-verbal behaviour that is central to attending, while the patient's non-verbal behaviour is critical to observing. Non-verbal behaviour conveys emotional and relational information (Henry et al 2012). For example, if nurses are trying to convey a sense of acceptance and a matter-of-fact attitude when undertaking particularly repulsive dressings, their behaviours and facial expressions can play a pivotal role.

Aspects of non-verbal communication behaviours include posture, facial expression, tone of voice, affect, eye contact and touch. In the nursing literature, the most frequently studied aspects of non-verbal communication of nurses are patient-directed eye gaze, affirmative head nodding, smiling, leaning forward and touch (Yu et al 2012). It is through these behaviours that a nurse conveys interest and warmth. Ratings of clinician warmth, as measured by non-verbal communication, is associated with greater patient satisfaction (Henry et al 2012).

When inconsistencies exist between the verbal and the non-verbal content of the message, there is a general tendency for the non-verbal aspects to be viewed as the more accurate or honest. For example, a nurse who is 'pretending' to listen, yet not attending, conveys a message of disinterest in relating to the patient. Likewise, a nurse may doubt that a patient who claims to be 'feeling fine', yet whose facial expression is a grimace, is really feeling fine.

However, non-verbal expression is particularly prone to cultural interpretation. For example, patients who are embarrassed because they don't know the answer to a nurse's question may avoid eye contact and stare at the ground. It is all too easy for a nurse to interpret this behaviour as 'non-cooperative', while the correct meaning is that the patient is trying to avoid the shame of not knowing.

A poignant reminder that non-verbal messages are open to misinterpretation is provided in the following scenario, which depicts the hospitalisation experience of a 12-week-old infant.

## SCENARIO

Oscar, a 12-week-old infant who had experienced child abuse, was admitted to a large children's hospital with a fractured left femur, seven fractured ribs and extensive bruising. Over the first two days of his hospitalisation he was given very few doses of an intramuscular narcotic for pain. As a result of his unrelieved pain, Oscar became withdrawn and unresponsive. Instead of alerting the staff who were caring for him to the fact that he was in pain, Oscar's behaviour was interpreted as a sign that he was pain-free: 'He wouldn't be so quiet if he was in pain'. When the attending doctor changed the analgesia orders to paracetamol on the third day after admission, not one member of the nursing staff challenged the assumption that Oscar's pain was resolving and therefore that the change in medication orders was appropriate.

It may be argued that interpreting Oscar's somewhat ambiguous behaviour as benign is in the 'best' interests of nurses who need to protect themselves from potentially overwhelming feelings. In other words, by interpreting Oscar's quietness as a sign that he was pain-free, those caring for him avoided the psychological distress that would be associated with caring for a severely abused infant.

It is perceived that one of the most common problems with non-verbal behaviour is the notion that the behaviour may be interpreted in a way that matches the needs, worldview and culture of the observer; however, this may or may not be an accurate interpretation.

# Perceiving messages

'Attending' demonstrates a nurse's interest in listening to the patient, and observing enables nurses to notice non-verbal cues presented by patients. Patients are now encouraged and free to tell their story to an actively interested nurse, and the nurse is in a position to receive the patient's messages.

There are many facets to patients' stories including the actual content of the story, the related feelings and the general theme of the story. Each facet comes together to create a picture of the patient – the whole story. While it is vital that the nurse receives the entire story, knowledge of the various facets of messages guides a nurse's perception throughout the listening process.

The following story, related by a female resident of a nursing home, serves as an example of the various facets of a story.

## A Patient's Story

Michael, the diversional therapist, never pushes you to participate in his activities. He takes one look at you and knows whether you feel like participating that day. He'll say, 'Come along and just watch today, okay?' He always has so many activities going, but you really don't have to do anything you don't feel like doing. That is what's so good about this place.

The content of this story revolves around the activities conducted by a diversional therapist. The feelings expressed are of contentment and satisfaction at not being forced to participate in these activities. The resident uses her discussion of the diversional therapy program as an illustration of the general manner in which residents of the nursing home are treated. The general theme is one of feeling respected by the way she is treated. The content (the diversional therapy activities) and its related feelings (happy and satisfied) come together to form the theme – the importance of having her wishes respected by others.

Notice how the resident speaks of herself in the second person, using the personal pronoun 'you' to indicate herself. When listening to patients it is important that nurses recognise use of the pronoun 'you' in patients' direct reference to themselves. In doing so, they are relating information about themselves, not another person. Perceptive nurses, who are in tune with patients' expressions, notice this use of language and can more fully understand the themes of patients' stories as a result.

At times, patients directly express the content, feeling and thematic facets of their stories, as in the example about the diversional therapist. At other times, however, any or all of the facets are expressed indirectly, through implications, hints and cues. Either way, the various facets of the patient's story must be received and perceived by a nurse who is listening.

# Perceiving content

The content of a message contains the objective, factual data about the topic being discussed and includes what is being discussed, who it involves and when and where an event occurred. The content of a message is the storyline. The following patient story, related by a female patient on an orthopaedic ward of a hospital, serves as an illustration.

## A Patient's Story

I had these pains in my Achilles tendon. I think it had something to do with playing tennis every day. At first I tried to ignore the pain, but it became so bad that I knew I had to do something. When I saw my local GP, he suggested cortisone injections, so I took the advice and had the injections. That was when the real trouble started. First my right leg started to give way, buckling on me. I fell a few times, and then the final time I fell, I really hurt myself. Now I'm told the right tendon has snapped, and here I am, needing to have it repaired. The whole thing has been going on for about six months now.

The content of this patient's story includes pain, falling, the local GP, cortisone injections, an injured Achilles tendon, the need to have the tendon repaired and a time frame of the past six months.

When nurses are listening, there is a tendency to make assumptions about what the patient is discussing. Sometimes these assumptions are accepted and even acted upon as if they were fact. When listening, it is important that nurses keep this tendency in check and recognise that further interaction is necessary to validate these initial assumptions (see Ch 7).

Activity 5.5 highlights some of the difficulties inherent in listening. First, there is a tendency for the listener to add elements that are not directly stated. For example, the assumption is often made that the person speaking in Patient story II is the mother of the child. It could be a primary caregiver of any relationship.

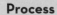

## ACTIVITY 5.5 Listening for content ⟳ 333

**Process**

1. This activity lists six patients' stories, as told by them. Read each one once only. Then cover it up and try to recall the content of the story. If possible, have someone else read the stories to you aloud (once only).

*cont.*

*Activity 5.5 continued*

2.  Record as much of the content of the message as you can recall. In recalling content, think about the following: 'who' is being discussed; 'what' is being discussed; 'when' and 'where' the 'what' occurred; and 'why' it is being discussed. Record the content on a piece of paper using the headings 'Who', 'What', 'When', 'Where' and 'Why'.

    **Patient story I**. I felt something really strange in my hip when I stood up yesterday. It began to really hurt and I was having trouble walking properly. Because it was Sunday afternoon I didn't want to bother anybody. So I took some aspirin, took it easy and went to bed early. Today when I woke up I rang my doctor. She said to go and have the hip x-rayed before I do anything else.

    **Patient story II**. The day started off as usual. I fed him breakfast and got him ready to go to kindy. I was getting ready to go to work when he suddenly began rolling on the floor, clutching his stomach and writhing in pain. It took me a while to work out what was happening. I felt panicked inside, although I didn't let on. I knew it was something major but had no idea what. I rang my GP's surgery and the receptionist said to bring him in straight away. I got into the car immediately and drove there.

    **Patient story III**. I was outside doing the gardening when I suddenly realised I could not move my left arm. I looked at it, saw it was still there, but couldn't make it move an inch. My beautiful left arm was just hanging there. I walked towards the house, not knowing exactly what I was going to do. I sat down on the sofa to think, when I realised that I could move my arm again. Then I really didn't know what to do.

    **Patient story IV**. I have been really worried about him. He hasn't been himself for months. When he comes home from work he has dinner and then just sits in front of the television. I can tell he's not really paying attention to it because he just stares. He doesn't even laugh at the funny bits of his favourite show. When I ask what's wrong, he just shrugs his shoulders.

    **Patient story V**. I know I should have regular Pap smears, but I never seem to find the time. What with the kids, my job and everything, I can't fit in a trip to my GP. Anyway, there's no cancer in my family. Maybe doing all those tests is just a way for the doctors to make money.

    **Patient story VI**. All that chemo and radiotherapy really takes it out of me. I try so hard not to give in to feeling so tired. I go to my room and think, 'Oh, I'll just close my eyes for a few minutes', and the next thing you know I've been asleep for a few hours. It's not fair on my kids because they need me to be there for them.

(Note: Suggested answers to this activity can be found at the end of this chapter.)

## Discussion

1.  In each story, which part of the content was easiest to recall? Which was most difficult? What difficulties did you experience in recalling the content of the stories?

*Activity 5.5 continued*

2. How accurate was your recall of content when you compare your results with those provided at the end of the chapter? (Don't become overly concerned if your answers don't exactly match the ones provided.)

3. Did you discover you 'read into' the stories and added content that was not originally there? Were there aspects of the content that you deleted? Or distorted?

4. What methods did you find yourself using as you attempted to recall the content of the stories?

# Perceiving feelings

When listening, nurses must perceive the feeling aspects of a patient's story, the emotional reactions and subjective responses that accompany the content. Patients often have strong emotional reactions to their health status and healthcare, and the importance of emotions in coping with demands such as those created by health events is increasingly recognised as central to understanding (Lazarus 2006). The connection of feelings to content begins to complete the picture that is the patient's experience. At times, patients express their feelings directly. For example:

- 'I'm really worried about the surgery.'
- 'I'm so pleased with the results of that MRI test.'
- 'I'm feeling a bit down and blue today.'

When expressed in a straightforward manner, patients' feelings are easy to perceive, as long as nurses are ready to listen and receive input. More often, feelings are not expressed so openly and directly. Feeling expression follows a more circuitous route, unlike content, which is often expressed in a straightforward manner. Feelings are often hinted at, implied, inferred and talked around, rather than talked about. It could be that patients are reluctant to share their feelings because of uncertainty about how the nurse will react. This is especially true when trust has not yet been established. It could be that patients are unaware of, and out of touch with, their feelings. These are possible explanations for why feelings are expressed indirectly.

A more probable reason is that adults often try to conceal emotions because they have learnt, through socialisation, which emotions are appropriate to express in various situations (Nelson-Jones 2013). It may be that patients believe it is not appropriate to share their feelings with nurses. But, no matter how much patients try to disguise or hide their feelings, their indirect expression is received by nurses whose perceptual antennae are ready to receive feeling messages.

There is, however, a word of caution about focusing on feelings. When nurses are perceptive to a patient's feelings, the patient's distress can increase. This could be because the patient is encouraged to express emotions to a nurse who is a good listener. This dynamic is not necessarily negative, as the patient may need time to express strong emotions. Another caution is that a nurse's perception of a patient's' emotional needs may not match the patient's perception of these needs (Florin et al 2005). That is, the patient may not perceive their feelings to be as important as the nurse thinks they are; conversely they may perceive them to be more significant. These interpersonal dynamics at play are important to bear in mind when listening for feelings.

In listening for feelings, it is vital for nurses to suspend their personal judgments about what is acceptable and appropriate. Feelings, by their very nature, are

---

## ACTIVITY 5.6  Listening for feelings  334

### Process

1. Participants in a group take turns reading each patient's statement aloud. Before each participant reads the statement they should think about a feeling to be conveyed along with the statement and then read it with the non-verbal cues that depict that feeling. Each participant records what they think the person reading the statement is feeling.

   **a.** 'I'm dying, aren't I?'

   **b.** 'Are you sure you know what you're doing?'

   **c.** 'That right leg won't ever be as strong as it used to be, no matter how hard I try.'

   **d.** 'I just wish I could be like I was before.'

   **e.** 'I've had enough. I just want to die.'

   **f.** 'Why can't anybody show me how to get out of this bed without pain?'

   **g.** 'I don't think my back will ever stop aching.'

   **h.** 'You have to be tough to be a nurse, don't you?'

   **i.** 'The surgery didn't go the way I expected.'

   **j.** 'Have you ever done this procedure before?'

   **k.** 'I'm not sure I should be taking all those tablets.'

   **l.** 'I should have known better than to leave the cleaning liquid sitting out on the benchtop. Now look what's happened.'

(Note: The answers to this activity can be found at the end of this chapter.)

### Discussion

1. Refer to the end of the chapter and compare your answers with those provided. Reflect on the differences between your answers and the ones provided.

2. If you are working in a group, compare your answers with those of the other participants after reading each patient's statement. Discuss any differences in perception of feelings and try to determine why they are different.

often irrational, illogical and difficult to control. In order for nurses to be open to the perception of a patient's feelings, they must hold the view that feelings are acceptable.

Open perception of feeling messages poses a challenge to nurses, not only because of the natural tendency to judge them but also because of the way in which they are indirectly expressed. As described in the section on observing, feelings are often expressed non-verbally, and an observant nurse will pick up these non-verbal cues. Feelings are also expressed indirectly, through verbal means, and a perceptive nurse will notice them.

While there is a tendency to jump to conclusions and make assumptions when listening for content, there is an even greater danger of this when listening for feelings. Listeners tend to project their own opinions about what feelings are being expressed. This is partly because feelings are subjective by nature. The tendency is for listeners to perceive feelings on the basis of what they would feel, given a similar set of circumstances. As with suspending judgment, nurses need to rely on their self-awareness and emotional intelligence (see Ch 3) in order to keep this tendency in check.

## Interpreting: listening for themes

The content of a patient's story and its accompanying feelings come together to form the general theme. Themes are the general point of the story – the consequences and implications of the content and feelings. It could be said that an understanding of the theme is the ultimate goal of listening, as once the point of each story is understood, the patient's entire experience comes into sharper focus. Nurses come to understand the theme of a patient's story by asking themselves the following questions:

- How is the patient experiencing a health event in terms of thoughts/content and feelings?
- What seems to be the most frequent topic/content brought up by the patient?
- What emotions are associated with the topic?
- What is 'triggering' the patient to bring up this topic at this time?
- How is this experience affecting the patient at the moment?
- What are the consequences of what the patient is experiencing?
- What are the implications for the patient in relation to effects of the health event on the patient's life?

Understanding themes requires interpretation. This is always tentative at first and needs to be validated with the patient. After nurses have listened and attempted to understand, they are ready to respond. Perhaps the nurse's current understanding, achieved through listening, needs to be clarified, explored or reflected back to the patient through paraphrasing. The skills needed to achieve any of these are covered in Chapters 6 and 7.

## ACTIVITY 5.7  Listening for themes

### Process

1. Form pairs for this activity. Each member of a pair is to relate a story of something that has recently happened in their life. The story need not be earth-shattering, but it should be meaningful to the person telling the story.

2. The other person is to listen, attend and say little during the telling of the story. At the completion, the listener should state what they think is the theme. The storyteller then validates (or invalidates) what the listener has interpreted as the theme.

3. Discuss any differences in interpretation.

### Discussion

1. How accurate were the interpretations of the theme? What accounted for any inaccuracies?

2. What interfered with listening? What enhanced it?

During Activity 5.7, it will probably be easier for the listeners to identify the theme if they have had a similar experience (i.e. when the story has a sense of familiarity about it). Repeated listening and identification of themes enables nurses to attain a sense of familiarity with common patient experiences. Listening with understanding becomes a valuable learning experience in accurately perceiving patients' stories.

# Recalling messages

Sometimes, the greatest challenge in listening is to recall what patients have said. Accurate recall is important if understanding is to occur. Themes often become apparent only after numerous interactions with a patient. Nurses must rely on their ability to recall previous interactions and put them together with current ones.

## ACTIVITY 5.8  Recalling messages

### Process

1. Four volunteers are needed for this activity. They will participate in recounting an incident that occurred during the night shift at a hospital. The details of the incident are provided below.

2. Two of the volunteers are to leave the room. The other two are to seat themselves in a place where all other participants can hear their conversation.

3. All other participants act as observers. They are to make notes of what is added, deleted and distorted each time the incident is reported.

4. The two volunteers who are in the room are to pretend they are in a handover report at the end of a night shift. One of them relates the following incident to the other by reading it aloud:

At about 2 am, Mr Smithers became confused and agitated. He got out of bed, went into the next room, over to Mrs Blue's bed and began to tell her about how to grow azaleas. Mrs Blue became frightened, rang her husband and asked him to come in immediately. She was so loud on the phone that all the other patients in the room were awakened. The patient in bed 18 reacted to Mrs Blue, tried to get out of bed and fell to the floor. In the meantime, Mr Smithers left the ward and headed towards the lift. Fortunately, another nurse was getting out of the lift and escorted him back to the ward. We contacted the RMO to come to see the patient in bed 18 and Mr Smithers. He ordered x-rays for the patient in bed 18 and a sedative for Mr Smithers.

Now everybody is settled and back in bed. There were no major injuries, but it was a real circus here for a while. In the midst of all of the chaos, Mr Blue arrived, in response to his wife's request. We let him visit her for about 20 minutes and now he's returned home. The incident report was completed and sent.

5. One of the volunteers, who is out of the room, is now called back in. The volunteer who received the report relates the incident to the volunteer who has come into the room, by retelling the story without reading it. No assistance is offered to the volunteer who is relating the story; they must rely on memory to recount the incident.

6. The remaining volunteer (who is still outside of the room) is brought back into the room, and the previous volunteer relates the incident to them by retelling the story. Again, no assistance is offered to this volunteer in retelling the story.

7. Each time the incident is retold, the observers are to record any additions, deletions and distortions made to the original story.

8. The incident report is now read aloud, as it was told originally.

### Discussion

1. The participants who observed the activity should now relate what was added to the original story. What was deleted? What was distorted when the story was retold?

2. What accounted for the alterations that were made to the original story?

3. Volunteers should report their reactions to having to retell such a complex story.

Patients' stories are usually not as complicated as the one told in Activity 5.8. Nevertheless, this activity does highlight how easily stories become diminished, embellished or distorted. Recalling patients' stories takes concentration and effort. If nurses find themselves asking patients to retell their stories many times, patients may not believe they have listened in the first place. When nurses listen and remember what they have heard, patients are comforted to know that somebody has taken the time to understand them.

## ACTIVITY 5.9  Responses that indicate listening

### Process

1.  Each of the following patient statements has a variety of possible responses. Evaluate each response in terms of whether it indicates that the nurse making the response has listened. Record on a piece of paper a YES or NO on the basis of your evaluation. Do not evaluate how good or bad the response seems to you, or base your decision on whether you would make the same response. Judge the response *only* in terms of listening by asking yourself: 'Does the listener's response indicate that the listener has heard the patient?'; and 'Does the response indicate an understanding of what the patient has expressed?'.

    **a.** *Patient*

    I don't think I'm going to make it. Am I going to die?

    *Responses*

    **i.**   The power of positive thinking can really help a lot. Many people in your situation have survived because they refused to give up. Keep fighting. Where there's life, there's hope.

    **ii.**  What has happened to make you worried about it?

    **iii.** I can't really say. You'll have to ask your doctor this question.

    **iv.**  We are all going to die sometime, but it's a frightening prospect when it stares us in the face.

    **b.** *Patient*

    Why is my blood pressure being taken so often?

    *Responses*

    **i.**   We have to check your blood pressure frequently.

    **ii.**  It's doctor's orders.

    **iii.** It's a general observation to keep a check on your vital signs.

    **iv.**  Is it worrying you?

    **c.** *Patient*

    How long will I be in here?

    *Responses*

    **i.**   As long as we think you need to be.

    **ii.**  Let's discuss it with the doctor. If you think you're ready to go home, and the doctor is happy for you to go, you can be discharged.

    **iii.** People who have the operation you are having usually stay in hospital for about three days. That's the usual routine, if there are no complications.

    **iv.**  What has your doctor said about this?

**d.** *Patient*

Why me? Why do I have to be the one who suffers like this?

*Responses*

**i.** It's a part of the usual course of this disease. If you tell me when you feel worse and better, I can help with the pain.

**ii.** We all suffer some kind of pain during our lifetime.

**iii.** It's just a bit of misfortune. You'll have better luck next time, I'm sure.

**iv.** I wish I could answer that question. I'm not sure there always is a reason.

**e.** *Patient*

I have contemplated suicide because I've hit rock bottom.

*Responses*

**i.** Are you thinking about suicide right now?

**ii.** Things can't be that bad.

**iii.** What's happened to you that you've hit rock bottom?

**iv.** What exactly have you contemplated?

**f.** *Patient*

What's going to happen when I come out of the operation?

*Responses*

**i.** We will look after you.

**ii.** There's nothing to worry about. You will feel better than you did before.

**iii.** Have you had a general anaesthetic before?

**iv.** You'll be drowsy for a few hours and, depending on your level of pain, you will receive regular pain relief.

**g.** *Patient*

I'm not sick, and yet I have to take all of these tablets every day.

*Responses*

**i.** It does seem a bit silly, doesn't it?

**ii.** It could be that you don't feel sick because you are taking the tablets.

**iii.** Which tablets are you taking?

**iv.** How long have you been taking the tablets?

**2.** Now review each response for which you recorded a YES. Evaluate each in terms of the major goal of listening – that is, the encouragement of patients to continue expressing their experiences. How encouraging is each?

**3.** Compare your answers with the ones provided at the end of the chapter.

# EVALUATION OF LISTENING

In the final analysis, nurses listen in order to respond in a way that matches the patient's experience. Listening is considered effective when the nurse's response reflects understanding of what the patient is expressing. This is not to say that initial understanding, achieved through listening, will be entirely accurate. The nurse's interpretation is always tentative, awaiting correction, validation or further explication from the patient. Responses that shift the focus, change the subject or miss the point entirely do not indicate active listening.

# SUMMARY

Meanings are derived and initial understanding is achieved through active listening. Listening enables nurses to perceive the patient's reality – the world as the patient is experiencing it. After listening effectively, nurses are in a position to respond according to what is perceived. Listening engages both the nurse and the patient. It is an essential and fundamental process in establishing effective relationships in nursing practice and actively demonstrating that nurses care about patients' wellbeing.

# REFERENCES

Barrett, C., Borthwick, A., Bugeja, S., et al., 2005. Emotional labour: listening to the patient's story. Pract. Dev. Health Care 4 (4), 213–223.

Browning, S., Waite, R., 2010. The gift of listening: JUST listening strategies. Nurs. Forum 45 (3), 150–158.

Chang, T., Lin, Y.P., Chang, H.J., et al., 2005. Cancer patient and staff ratings of caring behaviors. Cancer Nurs. 28 (5), 331–339.

Courts, N.F., Buchanan, E.M., Werstlein, P.O., 2004. Focus groups: the lived experience of participants with multiple sclerosis. J. Neurosci. Nurs. 36 (1), 42–47.

du Plessis, E., 2016. Presence: a step closer to spiritual care in nursing. Holist. Nurs. Pract. 30 (1), 47–53.

Egan, G., 2014. The Skilled Helper, tenth ed. Brooks Cole, Belmont CA.

Finfgeld-Connett, D., 2006. Meta-synthesis of presence in nursing. J. Adv. Nurs. 55, 708–714.

Florin, J., Ehrenberg, A., Ehnfors, M., 2005. Patients' and nurses' perceptions of nursing problems in an acute care setting. J. Adv. Nurs. 51 (2), 140–149.

Henry, S.G., Fuhrel-Forbis, A., Rogers, M.A.M., et al., 2012. Association between nonverbal communication during clinical interactions and outcomes: a systematic review and meta-analysis. Patient Educ. Couns. 86, 297–315.

Jonas-Simpson, C.M., Mitchell, G.J., Fisher, A., et al., 2006. The experience of being listened to: a qualitative study of older adults in long-term care settings. J. Gerontol. Nurs. 32 (1), 46–53.

Kagan, P.N., 2008a. Feeling listened to: a lived experience of human becoming. Nurs. Sci. Q. 21 (1), 59–67.

Kagan, P.N., 2008b. Listening: selected perspectives in theory and research. Nurs. Sci. Q. 21 (2), 105–110.

Kostovich, C.T., Clementi, P.S., 2014. Nursing presence putting the art of nursing back into hospital orientation. J. Nurses Prof. Dev. 30 (2), 70–75.

Kuis, E.E., Goossensen, A., van Dijke, J., et al., 2015. Self-report questionnaire for measuring presence: development and initial validation. Scand. J. Caring Sci. 29, 173–182.

Lazarus, R.S., 2006. Emotions and interpersonal relationships: toward a person-centered conceptualization of emotions and coping. J. Pers. 74 (1), 9–46.

Marshall, A., Kitson, A., Zeitz, K., 2012. Patients' views of patient-centred care: a phenomenological case study in one surgical unit. J. Adv. Nurs. 68 (12), 2664–2673.

McCabe, C., 2004. Nurse–patient communication: an exploration of patients' experiences. J. Clin. Nurs. 13, 41–49.

McMahon, M., Christopher, K.A., 2011. Toward a mid-range theory of nursing presence. Nurs. Forum 46 (2), 71–82.

Nelson-Jones, R., 2013. Practical Counselling and Helping Skills, sixth ed. Sage, London.

Papastavrou, E., Efstathiou, G., Tsangari, H., et al., 2012. Patients' and nurses' perceptions of respect and human presence through caring behaviours: a comparative study. Nurs. Ethics 19 (3), 369–379.

Penque, S., Kearney, G., 2015. The effect of nursing presence on patient satisfaction. Nurs. Manage. 46 (4), 38–44.

Shattell, M., 2005. Nurse bait: strategies hospitalized patients use to entice nurses within the context of the interpersonal relationship. Issues Ment. Health Nurs. 26, 205–223.

Stickley, T., 2011. From SOLER to SURETY for effective non-verbal communication. Nurse Educ. Pract. 11, 395–398.

Yu, X., Staples, S., Shen, J.J., 2012. Nonverbal communication behaviors of internationally educated nurses and patient care. Res. Theory Nurs. Pract. 26 (4), 290–308.

# ANSWERS TO ACTIVITIES

## Activity 5.5: Listening for content

**PATIENT STORY I**
WHO: self (speaker), doctor
WHAT: something happened to hip, difficulty walking
WHEN: Sunday afternoon
WHERE: not stated
WHY: reason for having the x-ray

**PATIENT STORY II**
WHO: speaker, child, GP's receptionist
WHAT: serious stomach pain, rang GP, drove to GP's surgery
WHEN: beginning of a day
WHERE: GP's surgery
WHY: explain the story, but not entirely clear

**PATIENT STORY III**
WHO: speaker
WHAT: unable to move left arm
WHEN: not stated
WHERE: garden, then house
WHY: don't know what to do

**PATIENT STORY IV**
WHO: speaker, 'him'
WHAT: he is not himself
WHEN: 'for months'
WHERE: home, in front of television
WHY: worried about 'him'

**PATIENT STORY V**
WHO: speaker, GP
WHAT: no time to have regular Pap smears
WHEN: not stated
WHERE: not stated
WHY: questioning whether regular Pap smears are necessary

**PATIENT STORY VI**
WHO: speaker
WHAT: chemo and radiotherapy, feeling tired
WHEN: now
WHERE: speaker's room
WHY: can't attend to children

## Activity 5.6: Listening for feelings

a.  fear, anxiety, worry
b.  fear, anxiety, worry
c.  frustration, anger, resignation
d.  sadness, anger, frustration
e.  sadness, anger, resignation
f.  anger, frustration
g.  sadness, anger
h.  fear, anxiety, apprehension
i.  disappointment, frustration
j.  apprehension, anxiety, fear
k.  uncertainty
l.  regret, guilt

## Activity 5.9: Responses that indicate listening

The answer NO indicates that the nurse responding has not understood/acknowledged what the patient is saying, while the answer YES indicates active reception of what the patient has said.

a.  *Patient:* I don't think I'm going to make it. Am I going to die?
    i.   NO – The power of positive thinking can really help a lot. Many people in your situation have survived because they refused to give up. Keep fighting. Where there's life, there's hope.
    ii.  YES – What has happened to make you worried about it?
    iii. NO – I can't really say. You'll have to ask your doctor this question.
    iv.  YES – We are all going to die sometime, but it's a frightening prospect when it stares us in the face.
b.  *Patient:* Why is my blood pressure being taken so often?
    i.   NO – We have to check your blood pressure frequently.
    ii.  NO – It's doctor's orders.
    iii. YES – It's a general observation to keep a check on your vital signs.
    iv.  YES – Is it worrying you?

c. *Patient:* How long will I be in here?

    i.    NO – As long as we think you need to be.

    ii.   YES – Let's discuss it with the doctor. If you think you're ready to go home, and the doctor is happy for you to go, you can be discharged.

    iii.  YES – People who have the operation you are having usually stay in hospital for about three days. That's the usual routine, if there are no complications.

    iv.   YES – What has your doctor said about this?

d. *Patient:* Why me? Why do I have to be the one who suffers like this?

    i.    NO – It's a part of the usual course of this disease. If you tell me when you feel worse and better, I can help with the pain.

    ii.   NO – We all suffer some kind of pain during our lifetime.

    iii.  NO – It's just a bit of misfortune. You'll have better luck next time, I'm sure.

    iv.   YES – I wish I could answer that question. I'm not sure there always is a reason.

e. *Patient:* I have contemplated suicide because I've hit rock bottom.

    i.    YES – Are you thinking about suicide right now?

    v.   NO – Things can't be that bad.

    vi.  YES – What's happened to you that you've hit rock bottom?

    vii.  YES – What exactly have you contemplated?

f. *Patient:* What's going to happen when I come out of the operation?

    i.    NO – We will look after you.

    ii.   NO – There's nothing to worry about. You will feel better than you did before.

    iii.  NO – Have you had a general anaesthetic before?

    iv.   YES – You'll be drowsy for a few hours and, depending on your level of pain, you will receive regular pain relief.

g. *Patient:* I'm not sick, and yet I have to take all of these tablets every day.

    i.    NO – It does seem a bit silly, doesn't it?

    ii.   NO – It could be that you don't feel sick because you are taking the tablets.

    iii.  YES – Which tablets are you taking?

    iv.   YES – How long have you been taking the tablets?

## CHAPTER OVERVIEW

- Empathy for patients is central to understanding patients and to good nursing care.

- Sympathy is a precursor to empathy, and compassion is a response to feelings of empathy.

- An analysis of how empathy is conceptualised in nursing helps to compare empathy with other related concepts such as sympathy and pity.

- There are a variety of ways in which nurses can verbally respond to patients, each differing in intent and impact on the patient–nurse relationship.

- Responses that promote understanding and empathy are viewed as the basis of the relationship.

- Understanding-based responses include paraphrasing, seeking clarification, reflecting feelings, connecting and summarising.

ⓔ Visit the Evolve site for video content to support the themes and skills explored in this chapter: http://evolve.elsevier.com/AU/Stein-Parbury/patient/

# INTRODUCTION

Understanding a patient's experience by viewing the world from the patient's perspective is one of the most central aspects of interacting and building relationships in nursing. Mutual understanding is the basis of meaningful interaction. In the patient–nurse relationship, it is the nurse's responsibility to facilitate this understanding. Mutual understanding requires time, effort, commitment and skill. It is challenging for one person to understand and appreciate another person's reality.

Effective attending and listening opens doors and aids a nurse's entry into a patient's world. The stage is set for a meaningful relationship because interpersonal contact has been established. Listening enables a nurse to develop an initial understanding of a patient's experience. It is important to recognise that an initial understanding remains tentative until it is either validated or corrected and altered through further interaction with a patient. The impressions formed in the process of listening are often partial, inaccurate and superficial. Nurses who act immediately, without checking the accuracy of these impressions, risk building a relationship that lacks mutual understanding and providing help that is not necessarily congruent with a patient's needs and desires. Taking time to understand a patient's experiences enables nurses to ground nursing care within the patient's reality.

Listening is largely an absorptive activity, as nurses take in and process patients' stories. But at some point during an interaction, verbal responses must be uttered; nurses usually have to say something. A variety of verbal responses are possible; however, a response that promotes greater understanding between the patient and the nurse is most beneficial, especially in the early stages of the relationship. Responses that promote understanding not only demonstrate that the nurse has listened but also convey a desire to comprehend the patient's experience more fully.

Effective listening demonstrates open acceptance of the patient and encourages the patient to interact. Effective understanding promotes further interaction because it openly acknowledges the patient's experience, confirming its reality. Understanding-based responses check how effectively a nurse's perceptions and interpretations correspond to the patient's meaning. Because they build meaning, understanding-based responses deepen the relationship between patients and nurses.

# THE CONCEPT OF EMPATHY

Empathy is the ability to understand the experiences of another; in the case of nursing, it involves understanding the experiences of patients. In this sense, empathy is the essence of 'knowing the patient' (see Ch 1). As such, it is often considered a prerequisite for nursing practice because it is difficult to comprehend how a nurse can be of help to patients without a clear understanding of how they perceive their situation and the circumstances surrounding it, including what they want to happen.

One of the most frequently cited conceptualisations of empathy is based on the work of Carl Rogers (1957). The humanistic philosophy that underpins Rogers' theory of counselling is consistent with patient-centred nursing care and the development of a therapeutic patient–nurse relationship as central to that care. Rogers (1957) viewed empathy as the ability to perceive the world from another person's view, and to take on the perspective of another, while not losing one's own perspective. In stressing the notion of not losing one's self, Rogers is referring to the sense of otherness that characterises a professional helping relationship.

For this reason, empathy relies on a strong sense of self, for without awareness of one's own perspective, attempts to enter another person's world may result in becoming lost in the world of the other. The strong sense of self that is required to fully appreciate the reality of another is related to emotional intelligence and therapeutic agency (Ch 3). The ability to understand others (i.e. to be empathic) is a core dimension of emotional intelligence (Goleman 1998), and it is one process that enables people to be competent communicators.

The process of developing empathy is complex and dynamic. Understanding how it is cultivated helps to unravel the complexity.

## The development of empathy

In understanding empathy, it is important to consider how it is aroused in humans and to appreciate the intertwining concepts of sympathy and compassion. The relationship between sympathy, empathy and compassion is depicted in Fig. 6.1.

How often have you heard statements such as, 'Looking at the car accident made me feel sick to my stomach' or 'I felt so sorry for her'? The first statement about feeling 'sick' at the sight of an accident is an example of an emotional contagion because it represents imagining what it would be like to be in the

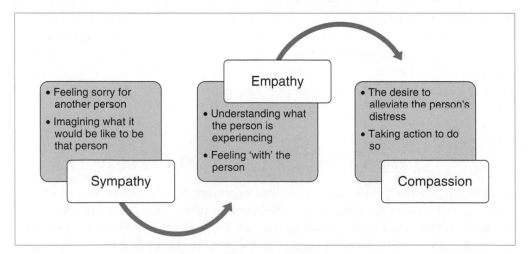

**Figure 6.1** Relationship between sympathy, empathy and compassion

collision. Neuroscientists have shown that this emotional arousal is anatomically based and therefore instinctual. There are actual neurological pathways that make such reactions automatic (Svenaeus 2015). These reflexive emotional reactions are then what spur feelings of sympathy or pity, feeling sorry for another's distress or suffering, as exemplified in the second statement.

## Empathy and sympathy

There has long been a tradition in nursing that sympathy, unlike empathy, is not helpful to the patient or the nurse because it is focused on how the nurse feels, thus shifting the focus away from the patient (Kalisch 1973). In contrast, Morse et al (2006) assert that sympathetic responses, such as commiseration, pity and consolation, *are* focused on the patient because responses such as these may be as comforting for patients as empathy. A contemporary understanding of the dynamic relationship between sympathy and empathy helps to resolve this inconsistency.

A contemporary understanding is that sympathetic sentiments arouse feelings of empathy; therefore, sympathy is the precursor to empathy (Svenaeus 2015). Sympathy is the driving force for empathy because it generates feelings of concern for the other person. While sympathy is imagining what it would be like to be that person in distress, empathy invokes an attempt to develop cognitive and emotional understanding – thoughts about what the person is actually experiencing. Sympathy is 'feeling for' another person, while empathy is viewed as 'feeling with' the other. The focus shifts from 'How would I feel if this was happening to me?' (sympathy) to 'How does this other person feel about what is happening?' (empathy).

At times, expressing sympathy or empathy is sufficient to alleviate distress and make an interpersonal connection with a patient. Expressions of sympathy can comfort and make interpersonal connection, while empathy conveys to patients that the nurse recognises their personal circumstances. When interpersonal engagement is the goal, then sympathy and empathy may be sufficient to help the patient.

The expression of empathy demonstrates that the nurse understands the patient's experience and provides an opportunity for patients to express their needs. Empathy has been shown to improve patients' outcomes such as decreased stress, anxiety, depression and complications; in addition, it helps them to feel valued thus increasing their self-esteem (Petrucci et al 2016). Empathy has also been shown to have other beneficial effects; when evaluated by patients themselves empathy increased satisfaction with care, assisted with psychosocial adjustment in illness and decreased their need for more information (Lelorain et al 2012). These outcomes demonstrate the value of empathy.

However, when patients are distressed or suffering, more is needed. In these circumstances nurses have a professional responsibility to take action to alleviate distress and suffering. Empathic understanding is necessary but not sufficient without a desire to assist the patient – a wish to relieve distress and suffering. This desire is the basis of compassion. Like the dynamic interplay between sympathy and empathy, there is a similar interaction between empathy and compassion.

### Empathy and compassion

Compassion is a process that involves a recognition of a patient's suffering, empathic understanding and the motivation to alleviate their distress (Ledoux 2015). Compassion is predicated on two conditions: the presence of suffering and the desire to relieve it. Currently, there is much interest in the development of compassion in nurses and other healthcare workers. For example, in a recent review of the concept, Sinclair et al (2016) reported that three-quarters of the reviewed papers were published in the five years preceding the review. This interest generates from a concern that an increasing emphasis on technology and evidence-based practice in healthcare has the potential to erode compassionate care.

From its inception compassion was viewed as an essential trait for professional nursing (Nightingale 1859/1992). The delivery of care that is compassionate is embedded into standards for nursing practice (Nursing and Midwifery Board of Australia 2016). In nursing, empathy is viewed as one component of compassion, along with: acting to alleviate suffering; being caring, approachable and open; connecting with and relating to patients; and involving patients in their care (Papadopoulos & Ali 2016). Because being empathic is an essential aspect of compassionate care, the ability to express empathy is a necessary skill.

# EMPATHY IN NURSING

Introduced to nursing science in around 1973, empathy has long been embraced as essential to effective nursing practice (Petrucci et al 2016). This was followed by a long tradition of continuing to view the process of empathy as fundamental to caring practices (Ward et al 2012; Wiseman 2007). As a result of being empathic, a nurse comes to know and understand a patient's experience. This absorption of a patient's reality is one way that empathy is realised in nursing.

Some of the first nursing theorists to discuss the view of empathy, although not necessarily using the term (Peplau 1952; Travelbee 1971; Zderad 1969), emphasised its purpose as promoting rapport between a patient and a nurse. Rapport is essential to building and maintaining a relationship with a patient that is based on mutual understanding. It is a reciprocal process of give and take, and it is important that patients feel understood by nurses, not just that nurses believe they feel empathic. Therefore, nursing theorists who first discussed empathy as a concept also stressed the importance of nurses communicating their understanding to patients (Gagan 1983; Kalisch 1973). In addition, it is important that patients perceive that nurses do indeed understand their health-related circumstances.

## Can empathy be learnt?

Because there is an innate aspect to the development of empathy – a sympathetic emotional arousal that is automatic – some nurses consider empathy to be an inherent personality trait. That nurses are innately empathic stems from an altruistic motivation to become a nurse (Eley et al 2012); it has been shown that beginning nursing students have higher empathy than other healthcare students (Petrucci et al 2016). While some studies have shown that empathy declines throughout nursing education, these results have been mixed (Ward et al 2012; Ward 2016). Although nurses may be naturally empathic, there is evidence that empathy is also learnt and developed (Hojat et al 2013; Richardson et al 2015). Nurses need self-awareness of their innate capacity for empathy so they can build on their basic empathy and learn to express it through a personal style (see Ch 3).

The development of empathy in nursing exists along a continuum that takes on different forms, beginning with incidents of empathy, which then leads to a way of knowing the patient, next developing into a process of care with repeated incidents and then finally becoming a way of being in nursing practice (Wiseman 2007). Rather than a single phenomenon it is a developmental process that occurs over time and is facilitated by experience and knowledge. In addition, Wiseman (2007) found that the context of care affected nurses' ability to be empathic, with the care environment needing to be supportive to the nurse.

Halpern (2003) critiques the idea of 'trained empathy' or 'clinical empathy', what has been termed a professional state that is promoted as a way of intellectualising patients' feelings rather than perceiving and experiencing them in an affective/feeling manner. She questions traditional views that the desired type of empathy in healthcare is one that stands apart and 'sees into' the patient's experience, in favour of an empathy that 'feels into' the experience. Halpern (2003) challenges a long-held view in healthcare that emotional detachment is necessary in medical decision making, claiming that grasping another's emotional state through empathic understanding and involvement enhances diagnosis.

# EXPRESSING EMPATHY

It is important that nurses be able to express empathic understanding because its use in nursing practice involves the ability to perceive the feelings of the other and the self and to convey to patients that the nurse understands their perspective. That is, empathy facilitates awareness and organises perceptions in addition to promoting mutual understanding. It is not simply the ability to label and name feelings in rote fashion (Halpern 2003). Empathy involves the ability to actually know what it feels like to experience a particular emotion. It is a perceptual activity; that is, empathy is not simply an intellectual activity or an interpersonal skill. It is a form of interaction that involves attitudes and perceptual skill.

Not only is empathy a perceptual skill, it is also a behavioural skill because the nurse must have the ability to express and convey their understanding to the patient. The skills in this chapter are designed to develop understanding and express empathy. Paraphrasing, seeking clarification and reflecting feelings are used prior to connecting and summarising. Expressing empathy is viewed as the sum total of all other skills that promote understanding (see Fig. 6.2). The

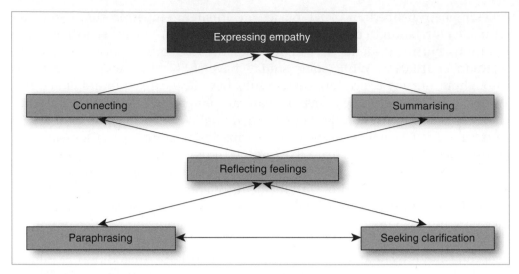

**Figure 6.2** Hierarchy of understanding skills

point at which the nurse can accurately express empathy is the point at which mutual understanding is achieved.

## Purpose of expressing empathy

When communicating empathy, nurses respond with a direct, clear and accurate statement that reflects their understanding of a patient's experience. Doing so promotes trust because patients are put at ease to disclose when they experience emotional attunement with the nurse (Halpern 2003). Expressing empathy is a skill that involves nurses sharing openly with patients that they understand their perspectives. Expressing empathy communicates this understanding, conveying both acceptance and confirmation of the reality of the patient's experience. In addition, empathy contributes to mutuality (described in Ch 2).

The purpose of expressing empathy should be borne in mind. Empathy is used to encourage a patient to continue expression, to provide direction to the nurse, to decrease the patient's sense of isolation and to bond the patient and nurse in understanding. Often, support and reassurance, direct aid and assistance, or advice or challenge follow the expression of empathy. At other times, empathy expression is an end in itself; it offers comfort and solace to patients – they know they are not alone because they are understood.

Empathic statements capture the essence of the patient's experience and move the relationship into a more intimate zone. For this reason, empathy expression, especially in relation to a patient's feelings, can be intrusive and prematurely intimate. Yet empathy expression in nursing is often equated with emotions. Knowing the patient (Ch 1) in such an intimate way may not be appropriate or desirable.

An empathic statement exposes patients, laying their reality in the open. It can expose areas of weakness, uncertainty and vulnerability. A patient may not want this exposure, and sensitivity to a patient's reaction to an empathic statement is needed. If a patient wants to appear strong or maintain control, a sensitive nurse will accept this and move out of the intimacy that empathy can bring.

It is for these reasons that timing is crucial when expressing empathy. If a nurse moves too quickly into empathic expression, a patient may feel invaded and inhibited. For these reasons, all the other skills of understanding should be used first in order to establish understanding and build the relationship. When a patient demonstrates comfort with discussing feelings, validates the nurse's paraphrases, confirms the connections made between thoughts and feelings and agrees with the summary, then the relationship is ready to move into the intimate zone of empathy. The point at which a nurse truly understands is the time to express empathy.

At first, it might feel awkward for nurses to express to patients what they believe the patient is experiencing. The awkwardness is based on a false notion that it is presumptuous and arrogant, if not downright impolite, to openly state what another person is experiencing. When empathy is expressed with an attitude of 'I know exactly what you are feeling', its basic nature has been violated. When employed in this manner, attempts at empathy expression will be met with defensiveness on the patient's part and will work against an effective relationship. Empathy expression is a confirmation, not an accusation. Nurses must remain sensitive and open to correction. When stated with too much certainty, empathy expression alienates rather than engages the patient.

The most congruent and compelling goal of empathy in nursing – that is, for nurses to come to understand a patient's experience – is that nurses' actions are based on their understanding of the patient's situation. In nursing, there is an obligation to act, not simply to understand; acting without understanding may result in actions that are not helpful to patients.

# PROMOTING UNDERSTANDING AND EMPATHY

After actively listening to a patient and forming an initial impression, it is natural for a nurse to respond verbally. While it is important that responses be spontaneous and sincere, it is equally important that they be thoughtful, developed with intention and skilfully employed. A nurse's initial verbal responses set the direction for further interaction. Because there is a variety of possible ways to respond, nurses must ensure their verbal responses move the relationship in a desired and intended direction. Choice of a response is based on insight into how it may affect the patient, the interaction and the relationship. A nurse who has this insight and awareness is in the best position to respond in a manner that both matches the current situation and realises the response's desired intent. In regard to intent, nurses should consider what they need to know about patients and why they need to know it.

## ACTIVITY 6.1  Your usual style of responding (I)

**Process**

1.  For each of the following statements/questions (a–o), write a response. Don't spend too much time pondering your response, but do try to be helpful to the person speaking. Record a response that is typical of how you would usually respond.

    **a.** A resident of a nursing home: 'I miss my wife. I don't know where she is. Where is she? Can you tell me?'

    **b.** A relative of an unconscious patient hospitalised in intensive care: 'Mum is really going to be upset when she wakes up. She is going to kill us for letting her be in here.'

    **c.** An adolescent patient during a routine health checkup: 'My folks keep pressuring me about the future. I don't have a clue about what I want to do.'

    **d.** A first-time mother about to be discharged from a postnatal unit: 'How am I ever going to be able to manage this baby on my own?'

    **e.** A client to a community nurse during a home visit: 'I'm so glad to see you. I haven't been at all well lately.'

    **f.** A patient, a young man, who is having haemodialysis at home: 'My girlfriend left me because she's afraid she might catch something and my best mate doesn't visit me anymore because he hates the sight of blood.'

    **g.** A resident of a hostel for the elderly: 'It's really boring in here. The days are so long and there's no one to talk to except the nurses, and they're always so busy.'

    **h.** A mother during a routine visit at an early childhood centre: 'My husband left and I'm having so much trouble managing on my own.'

    **i.** A resident of a nursing home: 'It's hard when you grow old and your friends and family start to die. My children are great, but they have their own lives.'

    **j.** A patient, a woman, during an outpatient clinic visit for a routine Pap smear: 'I'm not really sure about having any more children. I'm 39 now and reckon I've pushed my luck far enough. I have two healthy children. Perhaps I should just leave it at that.'

    **k.** A patient during a postoperative clinic visit: 'You know, I just take one day at a time. It's been two months since my surgery and I'm still not sure if I'll ever feel like my old self again.'

    **l.** A patient during an admission interview in hospital: 'I've lived with arthritis for years, but lately I'm having more trouble than usual. I can hardly get out of bed in the morning and the pain is becoming unbearable.'

    **m.** A resident of a hostel for the elderly: 'You can't possibly understand what it feels like. You've never had this problem. How would you understand?'

**n.** A client, a pregnant woman, during an antenatal visit: 'People are kind and concerned, but no one really knows what it's like to lose a child. It's the most painful experience imaginable. You never get over it.'

**o.** A patient, a man hospitalised for a myocardial infarction: 'I'm really worried about how my family will cope without my help. I have three small children, my wife works and we share all the household chores. Now that I've had this heart attack, I'm not sure how much assistance I can offer.'

2. Reflect on each of your responses:

   • What is your intention?

   • What do you hope to achieve by responding in this way?

   • How do you hope the patient will react to your response?

3. If you're working in groups, form pairs. One person now reads the statement or question (playing the role of the patient) and the other person reads their recorded response (playing the role of the nurse). The patient reflects after each response:

   • What is your impression of the nurse? And of the response?

   • How has the response affected you?

   • How encouraged are you to continue the interaction?

   • How much do you think the nurse understands your situation?

   The patient then shares these reflections with the nurse.

4. The nurse now shares their intention (step 2 of the process) with the patient. Make a note of the following:

   • How congruent is the nurse's intention with the effect on the patient?

5. Continue to read each statement or question followed by its response and share the reflections.

6. Switch roles and complete steps 3, 4 and 5.

**Discussion**

1. What differences are there between the nurse's intentions and the patient's impressions of the responses? How do you account for this?

2. Were some responses more encouraging than others? Which ones were encouraging? And discouraging?

3. Which responses resulted in a negative impression on the patient (e.g. 'the nurse does not understand', 'does not really care' or 'does not wish to discuss the topic')?

The initial phase of the relationship between a patient and a nurse is a particularly sensitive and critical time for responding because, more than likely, the trust required for full patient disclosure is not yet firmly established. Responses that work best at this time are those that validate patients by acknowledging their experiences. Validating and acknowledging responses convey a nurse's willingness to understand a patient. Patients will come to trust those nurses who can be relied on to understand. Inadvertently, nurses may respond in a manner that suggests a lack of desire to understand. The following response, which denies the patient's experience, is an example:

Patient: *I'm worried about how my family is going to manage without me.*

Nurse: *No need to worry; they'll survive without you. It'll do them good to realise how much you do for them.*

While the nurse may have wished to encourage the patient with this response, it is likely that the response indicates a rejection of the patient's perception of the situation. By failing to acknowledge the patient's reality, responses such as these engender the feeling that the nurse does not want to understand. Compare the preceding example with the following:

Patient: *I'm worried about how my family is going to manage without me.*

Nurse: *What is worrying you most about how they will manage?*

Here the nurse provides acknowledgment and confirmation of the patient's reality. Responses such as this deepen interpersonal engagement and promote understanding between a patient and a nurse; as such, they build trust.

Most nurses develop habitual, routine and even stylised ways of responding to patients. The intent is usually to be of help or assistance to patients, but this intent may not be fully realised if nurses overuse one type of response or lack awareness of the impact of their responses. Goodwill and desire alone are not sufficient in the absence of awareness and direction.

# Ways of responding

This section explores the various types of responses nurses might have to patients based on categories developed by Johnson (2013). In this scheme, responses are categorised according to their intent – what they are designed to do or their purpose. On this basis, the majority of responses fit into one of the following categories:

- questioning and probing
- paraphrasing and understanding
- reassuring and supporting
- analysing and interpreting
- advising and evaluating.

The categories include those responses that are significant – ones with the potential to have a critical impact on the interaction and the relationship. There are other possible responses, such as small talk about the weather, that do not fit into any of these categories. While social talk and chitchat are used by patients in making a connection with nurses, they are not included here because the intent of such conversations is not to directly assist the patient.

Each way of responding may be helpful in its own right and can be effectively employed within the context of the patient–nurse relationship. Nevertheless, each has a different intent, suggests a different type of relationship between a patient and nurse and therefore has a different impact on their interactions, especially in the sensitive early stages. Some responses facilitate interaction better than others, so timing and an awareness of each type of response are crucial.

## Questioning and probing

A response that questions and probes is one that attempts to gather more information and explore the situation further. It indicates a need for elaboration and may ultimately lead to greater understanding. Examples of this type of response include:

- 'What is worrying you most about the operation?'
- 'Where is your pain?'
- 'What methods have you tried to get to sleep?'
- 'What do you think?'

Responses that question and probe indicate that nurses are trying to understand but need more information to do so. Early in the course of the relationship, nurses frequently employ questions in an effort to get to know a patient. Throughout the course of the relationship, questions are further employed to develop an even greater understanding of the patient's experience. Unless they are overused, responses that question and probe are quite useful if they are stated correctly and timed appropriately. There are other ways to explore aside from questioning and probing, and effective exploration involves using a variety of skills that are fully covered in Chapter 7.

## Paraphrasing and understanding

When nurses paraphrase, they share their understanding with patients by rephrasing what patients have expressed, using their own words instead of the patients' words. Responses that paraphrase what the patient has expressed demonstrate that the nurse's intention is to understand the patient more fully. Examples in this category include:

- 'Seems like you can't sleep because of your uncertainty about the future.'
- 'You seem more relaxed here than you are in your own home.'
- 'Looks to me like it's frustrating for you to be asked the same questions over and over again.'

Responses that demonstrate understanding confirm and validate what patients have expressed, thus communicating a genuine interest in and acceptance of patients. Through paraphrasing, nurses share their understanding of patients' messages in order to ensure this understanding is correct. Paraphrasing and understanding responses demonstrate that the nurse wants to follow the patient's meaning and will check to ensure this happens. They convey the message: 'I won't assume I know what you mean or what you need until I am certain I know – and only you can tell me'. Early in the course of a relationship, this type of response is especially effective because it places the patient and nurse on equal footing and helps build trust.

All other categories of responses, except questioning and probing, are based on an assumption that nurses know what patients are experiencing and what is best for them. An understanding response attempts to validate or invalidate these assumptions. The meaning a nurse constructs from what a patient has expressed may not be what the patient actually meant. An understanding response is of value in preventing such lack of congruency; it addresses one of the most common problems in communication, which occurs when people do not realise there is sometimes a difference between what is meant and what is said and consequently misunderstand what is meant.

## ACTIVITY 6.2  Recognising the types of responses  334

### Process

1. For each statement below (a–l), five possible responses are provided. Read all five responses to the statement and decide on the response that most closely matches what you would say under the circumstances.

2. For each set of five responses, determine which of the following categories best represents each response. There is a response from each category in each set. The answers to this activity can be found at the end of the chapter.

   E – Advising and evaluating

   I – Analysing and interpreting

   S – Reassuring and supporting

   P – Questioning and probing

   U – Paraphrasing and understanding

   a. 'I'm just so fed up with being sick and in pain. I'm tired of having to rely on the nurses all the time.'

   **Responses**

   1) 'It's okay to rely on us. That's why we're here.'

   2) 'You're an independent type of person who prefers to do things for yourself.'

   3) 'All of this is really starting to get you down.'

   4) 'Just relax and let us help you.'

   5) 'What is bothering you the most?'

**b.** 'I never really looked after myself. Now look how I am suffering.'

**Responses**

**1)** 'I don't know what you mean.'

**2)** 'Lots of people say the same thing.'

**3)** 'Well, you would have looked after yourself if it mattered to you.'

**4)** 'It's hard to look back with regrets, isn't it?'

**5)** 'Sounds as if you're angry with yourself.'

**c.** 'Don't bother with me. I am going to die anyway.'

**Responses**

**1)** 'That sounds sad and depressing.'

**2)** 'Don't talk like that. You're not going to die.'

**3)** 'What makes you say that?'

**4)** 'It's not a bother to look after you. I'm here because I want to help you.'

**5)** 'You've given up hope because you're getting on in age.'

**d.** 'I'm in so much pain all the time. I manage to get through the day all right because I keep busy, but my backache prevents me from getting a good night's sleep. So I keep busy during the day, end up really tired, but then can't get the rest that I need. I'm getting more and more tired all the time.'

**Responses**

**1)** 'Why don't you try some relaxation exercises to get to sleep?'

**2)** 'How often do you have a bad night?'

**3)** 'Keeping busy during the day helps with the pain, but getting enough sleep at night is more of a worry for you right now.'

**4)** 'Sounds as if you're letting the pain control your life.'

**5)** 'I'm sure you'll be able to work something out once you become accustomed to living with the pain.'

**e.** 'People think they want to live a long time, but I'm telling you, don't ever grow old. You'll end up in a place like this. It's boring and depressing. Look at everybody here. Do they look happy to you?'

**Responses**

**1)** 'Everybody feels a bit blue sometimes. Things will get better – you'll see.'

**2)** 'Come on, let's go for a walk. It's a beautiful day today.'

**3)** 'What's so boring and depressing about this place?'

**4)** 'You are approaching things with a negative attitude so, naturally, the whole world looks grim.'

**5)** 'You're really not happy about being here, are you?'

*cont.*

*Activity 6.2 continued*

**f.** 'My wife died recently. I don't want to talk about it.'

**Responses**

**1)** 'It does help to talk about these things.'

**2)** 'What do you want to talk about instead?'

**3)** 'You'll get over it in time, I'm sure.'

**4)** 'Maybe you're the type of person who has difficulty letting people help you.'

**5)** 'You don't feel like talking to me?'

**g.** 'I know I should change my diet and alter my lifestyle. The doctor said I'm a high risk for a heart attack. I've always been a bit of a go-getter – take after Dad in that respect. He had a heart attack at 50, so I guess I should do something – but I really don't know where to start.'

**Responses**

**1)** 'Sounds as if you have been avoiding the inevitable. You know what to do but don't want to face it. You could change if you really wanted to.'

**2)** 'Just try a bit harder to slow down and eat the right foods.'

**3)** 'You have an idea about what you should do but are having trouble getting started.'

**4)** 'What do you think you should change first?'

**5)** 'Worrying about it will only make things worse. I'm sure you can change.'

**h.** 'I get so tired looking after David day after day. There's all the physical care, but I think the mental strain is the worst. I worry constantly about where he is and what he's doing. I think he gets a bit annoyed with my constant hovering over him. The worst thing is that I get no relief – it's so constant.'

**Responses**

**1)** 'The constant worry is really getting to you and wearing you down. You just can't seem to get away from it.'

**2)** 'People in your situation often feel this way. It's a difficult problem to come to terms with.'

**3)** 'Try to put the worry out of your mind at least once each day. Make yourself a cup of tea, sit down and just relax.'

**4)** 'Is there ever an opportunity for you to get away?'

**5)** 'There may be a bit of guilt in what you're saying. You probably keep thinking about the times in the past when you could have been more understanding and supportive towards David.'

**i.** 'The least they could have done was warn me that Dad was going to be sedated. Those doctors didn't even tell me beforehand so I could have a quick visit with him. Now I need to leave the hospital without even speaking to Dad.'

**Responses**

1) 'You sound like one of those people who likes to be in control.'

2) 'The doctors were really busy. Otherwise, I am sure they would have told you.'

3) 'I can see you're frustrated and angry about not getting to talk to your dad.'

4) 'If this happens again, I would say something if I were you.'

5) 'What exactly did they tell you?'

j. 'Mum was always there to look after us when we needed something. Now that she's sick, I guess it's our turn to look after her. It feels so strange and I'm not sure she'll even let us do much for her.'

**Responses**

1) 'Because you always had her to look after you, you wonder if she'll let you look after her.'

2) 'Of course she will. Your mother is a sensible woman.'

3) 'You feel scared that you won't be able to switch roles with your mum.'

4) 'Tell me more about it.'

5) 'Just tell her she needs you now and she will have to let you take care of her.'

k. 'What will happen to me if Carmelo dies? I don't know what I'd do. I couldn't go on without him.'

**Responses**

1) 'No need to worry about things before they happen.'

2) 'You're scared because you've allowed yourself to become too dependent on Carmelo and can't see how you'll make it on your own.'

3) 'What makes you think he won't make it?'

4) 'I suppose it's frightening to think you can't survive without Carmelo.'

5) 'There's plenty of help around. You can join a social club in your area.'

l. 'That surgeon explained everything about the operation, but I couldn't understand what was being said. I didn't even know what to ask.'

**Responses**

1) 'You're scared to ask questions of the doctors because they're so powerful.'

2) 'So the surgeon's explanation was not quite enough for you to understand?'

*cont.*

*Activity 6.2 continued*

**3)** 'What questions do you still have?'

**4)** 'The next time you see the surgeon, tell him you want some answers.'

**5)** 'Don't worry too much. Most people don't really understand the technical aspects of surgery.'

### Discussion

1. Compare your answers with those provided at the end of the chapter. Are there any types of responses that were difficult to recognise? Which ones? Review the section of the text that pertains to these.

2. In groups of five or six, discuss your answers. Are there any types of responses that other members had difficulty recognising? Which ones? Discuss these until understanding of each type of response is achieved.

3. Review your responses to step 1 of the process and determine whether there are some types of response you seem to provide naturally. Compare these results with the other participants in the group.

4. Discuss the reason(s) you tend to provide some types of response more than others.

## ACTIVITY 6.3  Your usual style of responding (II)

### Process

1. Refer to the responses you recorded for Activity 6.1, 'Your usual style of responding (I)'.

2. For each of your responses, determine which type of response you used (i.e. advising and evaluating; analysing and interpreting; reassuring and supporting; questioning and probing; or paraphrasing and understanding) and mark each accordingly. You may have used more than one category in a given response. If this is the case, include all categories used.

3. Tally the total number of times you used each type of response. Is there one type you used more than others? Reflect on the reasons for your apparent preference.

4. Have someone else determine which types of responses you used. Discuss any discrepancies and make a final determination about which type of response was used.

### Discussion

1. Compare your tally with those of other participants. Is there a type of response that was preferred by a majority of participants? Discuss the results.

2. Which ways of responding seem to fit the perceived role of the nurse? Which do not?

3. How frequently was the paraphrasing and understanding response used? Discuss why this is the case.

## Reassuring and supporting

There is a definite place for realistic reassurance and support (see Ch 8) in the course of patient–nurse relationships, and a nurse's approach needs to convey an overall attitude of support whenever interacting with patients. Nevertheless, a falsely reassuring response (the type discussed here) is one that glosses over and minimises the importance of a patient's experience before that experience is entirely acknowledged and understood.

### *False reassurance*

A falsely reassuring response is one that attempts to smooth a patient's discomfort by making everything sound 'all right', regardless of the objective or subjective reality of the situation. It may convey a patronising attitude or present a patient with a sense of unrealistic assurance. Examples of responses that falsely reassure and support include:

- 'A good night's sleep will do wonders for you.'
- 'There is nothing to worry about. It's only a minor procedure.'
- 'Don't be silly, Mrs Amari, nothing will go wrong.'
- 'You'll feel better after the surgery and will get well soon.'

False reassurance may sound good on the surface but, more often than not, it is dismissive of the patient's reality; it lacks understanding. Reflect for a moment on how you feel whenever someone tells you not to worry about something that is causing you concern. Do you have an impression that this person is genuinely interested? Does this person demonstrate a desire to understand your concern?

The use of clichés is another example of responses that attempt to support and reassure. Some examples include:

- 'It's always darkest just before a storm.'
- 'Every cloud has a silver lining.'

Responses such as these, often said whenever patients express anxieties and concerns, fail to acknowledge the subjective reality of patients' experiences. They carry an implied judgment that patients' concerns are unfounded, and even foolish. Because they discount the validity and significance of patients' feelings and perceptions, falsely reassuring responses sound as if the nurse is not really interested. Like premature advice, reassuring responses and clichés attempt to 'fix things' before they are fully clarified and understood.

## Analysing and interpreting

A response that analyses and interprets reaches beyond what the patient has expressed into a deeper level of meaning. An interpretive response reads into patients' messages, giving the impression that the nurse knows how patients *really* feel or what they *really* think. Interpretations imply that a nurse knows more about patients than they know themselves (Johnson 2013). Examples of analysing and interpreting responses include:

- 'You really don't want to assume responsibility for your own health.'
- 'You are acting like most new mothers, worrying too much and being overprotective of your baby.'
- 'You are afraid that if you tell the surgeon how you feel about the operation, he will reject you entirely and drop you as a patient.'

Responses such as these delve beneath the surface and open up areas that the patient has not expressed directly. As with advising, interpreting may have a legitimate place, but as an initial response it is often too threatening to be effective in building the relationship. An interpretation, regardless of its accuracy, can be threatening because it confronts patients with another reality – one that they may not be willing or able to face. Because such interpretations have a confronting edge, they are better left until the relationship has been established and the nurse has 'earned the right' to challenge in this way (see Ch 8).

Patients are more likely to accept interpretations from a nurse who has taken the time to fully understand their situation. It is unlikely that a nurse would know a patient well enough to make interpretations early in the course of their relationship. As an initial response, interpretations are intrusive and invasive and may impede the development of trust.

## Advising and evaluating

This category includes responses that offer an opinion or advice, ranging from a mild suggestion to a directive about what the patient should do. Such responses are based on the nurse's opinions and ideas and therefore have an evaluative edge. Examples in this category include:

- 'It's best not to dwell too much on such things.'
- 'Try to relax and stop worrying so much; it doesn't really help.'
- 'Ask the doctor these questions.'
- 'Just tell your mother it's your life and you'll do with it what you want.'

Responses such as these are among the most common made by people who are trying to help. When nurses use this type of response, they convey the message that they 'know best' and are in a position that is superior to the patient (Johnson 2013). Advice and evaluation carry the implication that patients are unable to know what to do, thus increasing their sense of vulnerability. For this reason, advising and evaluating responses run the risk of being met with a defensive reaction or a rejection of the advice. Have you ever told a friend what you think they should do to resolve a problem, only to be met with 'Yes, but ...', or 'That's easy for you to say', or 'I already tried that and it didn't work'? When given as an initial response, advice rarely works because of its potential to produce a sense of inadequacy in the patient and the patient's need to defend against this feeling.

Responses that advise offer solutions about what ought to be done. As a general rule, it is better to reach a sound understanding of a patient's situation before launching into solutions. An advising response gives the impression that a patient's difficulties and problems are easily solved – that there is a 'quick fix'. Some situations are easily resolved but, more often than not, further elaboration is needed before answers are found (if any *can* be found). Advice-giving is better left until the nurse fully understands the patient's experience.

Just as it is difficult to listen without judging, it is equally difficult to curtail the tendency to evaluate and advise. The tendency of nurses to give advice reflects the perception of many nurses that their role involves possessing knowledge and expertise. This perception often leads nurses to attempt to help patients by telling them what to do and providing answers.

While there are times when nurses offer expert advice to a patient, it is important that the patient's need and desire for such advice is established beforehand. Likewise, if advice is to be effective, it must be based on a clear understanding of the patient's experience. For example, explaining the usual course of events following anaesthesia and advising how to cope with 'waking up' is advice based on understanding of the situation. This is objective 'case knowledge' (see Ch 1), which does not necessarily require interaction with the patient. In a more subjective situation, such as anxiety about impending surgery, telling a patient to relax is of little use unless the nurse takes the time to understand the nature of the patient's worry. Advice given without understanding runs the risk of being ill-timed or irrelevant.

Giving advice is sometimes confused with sharing information. While they are similar, sharing information is not the same as telling patients what to do. When they share information (Ch 8), nurses provide knowledge, alternatives and facts. When they offer advice, nurses provide specific actions to perform, based on what the nurse thinks the patient 'should' do. Therefore, advice is often based on the nurse's personal value judgments, while sharing information is free of such judgments.

## Most common ways of responding

The 'advising and evaluating' type of response is one of the most frequently used when people are trying to be helpful (Johnson 2013). This is probably due to people's natural tendency to make judgments and offer opinions, especially when they are trying to be of help. There are times when being directive and prescriptive will be helpful to patients, but there are risks if this approach is used exclusively or too extensively. When using advising and evaluating responses, nurses place themselves in the position of expert and fail to acknowledge patients' expertise and capabilities in managing their own lives. Patients are not encouraged to seek solutions that fit their unique experience but rather are offered solutions and answers.

Nurses often show a strong preference for the 'reassuring and supporting' type of response. This is understandable because nursing care is best given in a reassuring and supportive atmosphere. Nevertheless, a truly reassuring and supportive manner differs from glossing over a patient's experience with a reassuring cliché. Falsely reassuring statements may negate the reality of patients' experiences. Because of their failure to acknowledge and affirm the patient, such responses interfere with effective interaction between patients and nurses.

It is important to recognise that none of the categories is inherently good or bad. Each is appropriate at different times in the relationship and under different circumstances. The ultimate aim is for each nurse to develop as wide a repertoire as possible and to use each type of response with awareness of its appropriateness and consequence. (Subsequent chapters cover the various types of responses, except the understanding type, which is the subject of this chapter.)

Understanding-based responses are most appropriate for building a relationship based on mutual meaning. They are effective in the early stages of the relationship and are also used throughout as a natural reaction to active listening (see Ch 5). Regardless of how effectively a nurse has suspended judgment during listening, the patient's messages are still processed through personal, interpretive filters. In processing patients' messages, nurses form impressions and reach conclusions about what patients are expressing and experiencing. These interpretations may not be entirely correct. If a nurse's interpretation of what a patient is saying is not shared actively and openly with the patient, potential misunderstandings are likely to go unchecked. In using an understanding response, nurses share their interpretations so they can be validated or corrected. Such responses enable nurses to build meaning that is congruent with a patient's experience.

## RESPONDING WITH UNDERSTANDING

In order to be helpful to patients, it is best if nurses operate from a vantage point within patients' experiences. When responding with understanding, nurses should attempt to view the world from the patient's point of view. Nurses reach for meaning by asking, 'What is this patient experiencing?', 'What is the meaning of the experience for the patient?', 'Am I following ... do I get the drift?'. Understanding-based responses check the answers to such questions. The following scenario serves as an illustration.

### SCENARIO

Patient: *It doesn't seem right that I'm still in so much pain. My hip surgery was six weeks ago, and I still can't seem to get comfortable. Is it just me? I asked my doctor and she said, 'No, this is not unusual, so don't worry.' But I really don't know.*

> Nurse: *It doesn't seem right to you that you're still in so much pain six weeks after the surgery?*
>
> Patient: *Yes and no, because I really didn't know exactly what to expect.*
>
> Nurse: *So, it's more that you don't know the usual course of events following hip surgery?*
>
> Patient: *Yes, I mean the only thing the doctor said was this is not unusual, so I'm still in the dark. I think I'm getting a bit neurotic about the whole thing.*
>
> Nurse: *So, what you really want to know is how much pain is reasonable and to be expected six weeks after the surgery?*
>
> Patient: *Yes, if I knew for sure that this is expected, I wouldn't be so worried. What do you think?*

In this scenario, because understanding is achieved, the nurse can now proceed to act. The nurse can provide the patient with concrete information (see Ch 8) about recovery after hip surgery. Exploration (Ch 7) into the exact nature of the patient's pain may also be warranted. Perhaps support (Ch 8) in pain management can be provided. The key is that the nurse is guided by the understanding that, for *this* patient, fear of the unknown is the central meaning in the expression.

Notice how the nurse's initial understanding response was not entirely accurate. The patient took the opportunity to clarify the meaning because the nurse's response indicated a desire to understand. The patient's final question, 'What do you think?', is indicative of the beginning of trust in the nurse. The patient feels able to rely on this nurse because the nurse has taken the time to understand the situation.

Because each patient's experience is unique, another patient may have expressed similar thoughts for an entirely different reason.

This next scenario is a similar example of an interaction, with a different patient.

## SCENARIO

Patient: *It doesn't seem right that I'm still in so much pain. My hip surgery was six weeks ago, and I still can't seem to get comfortable. Is it just me? I asked my doctor and she said, 'No, this is not unusual, so don't worry.' But I really don't know.*

Nurse: *It doesn't seem right to you that you are still in so much pain six weeks after the surgery?*

Patient: *It's not the pain so much but the amount of medication I'm taking.*

Nurse: *You think it might be too much?*

Patient: *Well, yes, I take those tablets every four hours. Could I be taking too many?*

As with the first scenario, the nurse may need to explore this situation further, or offer concrete information about the likelihood of taking too much pain medication. The illustrations show how different patients experience the same event. These scenarios exemplify the importance of achieving understanding that is based on the patient's view of the situation. While the situation is similar, each patient's experience of it is different. In both scenarios, the nurse listens to the patient's view, comes to understand it and is then able to operate from a vantage point within the patient's experience. The nurse can now offer help, in the form of advice, information or reassurance that is specific to the patient.

## Internal and external understanding

The understanding that is emphasised here is termed 'internal' because it is grounded in the patient's subjective world and personal view of a situation. External understanding, on the other hand, is an objective view of a situation. In nursing, these external understandings are based on clinical information that is devoid of any specific patient, for example, a textbook case based on standardised knowledge such as case knowledge (see Ch 1).

Nurses often become so focused on having the answers that they rely exclusively on an external understanding of the situation. Becoming overly concerned with 'What can I do?' often prevents nurses from asking, 'What is this like for this patient?'. Focusing solely on what can be done keeps nurses externally focused. There is a danger that nursing care based solely on external understanding will be misguided and will not take into account the uniqueness of the patient. In the first two scenarios, the nurse could have relied on an informed understanding of recovery following hip surgery and not taken the time to understand this patient's experience of recovery.

Focusing externally can lead to premature and automatic solutions that look to results and outcomes. Focusing internally meets patients where they are and offers a way of operating from within their experiences before moving to solutions and outcomes. Advising, evaluating, interpreting and falsely reassuring, in the absence of internal understanding, usually arise from an externally focused approach. Both external and internal understandings are necessary. They can be combined to provide guidance in appreciating what is appropriate in caring for a particular patient.

## Barriers to understanding

Many potential barriers exist when nurses are trying to understand a patient's perspective and frame of reference. The interferences that affect listening (see Ch 5) are still active. The natural tendency to judge and evaluate must still be kept in abeyance. An even greater barrier that exists is the tendency to jump to conclusions about what the patient is experiencing. Unless the patient validates these conclusions, they remain assumptions. Unshared assumptions lead to unshared meaning.

# THE SKILLS OF UNDERSTANDING

Interpersonal skills related to the art of understanding are paraphrasing, seeking clarification, reflecting feelings, connecting thoughts with feelings, and summarising. Paraphrasing is listed first because it is essential to building meaning. Seeking clarification, reflecting feelings, connecting thoughts with feelings, and summarising are presented as related skills in the process of developing understanding.

# Paraphrasing

Paraphrasing is the backbone of the skills of understanding because doing so acknowledges what the patient has said and demonstrates the nurse has listened. They encourage further patient expression because they are confirming and accepting. Paraphrases, although statements, contain an implied question: 'Is my understanding of what you are saying the same as what you mean to say?' They often begin with phrases such as:

- 'So, what you're saying is …'
- 'Would I be correct in saying that you …'
- 'In other words …'
- 'Let me see if I understand correctly …'

Beginning a paraphrase with phrases such as these brings the implied question into the open. However, it is not essential that paraphrases begin in this manner. A nurse may simply rephrase what the patient has expressed.

The value of the paraphrase is that nurses can check the accuracy of their understanding of what the patient means against the patient's intended meaning. Use of the paraphrase is an effective way to prevent misunderstandings. Because patients hear the nurse's interpretation, they are afforded an opportunity to confirm or deny its accuracy.

## Interchangeable responses

When paraphrasing, a nurse attempts to produce a response that is interchangeable with what the patient has expressed. An effective paraphrase neither adds to (additive response) nor detracts from (detractive response) what the patient has said.

Additive responses include comments on, explanations of and opinions about what the patient is expressing. Analysing and interpreting responses are examples of additive responses. Although quite helpful when the goal is to increase the patient's awareness, additive responses do not necessarily facilitate the nurse's understanding.

Responses that detract are those that shift the focus away from the patient or focus only on what the *nurse* thinks is important. Offering premature solutions and advice are examples of detractive responses. Paraphrases neither add nor detract; they are interchangeable with what the patient has expressed and do not attempt to alter the meaning of that expression.

## Accuracy in paraphrasing

Even though nurses attempt to make paraphrases interchangeable, there is still no guarantee they will be entirely accurate. The meaning a nurse derives from a patient's expression may not be what the patient intended. This does not signal failure because an inaccurate paraphrase allows the patient to correct the nurse's misinterpretation before progressing further in the interaction. In responding to a paraphrase, a patient has an opportunity to restate the meaning of an expression, amplify it or reiterate what was originally expressed. As long as the nurse does not detract completely from the meaning, understanding can still be achieved through further interaction.

For this reason, it is important to state a paraphrase in a tentative manner and closely observe the patient's response to it. Even when it is inaccurate, a paraphrase still conveys a nurse's desire to understand and a willingness to engage in interactions that build meaning. The ultimate aim is to achieve congruence between what the patient means and what the nurse understands the patient to mean. This requires effort, time and the use of responses that work towards this aim. Mutual understanding must be negotiated between patients and nurses. Paraphrasing works towards the goal of mutual understanding because it enables meaning to be negotiated.

---

### ACTIVITY 6.4  Paraphrasing: have I got it right?

**Process**

1. Form pairs for this activity, and designate one person as A and the other as B.

2. A makes a statement about a recent interaction with a patient that was significant.

3. B responds with a paraphrase and begins with, 'So, in other words, what you are saying is ...'. B is not to advise, judge, evaluate or probe. At the end of the paraphrase, B asks, 'Have I got it right?'

4. A confirms or denies B's paraphrase and then continues to discuss the situation. B continues to paraphrase each of A's statements, asking each time, 'Have I got it right?' This process continues until A is able to say to B, 'Yes, you have got it right, that's exactly what I mean.'

5. Reverse roles, with B relating a story and A paraphrasing.

**Discussion**

1. How accurate were the initial paraphrases? What was the response to an inaccurate paraphrase? How long did it take to achieve accuracy?

2. What were the effects of paraphrasing in the interaction? How did each participant feel during the interaction?

3. How was listening affected when you knew you had to paraphrase?

Paraphrasing is effective in building meaning and, when used to this end, results in greater understanding between patients and nurses. As with any skill, nurses must pay careful attention to how patients respond to paraphrasing. A paraphrase works towards its desired end when it encourages patients to elaborate on their experiences, thus enabling nurses to understand these experiences more fully.

## Overuse of paraphrasing

Overuse of paraphrasing, in the absence of other skills, can be frustrating for a patient because the interaction may seem to be going in circles, with little progress. Continuous rephrasing of what a patient has said gives the impression that the interaction is 'going nowhere'. To prevent this, paraphrases need to be used with a mixture of other skills.

The aim and intention of paraphrasing must be borne in mind. An accurate paraphrase is a direct acknowledgment of what a patient has expressed. It serves to deepen the relationship and encourage further interaction. When paraphrases stifle interaction, they do not meet their intended aim.

## Reluctance to use paraphrasing

Despite the value of paraphrasing in building and negotiating meaning, sometimes there is a lack of appreciation of its use. Nurses may be reluctant to paraphrase out of a fear of appearing inept or poorly informed. They often think they 'should' automatically understand what patients are experiencing and may feel foolish in not knowing. It is virtually impossible for nurses to fully appreciate what patients are experiencing until an effort is made to understand. Each patient's experience is unique, and subjective. To believe there is an objective reality that is applicable to all patients is unrealistic.

At other times, reluctance to paraphrase stems from a fear of reinforcing a patient's negative state. For example, when patients express unpleasant emotions or self-destructive thoughts, nurses may fear that restating such negative experiences elevates them, giving them more status than they deserve. Nurses may believe that it is better to deny or dismiss them, avoid further discussion of them or try to talk the patient out of them. But avoidance alienates patients, giving the impression that nurses do not really care.

Paraphrasing acknowledges the patient's reality, demonstrates acceptance of it and conveys the nurse's desire to understand that reality. This is not the same as agreement and reinforcement; eventually, a nurse may challenge a patient and encourage them to adopt an alternative perspective (see Ch 8). However, another perspective cannot be introduced until the nurse shares the patient's current perspective and paraphrases work towards this shared understanding.

# Seeking clarification

The skills of clarification are used whenever nurses are uncertain or unsure about what patients are saying. Under these circumstances paraphrasing is not possible because the nurse is unable to get an adequate sense of what the patient means. Through clarification, nurses convey that they are trying to understand and will not proceed until they are able to do so. Statements that clarify could begin with:

- 'I'm not sure I follow you.'
- 'That's not clear to me.'
- 'I'm not certain what you mean.'
- 'I'm having difficulty understanding that.'
- 'I'm a bit confused about …'

Notice how the nurse takes responsibility for the lack of clarity and understanding. The intent and effect would be very different if statements such as 'You're not expressing yourself clearly' or 'That's not clear' were made. A properly phrased clarification is focused on a desire to receive a clearer message from the patient – a rephrase, an illustration and/or amplification. It should not put patients on the defensive or lead to discomfort by creating the feeling that they have to justify themselves or provide rational explanations to nurses (see 'Assertive skills' in Ch 10).

## Clarification through questioning

Clarification is often achieved through using probing skills (see Ch 7); however, the intention is not focused as much on exploration as it is on clearing an area of confusion or ambiguity. An open question such as 'What do you mean?' is a direct clarification. Nurses must use such a question with care and caution because of its potential to sound critical and accusatory (it could imply 'You are not making sense'). Intonation and other non-verbal aspects make the difference.

## Restatement

Sometimes a restatement of what a patient has said is an effective means of clarifying. The nurse simply parrots the patient's exact words, usually switching from the first person to the second person. The accompanying non-verbal intonation should indicate that the restatement is really a prompt, which is aimed at further amplification. Restatement is similar to one-word or phrase accents (see Ch 7) except that, in restatement, the entire message is reiterated. An example of a restatement is:

Patient: *I can't move my right arm.*

Nurse: *You can't move your right arm?*

Sometimes, nurses overuse restatement because they do not know what else to say. Overuse of parroting can lead to frustration on the part of the patient, so its use should be kept to a minimum. It should be used with the intention of reaching greater clarity and understanding, not as a substitute for lack of words.

## Clarification through self-disclosure

At times, nurses clarify what a patient has said by sharing how they might feel, think and perceive the situation if they were the patient. An example is: 'I'm not sure I entirely follow what it's like for you, but if I were you I'd be …'. Care must be exercised when using self-disclosure because of the potential to shift the focus from the patient to the nurse. In using self-disclosure in this manner, the nurse is attempting to clear an area of confusion, not detract from what the patient is expressing.

# Reflecting feelings

Reflection is the mirroring of feelings expressed by patients. Because feelings are often expressed indirectly, nurses translate the feeling aspects of a patient's message into other words. In this sense, reflecting feelings is similar to paraphrasing. Instead of rephrasing the actual words of the patient, the nurse rephrases an indirectly expressed emotion. An example of reflecting feelings is:

Patient: *This darn leg won't get any stronger, despite all the physio.*

Nurse: *That leg is frustrating you, isn't it?*

Reflecting feelings is useful because it conveys the nurse's recognition of feelings and confirms the existence of emotions. More than any other area of the patient's experience, feelings must be accepted as valid and real. Like paraphrasing, the reflection of feelings must be stated tentatively, awaiting feedback from the patient that either confirms or denies the accuracy of the nurse's perception.

Reflecting feelings is verbalising what a patient has implied, but this is not the same as interpreting the patient's feelings. An interpretation involves adding to the patient's expression, rather than bringing into the open what was expressed indirectly. The nurse is still working with what the patient has communicated, not providing an explanation of, or judgment about, the patient's feelings.

In reflecting feelings, as in paraphrasing, nurses attempt to respond interchangeably with what patients have expressed. An interchangeable feeling reflection matches both the type of feeling and its intensity. Frustration is different from anger; feeling a bit blue is not the same as feeling despondent; happiness is not equivalent to elation. Making the distinction between different emotions and feelings requires an extensive vocabulary. A major difficulty in reflecting feelings is a limitation of the language the nurse possesses for describing feelings. Activity 6.5 is designed to increase your feeling-word vocabulary.

When nurses are reflecting feelings, they must first identify the appropriate feeling category. Most feelings will fit into one of the categories used in Activity 6.5. Second, the intensity of the feeling expressed must be determined. Once the correct feeling and its intensity have been decided, a word or phrase that accurately describes the feeling is selected. The choice of words must suit the age (see Ch 10) and cultural background (Ch 4) of the patient.

## ACTIVITY 6.5  Building a feeling-word vocabulary

**Process**

1. Divide a blank piece of paper into seven vertical columns. Place the following 'feeling' categories at the top of the columns:

   Happy   Sad   Angry   Confused   Scared   Weak   Strong

2. In each column, record as many words as you can that express the emotion. Phrases such as 'over the moon' can also be used.

3. Form groups of five to six and compare lists. Add words from other participants' lists that you have not already recorded.

4. Evaluate each feeling word on the list according to its intensity. Label each as *high*, *medium* or *low* intensity. For example: elated = high; happy = medium; pleased = low.

**Discussion**

1. In which feeling categories was it easy to develop words and phrases? Which were difficult? Why are some categories easier to describe than others?

2. Which feeling category has the most words and phrases? Which has the least? What do you make of this?

3. Compare the feeling categories that were hard and easy with the ones that have the most and least words and phrases. Is there any relationship? Explain.

4. Look at the language used in each of the categories. Are some feeling words and phrases more appropriate with patients in different age groups and from different cultural backgrounds?

5. What role does culture play in evaluating feeling-word intensity?

6. Are there some words and phrases that you would not personally use under certain circumstances? What are they and why would you not use them?

Source: Reprinted from *The art of helping student workbook*, 2nd edn, by Robert R Carkhuff. Copyright © 1983. Reprinted by permission of the publisher, HRD Press, Inc. Amherst, MA, (800) 822-2801, www.hrdpress.com.

A nurse's feeling-word vocabulary can be further built through interactions with patients by paying careful attention to the language used when patients express various emotions and feelings.

Before attempting to reflect the feeling, nurses may first need to check their perceptions (Ch 7) of how they think the patient is feeling because feelings are often expressed indirectly, through non-verbal means, cues and innuendo. Frequently, it is better to check perceptions of feelings before proceeding to reflect them.

## A word of caution about reflecting feelings

Some patients are more comfortable than others in discussing their feelings. Additionally, a discussion of feelings may enhance a patient's sense of vulnerability because feelings are difficult to control and contain. When a patient is working hard at containing emotions, and prefers to keep doing so, it is insensitive for a nurse to proceed into a discussion that uncovers these feelings and focuses on them. Nurses must pay careful attention to a patient's reaction to the discussion of feelings.

Likewise, discussion of feelings should be left until trust has formed between a patient and a nurse. The extent to which a patient is relaxed and at ease with a discussion of feelings demonstrates the degree of trust that has been established. Nurses can use a feeling discussion as a means of determining how much trust has been established. This requires acute awareness and sensitivity to a patient's response.

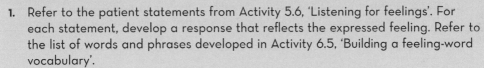

## ACTIVITY 6.6  Reflecting feelings

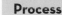

### Process

1.  Refer to the patient statements from Activity 5.6, 'Listening for feelings'. For each statement, develop a response that reflects the expressed feeling. Refer to the list of words and phrases developed in Activity 6.5, 'Building a feeling-word vocabulary'.

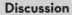

### Discussion

1.  Which feelings were easy to reflect? Which were difficult? What do you make of this?

2.  Are there any feeling reflections you would find personally difficult to express? Why?

# Connecting thoughts and feelings

Chapter 5, on listening, differentiated listening for content and listening for feelings. In this chapter, the skill of paraphrasing is used predominantly to respond to content while reflecting feelings responds to emotional states. Although it is possible to perceive them separately, and even respond to them separately, patients' experiences include both content and feelings. Initially, nurses may choose to focus on one or the other when responding; eventually, thoughts (content) and feelings (emotion) must be put together. Connecting skills are used for this purpose. When connecting, nurses can use the following format: 'You feel … when …'.

Connecting thoughts and feelings adds depth to a nurse's understanding and moves the interaction in a forward direction. Through this response, a nurse is moving into the area of fully understanding a patient's experience. Listening attentively and clarifying enables nurses to make the connection between patients' thoughts and their feelings. Again, it is necessary for the nurse to await feedback from the patient that confirms, denies or expands on the nurse's understanding.

## ACTIVITY 6.7  Connecting thoughts and feelings  335

### Process

1. Refer to each patient statement in Activity 6.2: 'Recognising the types of responses'. Ignore the responses that are provided and develop one of your own that connects the patients' expressed thoughts to their feelings. Use the format: 'You feel ... when ...' as a guide. Refer to your feeling-word vocabulary, developed in Activity 6.5, for ways to describe feelings.

2. Compare your responses with those of other participants.

### Discussion

1. What differences are there in responses developed by various participants? Are there some responses that are the same?

2. In comparing connecting responses, how similar are the feeling portions? How different are they?

3. In comparing the connections between feelings and content, did some participants focus on content that was different from that of other participants?

# Summarising

Summarising is the skill of responding in a way that reviews what has been discussed between a patient and a nurse. It is a brief, concise collection of paraphrases and feeling reflections that are accurately connected. Like other skills of understanding, a summary allows nurses to check understanding by verbalising it, then awaiting feedback from the patient. Summaries often begin with phrases like:

- 'So, to sum it up ...'
- 'We have discussed so much; let me see if I can pull it together ...'
- 'Overall, I get the picture that ...'

Summarising is used most often to bring closure to an interaction and serves as a final check of a nurse's understanding. When a nurse uses summarising to bring closure to an interaction, it is important that they allow adequate time for the patient to respond. As with other understanding skills, patients need an opportunity to clarify, expand on an idea or correct the nurse's misinterpretation.

There is an even more important reason for allowing adequate time following a summary. Frequently, patients present the most significant aspect of their experience just as the time draws near to close an interaction. In this case, patients perceive a nurse's summary as a signal that time is of the essence and use the remaining time as a final opportunity for expression. This is not at all uncommon during patient–nurse interactions. An aware nurse recognises and accepts this interpersonal dynamic and allows time for its occurrence.

While closure is the most common reason to summarise, a summary is also effectively used either in the middle or at the beginning of an interaction. When used in the middle of an interaction, a summary serves to open new areas of discussion by clearing the way for new ideas to be expressed. When it is used at this point, summarising serves as an exploration skill that encourages patients to bring forward new thoughts and feelings. When it is used at the beginning of an interaction, summarising serves to orient both the patient and the nurse to the current interaction by reviewing previous interactions.

---

## ACTIVITY 6.8 Expressing empathy

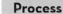

**Process**

1. Refer to Activity 6.1: 'Your usual style of responding (I)'.

2. For each statement or question, develop a response that expresses empathy with the experience of the 'patient'. Assume you have validated your understanding and have accurately understood the patient.

3. Compare these responses with the ones you originally developed when completing Activity 6.1.

**Discussion**

1. What differences are there between the responses you originally developed and the ones you have now developed?

2. Which took more time to develop?

3. What risks are there in expressing empathy to patients?

4. What benefits are there in expressing empathy?

---

# SUMMARY

Understanding-based responses are used after nurses have received meaningful input from patients during the process of listening. Once initial impressions are formed, understanding-based responses are employed to build meaning between patients and nurses. The skills of understanding are used to bring nurses in touch with patients' private and personal worlds. They allow nurses to be 'in tune' with patients and therefore empathic.

Attending and listening to patients' reactions to understanding-based responses is essential and highlights the need for constant listening. Patients may react to an understanding response by validating it, denying it, altering it or expanding on it. Each of these patient reactions provides an opportunity for nurses to deepen their level of understanding.

When nurses employ the skills of understanding (paraphrasing, seeking clarification, reflecting feelings, connecting and summarising) in conjunction with effective exploration (see Ch 7), they are in a position to know what a patient is experiencing from the personal perspective of the patient. This inside understanding involves knowing what is happening to that person and even feeling what it is like to be that person. Knowing and feeling through vicarious experiences such as these are the backbone of empathy. It requires time and effort to truly understand another's reality. Nurses need to allow themselves time to think and reflect on how effectively they are understanding patients' experiences. They need to allow themselves enough time to respond to patients with understanding. This may also involve 'letting go' of familiar ways of responding, in favour of responses that reflect understanding.

# REFERENCES

Carkhuff, R.R., 1983. The Student Workbook for the Art of Helping, second ed. Human Resource Press, Amherst, MA.

Eley, D., Eley, R., Bertello, M., 2012. Why did I become a nurse? Personality traits and reasons for entering nursing. J. Adv. Nurs. 68 (7), 1546–1555.

Gagan, J.M., 1983. Methodological notes on empathy. Adv. Nurs. Sci. 5 (2), 65–72.

Goleman, D., 1998. Working With Emotional Intelligence. Bloomsbury, London.

Halpern, J., 2003. What is clinical empathy? J. Gen. Intern. Med. 18, 670–674.

Hojat, M., Louis, D.Z., Maio, V., et al., 2013. Empathy and health care quality. Am. J. Med. Qual. 28 (1), 6–7.

Johnson, D.W., 2013. Reaching Out: Interpersonal Effectiveness and Self-Actualization, eleventh ed. Allyn and Bacon/Merrill, Boston, MA.

Kalisch, B.J., 1973. What is empathy? Am. J. Nurs. 73, 1548–1552.

Ledoux, K., 2015. Understanding compassion fatigue: understanding compassion. J. Adv. Nurs. 71 (9), 2041–2050.

Lelorain, A., Brédart, A., Dolbeault, S., et al., 2012. A systematic review of the associations between empathy measures and patient outcomes in cancer care. Psychooncology 21, 1255–1264.

Morse, J.M., Bottoroff, J., Anderson, G., et al., 2006 (originally 1992). Beyond empathy: expanding expressions of caring. J. Adv. Nurs. 53 (1), 75–90.

Nightingale, F., 1859. Notes on Nursing: What It Is and What It Is Not. Reprinted 1992, Lippincott, Philadelphia, PA, originally published by Harrison & Son, London.

Nursing and Midwifery Board of Australia, 2016. Registered Nurse Standards for Practice. NMBA, Melbourne.

Papadopoulos, I., Ali, S., 2016. Measuring compassion in nurses and other healthcare professionals. Nurse Educ. Pract. 16, 133–139.

Peplau, H., 1952. Interpersonal Relations in Nursing. GP Putnam & Sons, New York.

Petrucci, C., Le Cerra, C., Aloisio, F., et al., 2016. Empathy in health professional students: a comparative cross-sectional study. Nurse Educ. Today 41, 1–6.

Richardson, C., Percy, M., Hughes, J., 2015. Nursing therapeutics: teaching student nurses care, compassion and empathy. Nurse Educ. Today 35, e1–e5.

Rogers, C., 1957. The necessary and sufficient conditions of therapeutic personality change. J. Consult. Psychol. 21, 91–105.

Sinclair, S., Norris, J.M., McConnell, S.J., et al., 2016. Compassion: a scoping review of the healthcare literature. BMC Palliat. Care 15, 1–6. doi:10.1186/s12904-016-0080-0.

Svenaeus, F., 2015. The relationship between empathy and sympathy in good health care. Med. Health Care Philos. 18, 267–277.

Travelbee, J., 1971. Interpersonal Aspects of Nursing. FA Davis, Philadelphia, PA.

Ward, J., 2016. The empathy enigma does it still exist? Comparison of empathy using students and standardized actors. Nurse Educ. 41 (3), 134–138.

Ward, J., Cody, J., Schaal, M., et al., 2012. The empathy enigma: an empirical study of the decline in empathy among undergraduate nursing students. J. Prof. Nurs. 28, 34–40.

Wiseman, T., 2007. Toward a holistic conceptualization of empathy for nursing practice. Adv. Nurs. Sci. 30 (3), e61–e72.

Zderad, L.T., 1969. Empathic nursing: realisation of a human capacity. Nurs. Clin. North Am. 4 (4), 655–662.

# ANSWERS TO ACTIVITIES

## Activity 6.2: Recognising the types of responses

2    a
  1)   S (reassuring and supporting)
  2)   I (analysing and interpreting)
  3)   U (paraphrasing and understanding)
  4)   E (advising and evaluating)
  5)   P (questioning and probing)

2    b
  1)   P (questioning and probing)
  2)   S (reassuring and supporting)
  3)   E (advising and evaluating)
  4)   U (paraphrasing and understanding)
  5)   I (analysing and interpreting)

2    c
  1)   U (paraphrasing and understanding)
  2)   E (advising and evaluating)
  3)   P (questioning and probing)
  4)   S (reassuring and supporting)
  5)   I (analysing and interpreting)

2    d
  1)   E (advising and evaluating)
  2)   P (questioning and probing)
  3)   U (paraphrasing and understanding)
  4)   I (analysing and interpreting)
  5)   S (reassuring and supporting)

2    e
  1)   S (reassuring and supporting)
  2)   E (advising and evaluating)
  3)   P (questioning and probing)
  4)   I (analysing and interpreting)
  5)   U (paraphrasing and understanding)

2    f
  1)   E (advising and evaluating)
  2)   P (questioning and probing)
  3)   S (reassuring and supporting)
  4)   I (analysing and interpreting)
  5)   U (paraphrasing and understanding)

2　g
    **1)**    I (analysing and interpreting)
    **2)**    E (advising and evaluating)
    **3)**    U (paraphrasing and understanding)
    **4)**    P (questioning and probing)
    **5)**    S (reassuring and supporting)

2　h
    **1)**    U (paraphrasing and understanding)
    **2)**    S (reassuring and supporting)
    **3)**    E (advising and evaluating)
    **4)**    P (questioning and probing)
    **5)**    I (analysing and interpreting)

2　i
    **1)**    I (analysing and interpreting)
    **2)**    S (reassuring and supporting)
    **3)**    U (paraphrasing and understanding)
    **4)**    E (advising and evaluating)
    **5)**    P (questioning and probing)

2　j
    **1)**    U (paraphrasing and understanding)
    **2)**    S (reassuring and supporting)
    **3)**    I (analysing and interpreting)
    **4)**    P (questioning and probing)
    **5)**    E (advising and evaluating)

2　k
    **1)**    S (reassuring and supporting)
    **2)**    I (analysing and interpreting)
    **3)**    P (questioning and probing)
    **4)**    U (paraphrasing and understanding)
    **5)**    E (advising and evaluating)

2　l
    **1)**    I (analysing and interpreting)
    **2)**    U (paraphrasing and understanding)
    **3)**    P (questioning and probing)
    **4)**    E (advising and evaluating)
    **5)**    S (reassuring and supporting)

# Collecting information: exploring

- Exploration of patients' experiences are both planned and spontaneous.

- An example of planned or focused exploration is a formal interview conducted as an initial patient assessment, while spontaneous exploration occurs as a result of a trigger or cue from a patient.

- Both types of exploration rely on using the same skills, and these skills are divided into the broad areas of prompting and probing.

- Prompting techniques include minimal encouragement, one-word/phrase accents, gentle commands, open-ended statements, finishing the sentence and self-disclosure.

- Probing techniques include open-ended questions and closed questions.

- In both planned and spontaneous exploration the nurse needs to be mindful of taking the lead and following the patient's lead in order to share control with patients.

e Visit the Evolve site for video content to support the themes and skills explored in this chapter: http://evolve.elsevier.com/AU/Stein-Parbury/patient/

# INTRODUCTION

The skills covered in Chapters 5 and 6 – attending, listening and understanding – laid the foundation for effective interaction between patients and nurses because their use enables nurses to hear, perceive and reflect what patients are expressing. Exploration, the subject of this chapter, moves the interaction beyond absorption and reiteration of patients' messages. Exploration opens new areas, focuses on selected themes and delves more deeply into a patient's total experience.

The process of exploration is one of searching, carried out for the purpose of discovery, detection, recognition and identification. Successful exploration results in greater understanding between patients and nurses; it can be directed towards something in particular or it can be open-ended, leading to discovering something unexpected. Collecting specific information from patients (the directed type of exploration) is necessary. Is Mr Sardo allergic to any medications? How long did Ms Geraghty sleep last night? Does Mr Nguyen understand his special low-fat diet? Answers to such questions help guide nursing approaches and actions, and nurses need to know how to collect pertinent information from patients.

Nevertheless, effective exploration in the nursing context involves more than merely collecting specific facts from patients. Open-ended, spontaneous enquiry, the other type of exploration, is also needed because it is the means by which a nurse can come to understand how a patient interprets health and illness. What are Mr Sardo's expectations about his pending surgery? What is interfering with Ms Geraghty's sleep? How different is Mr Nguyen's special diet from his usual one? Exploration into areas such as these is aimed at discovering ideas, thoughts, perceptions, feelings and reactions experienced by patients. It is important that nurses come to understand patients' responses to health and illness, and effective exploration assists in this understanding.

Now consider the following patient's story.

## A Patient's Story

Martin spent his life in a rural part of the country. He felt very much at home 'on the land'. He disliked city life and avoided 'the big smoke' at all costs. Martin also had another aversion: visiting the doctor. He always put that off as long as he could. However, the obvious problems he was experiencing with his throat made it impossible to ignore his need for medical attention.

When he was finally admitted to a large metropolitan hospital for major surgery, Martin felt very much out of place. However, coping with being in the city seemed minor in comparison with his worry about being ill and in hospital. He didn't ask many questions of the surgeons when they came to explain his surgery, which included possible removal of his larynx (voice box). Martin listened as the surgeons explained what they would do but didn't think too much about what it meant. Being a man of few words, he didn't ask for clarification.

The night before his surgery, Lucille was the nurse caring for Martin. She felt an instant rapport with him, despite his quiet nature and the paucity of words between them. As she explained to him what he could expect following the surgery, she slowly came to the alarming realisation that he didn't understand that the surgery would affect his ability to speak. In fact, if the surgeons performed the laryngectomy, he would not speak again. Although he had consented to the surgical procedure, he didn't seem to appreciate the potential consequences for his life. Through exploring his understanding and desires, Lucille discovered that Martin preferred a shorter life with the ability to speak rather than a longer life and the inability to speak. As a result of her exploration and understanding, Martin's surgery was cancelled and other treatment options were explored.

While this story might raise questions as to whether Martin's consent to the surgery was adequately informed, imagine what might have happened had the nurse *not* taken the time to understand the patient's point of view. And understanding the patient's point of view is contingent on effectively exploring a patient's perceptions and interpretation.

## ACTIVITY 7.1 Developing exploratory responses (I)

### Process

Record how you would respond to each of the following patients' statements. Do not concern yourself with how 'right' or 'wrong' your responses are, but do try to make them helpful to the patient. Assume that all statements are made to you, the nurse caring for the patient making the statement.

1. A hospitalised 65-year-old woman, who has recently undergone a total hip replacement: 'How am I ever going to manage on my own when I return home?'

2. A hospitalised patient speaking to a first-year nursing student: 'Do you know what you are doing? How much experience have you had?'

3. A 20-year-old woman who is undergoing diagnostic tests on an outpatient basis: 'The doctor keeps evading my questions. What is really going on?'

4. A mother of a five-week-old baby during a routine visit to an early childhood centre: 'I wish I could get a decent night's sleep like I used to.'

5. A long-term resident of a nursing home: 'I can't stand being here. There's nothing to do and no one ever comes to visit me.'

6. A 20-year-old man who is hospitalised with a fractured femur following a motor vehicle accident: 'Why do these things always have to happen to me? Bad things always happen to me.'

7. A hospitalised patient during medication rounds in hospital: 'I think all these tablets are really making me sleepy.'

8. A hospitalised patient during morning care: 'I have asked the doctors how long they think I have to live, but they keep avoiding the question. Will you tell me, please?'

*cont.*

*Activity 7.1 continued*

9. A hospitalised patient during morning nursing rounds: 'I'm so glad to see you. Those nurses on the night shift just don't help me.'

10. A 70-year-old man in an outpatient clinic following consultation with a doctor: 'If what the doctor says is true, I don't see the point in going on and suffering ... better to just end it now.'

**Discussion**

1. Each of the statements presented indicates a situation that requires further exploration by the nurse – more information, clarification and/or elaboration is required. Review your responses and decide which of your responses do explore the patient's statement. Mark these with a tick.

2. Write a new response for those not marked. Try to make this revised response an exploratory one.

(Note: This activity will be further developed in Activity 7.8: 'Developing exploratory responses (II)'.)

# PLANNED VERSUS SPONTANEOUS EXPLORATION

Planned exploration is directive because the nurse controls the interaction by guiding the flow and content of the patient's response. A good example of planned exploration is a formal interview conducted for the purpose of an initial health assessment. Spontaneous exploration is responsive because the nurse reacts to something the patient has said or done. In planned exploration, nurses assume the lead and introduce the topics; in spontaneous exploration, nurses follow the patient's lead. The distinction between planned exploration and spontaneous exploration is somewhat artificial because similar skills and techniques are used for both types of exploration. The distinction is drawn to highlight the different contexts in which nurses use exploration skills and techniques.

A common context in which nurses use exploration skills is when they conduct a health assessment. Most often, nurses conduct health assessments when they encounter a patient for the first time (e.g. on admission to hospital). It is important to clarify the purpose of a health assessment. If the purpose is to collect data about the history of a patient's health status, then planned exploration is appropriate. If the purpose is also to explore personal meaning of a patient's health status, then a less formalised, spontaneous exploration is appropriate. In nursing, both purposes are relevant. Nurses need to collect factual data about a patient's health as well as understanding the meaning of the health experience for the patient. As a result, exploration is most effective when it is both planned and spontaneous. In this way the interview takes on the characteristics of a conversation, which closely mirrors the balanced give and take of everyday exchanges, rather than an interrogation. A conversational style of interviewing helps put the patient at ease, as compared with the one-way, controlled structure of a formal interview in which questions impose an obligation to answer.

# Planned exploration

During planned exploration, the nurse directs and leads the search for information regarding pertinent aspects of a patient's 'health story' and current needs for nursing care. Specific data collection is the primary purpose of planned exploration, and topic areas are introduced and explored on the basis of what the nurse needs to know in order to care for the patient. Nurses direct and often control this type of exploration.

Structured, planned exploration occurs in the beginning phase of the patient–nurse relationship, usually upon initial contact. The manner in which exploration occurs during these initial contacts sets the stage for subsequent interactions and further development of the relationship by establishing the conditions for trust and openness. A nurse whose approach is authoritarian and rigid may convey a message to a patient that the nurse is in control and obedience in answering the questions is expected. This might happen when the nurse becomes so focused on filling out a nursing history form that patients are left with the impression that completion of the record is more important than them as people. Likewise, an overconcern with the techniques of exploration may interfere with a nurse's ability to fully attend and listen to patients' replies.

# Spontaneous exploration

Spontaneous exploration occurs when nurses notice and follow through in exploring what a patient has expressed. This type of exploration is patient-controlled and patient-led; the nurse follows the patient's lead, instead of the patient following the nurse's lead. A patient's expression may take the form of a direct expression of need or emotional distress, referred to as a concern, or it can take the form of an implied need or emotion, referred to as a cue (Zimmermann et al 2007).

Cues are more common than concerns, as patients frequently communicate their needs, desires and feelings through indirect messages, indicating what they are experiencing by hints, suggestions and implied questions (Griep et al 2016). Patients report that they perceive barriers in relation to directly expressing their concerns. They perceive that the healthcare providers who do not actively invite them to express their concerns are not understanding and empathic, and that there is a lack of time to discuss concerns (Brandes et al 2015). Indirectly, patients are requesting a response from a nurse by presenting these communication cues.

How nurses respond to cues from patients helps shape the direction of their continuing relationship. Spontaneous exploration is important to the continuing relationship between a patient and a nurse because it affirms that the nurse is attending and listening to the patient. It deepens the relationship and communicates the nurse's continued interest in the patient's welfare because it is a concrete demonstration of the nurse's ongoing concern for the patient (see *Research highlight*).

**RESEARCH HIGHLIGHT** Responding to patient cues

*Griep, E.C.M., Noordman, J., Vandulmen, S., 2016. Practice nurses mental health provide space to patients to discuss unpleasant emotions. J. Psychiat. Ment. Health Nurs. 23, 77–85.*

### Background

Practice nurses are specialists who work alongside general practitioners (GPs) in a general practice setting. Mental health practice nurses are employed by GPs to undertake assessment and care for patients who present to the GP with psychosocial or psychological concerns.

### Purpose of the study

The aims of this study were to examine how patients express mild psychosocial or psychological problems to mental health practice nurses and to evaluate how the nurses respond to these expressions.

### Method

The design of the study was observational and exploratory. Data were collected by videotaping consultations between 15 practice nurses and 116 different patients with mild psychosocial or psychological problems. The video recordings were analysed using a standardised coding sheet to determine the types of responses that nurses made to patients' cues and concerns.

### Key findings

During the majority of consultations (94 per cent) the patients expressed at least one concern or cue. Nurses responded by providing space for the patient to further discuss their distress. However, the space was provided passively by using minimal prompts, such as 'uh huh' and 'mm hum'. The exploration was implicit as they rarely responded actively in further exploring the patient's problems.

### Implications for nursing practice

Even though the nurses in this study were specialists in mental healthcare and therefore skilled interpersonally, they tended to respond passively to patients' cues and concerns. This highlights the importance of active exploration because being active in exploration demonstrates interest in the patient and encourages further interaction. It is only through further interaction that nurses will come to understand a patient's situation.

# Patient-cue exploration

Cues are small units of information that are part of a larger, more complex phenomenon. They indicate a need for further exploration into the phenomenon. They signal the need for exploration much like a green light at a traffic intersection signals that drivers may proceed. Effective exploration of patient cues, like all exploration, leads to further data collection and greater understanding between a patient and a nurse. It has been shown that nurses do passively acknowledge patient cues, for example, by nodding their heads, but they also distance themselves, for example, by changing the subject (Chan 2014; de Leeuw et al 2014; Griep et al 2016; Sheldon et al 2011). However, they are more likely to provide space for the patient to discuss their concerns when these concerns are expressed directly, rather than indirectly in the form of a cue (Finset et al 2013).

In contrast with the previously cited studies, Grimsbø et al (2012) found that nurses did respond directly to patients' cues and concerns. But rather than face-to-face interactions, their communication was via email conversations. Patients were more explicit in their expressions of emotional concerns, and nurses responded with empathy and information. The authors speculated that their findings differed from other studies because the patients' concerns were more visible when in writing. In addition, nurses may not have felt hurried and under time pressure because they had the opportunity to re-read the patients' messages and reflect on them before responding.

## ACTIVITY 7.2 Exploring patient cues

### Process

1. Think of an instance, real or imagined, in which a patient presents a cue that indicates the need for further exploration or elaboration (e.g. a facial grimace, possibly indicating pain). Record this patient cue on a slip of paper, providing any information that would be of assistance in understanding the situation (the setting and circumstances).

2. Collect the slips of paper and redistribute them to other participants in the activity.

3. The contents of the slips of paper are then read aloud to all participants. Each participant develops and records an exploratory response, using any type of exploration technique.

4. Form groups of five to six and share exploratory responses in these groups. Each small group discusses the various exploratory responses and selects the one that is most appropriate as an exploration technique. These are then read aloud to the rest of the participants.

### Discussion

Discuss each cue and responses selected by the small groups. During the discussion, use the following questions to evaluate the responses, bearing in mind that the purpose of the response is to explore the cue presented by the patient.

*cont.*

*Activity 7.2 continued*

1. Which exploration technique was used?
2. How effective is the response in exploring the cue?
3. In which context would this response be most appropriate?
4. What purpose does the exploration serve? Is it helpful? How?
5. Could you actually say this to a patient? If not, why not?

## Cues and inferences

A cue is a unit of sensory input – a sight, sound, smell, taste or touch that is perceived as important to be noticed. For example, during an interaction, a nurse notices that a patient keeps fidgeting with the bedclothes. By noticing this piece of information, the nurse has perceived a cue.

Almost without awareness, meanings are assigned to perceived cues as a way of making sense of what is experienced. The meanings attached to cues are inferences – conclusions drawn from the cues. Inferences are based on knowledge, previous experience, expectations and needs. For example, fidgeting with the bedclothes may be interpreted as a sign of general anxiety or discomfort with the interaction. Nevertheless, inferences are usually formed on the basis of more than one cue. The combination of fidgeting with the bedclothes, startling easily, pressured speech, non-stop talking and foot tapping are cues that may lead to an inference that a patient is anxious.

It is impossible not to make such interpretations about what is perceived; inferences are automatic. What is possible is to differentiate a cue (concrete data) from an inference (the interpretation of the data).

Once inferences are recognised by the nurse, they need to be validated with the patient in order to determine if they are correct. In the example of fidgeting with the bedclothes, if the patient admits to feeling anxious, the inference is validated. It is important not to jump too quickly to a conclusion about patient cues. Further exploration is usually the most appropriate initial response to a patient cue.

### ACTIVITY 7.3 Cues and inferences  335

**Process**

Determine whether each of the following statements is a cue or an inference:

1. Answered interview questions completely.
2. Uninterested in the interview.
3. Changed the topic when asked about her family.

4. An open person.

5. Sleeping quietly.

6. Shallow, rapid respirations.

7. Doesn't understand prescribed medications.

8. Keeps asking questions about diagnostic tests.

9. No eye contact during the interview.

10. Speech is pressured.

11. Puzzled expression on his face when I asked him about the surgery.

12. Doesn't know what to expect.

13. No visible signs of distress.

(Note: The answers to this activity can be found at the end of this chapter.)

**Discussion**

1. Compare your answers with those of other class participants. Are there any differences in the answers?

2. If differences exist, discuss the item(s) and decide what makes them inferences or what makes them cues.

3. Compare your answers with those provided at the end of this chapter.

## Communication cues

When nurses prompt and probe during the process of exploration, many verbal and non-verbal cues are elicited because the exploration itself triggers the cues. A straightforward, closed question such as 'Have you ever been in hospital before?' may elicit numerous cues about the patient's experience in hospital. The patient's tone of voice may change, their rate of speech may accelerate or they may disclose feelings and reactions to previous hospitalisations. In this instance, the exploration triggered the cues, and the cue is a trigger for further exploration. This spiralling effect is common in effective exploration.

## Patients' questions as cues

Often patient cues come in the form of questions asked of the nurse. Patients' questions that are difficult to answer, yet require a response from the nurse, are examples of cues needing further exploration. For example:

- 'Am I going to die?'
- 'Is Dr Murthy a good surgeon?'
- 'What would you do if you were in my place?'

Questions such as these, which put nurses on the spot, are difficult to answer and are equally difficult to ignore. Perceiving patients' questions as cues for exploration is useful because this enables nurses to respond effectively. Further exploration helps to uncover what is really on the patient's mind. The first example, 'Am I going to die?', can be explored by stating, 'That's difficult for me to answer, but I am curious about the question'. This open-ended statement indicates the nurse's willingness to hear more about what the patient is experiencing. Think 'exploration' whenever patients pose questions that either have no answer or are difficult to answer. It is preferable to do this rather than ignoring the question or changing the subject, which could happen when nurses feel put on the spot and uncomfortable.

## Cue perception

Patient cues must be noticed and perceived if they are to be of use in exploration. Attending and active listening keep nurses open and receptive to cue recognition. Observing how a patient reacts and responds to the environment, and the situation at hand, is a skill in itself (see Ch 5).

Often, nurses perceive subtle communication cues from patients on the basis of a 'gut' feeling, a hunch or an intuition that the patient is trying to tell them something. Cue perception involves not only noticing how the patient is responding but also trusting a 'gut' reaction about what might be going on. In the following situation, a nursing student relates such a hunch in discussing her observations of a young man, close to her own age, who had recently become a paraplegic.

### A Student Nurse's Story

He kept joking around all morning about the MRI that was scheduled that day. I was quite comfortable with the banter because I like to joke around a lot too. He kept asking me, in a silly, almost childlike way, if I would be coming with him to 'hold his hand' when he had the procedure. Although I joked back about him being a 'big boy' now and stuff like that, I had the feeling he might have been scared about the test. I wondered how much he really understood about what was going to happen. I guess I am especially sensitive to this because, as I said, I often joke around, especially about things that are really upsetting me.

A hunch such as this is often an indication of a need, however well disguised it is by a patient. The nursing student perceived the possibility that this patient was trying to express a need by interpreting the cues he was presenting. She identified an opportunity for further exploration.

## Cue exploration: sharing perceptions

Patient cues can be explored using any of the skills described in this chapter, but one of the most effective ways to explore cues is through open-ended statements in which nurses state their own perceptions. Open-ended statements allow nurses to validate their observations and interpretations of the cue by sharing them with the patient. In the preceding scenario, an effective way for the nursing student to explore her hunch would be to say, 'Hey, all joking aside, I get the feeling you may be a bit anxious about the MRI'. This open-ended statement shares the student's perception with the patient, attempts to validate the perception and therefore opens the interaction to exploration of the cues. Open-ended exploratory statements, which share the nurse's perceptions, usually begin with:

- 'I notice that …'
- 'I get the feeling that …'
- 'I'm wondering if …'

These sentences are then completed by a concrete description of what the nurse has observed, perceived or interpreted from the patient's messages. This is an effective way to validate a cue and explore it further because it acknowledges the patient's message, encourages further discussion of the patient's experience and demonstrates the nurse's willingness to listen.

## A word of caution about sharing perceptions

The danger in exploring in this manner is that a nurse may fall into the trap of being a pseudo-psychoanalyst, always looking for hidden meanings and motives. Patients present cues in an attempt to communicate with nurses, so the question nurses must ask themselves is, 'Do I get the feeling this patient is trying to tell me something?', rather than, 'What's really behind this patient's behaviour?'. It is a subtle yet important distinction.

**ACTIVITY 7.4  Ways of exploring: questions versus statements**   **335**

### Process

1. Form pairs for this activity. The participants in a pair should not be well known to each other. Designate one person as the interviewer and the other as the interviewee. If the number of participants is uneven, form a group of three, with the third person acting as an observer.

#### Interview I

1. The interviewer is to find out as much as possible about the interviewee by asking questions only. The interviewer is not to make any statements during the interview. This interview is to last five minutes.

2. After the interview, each of the participants records a summary of the information discussed, as well as the reactions and feelings experienced during the interview. Observers (if used) record what type of information (e.g. factual, opinions, feelings) the interviewer actively solicited, as well as general impressions about the comfort level of participants in the interview.

#### Interview II

1. The interviewer and the interviewee now reverse roles. Conduct a second interview, only this time the ground rule is that no questions are to be asked

*cont.*

*Activity 7.4 continued*

during the interview. The interviewer is to learn as much as possible about the interviewee by making statements only. This interview is to last five minutes. The observer records the specific strategies used by the interviewer during the interaction.

2. After the interview, each of the participants records a summary of the information discussed, as well as reactions and feelings during the interview. Observers (if used) record the type of information that was solicited during the interview, as well as general impressions about the comfort level of participants in the interview.

3. Before proceeding to the discussion section, participant pairs should discuss their reactions to the activity with each other.

## Discussion

On a board visible to all participants, record the answers to the following discussion questions, using the grid (at Fig. 7.1) as a format.

**Discussion questions for interview I**

1. What were the reactions of the interviewer to the first interview?

2. What were the reactions of the interviewee to the first interview?

3. What kind of information was discussed during the interview? How much was learnt about the interviewee during this interview?

4. Observers (if used) report their general impressions of interview I.

**Discussion questions for interview II**

1. What were the reactions of the interviewee to the second interview?

2. What were the reactions of the interviewer to the second interview?

3. What kind of information was discussed during the interview? How much was learnt about the interviewee during the interview?

4. Observers (if used) report their general impressions of interview II.

5. What strategies were used in interview II to promote and sustain the interaction?

| | Interview I: all questions | Interview II: no questions |
|---|---|---|
| Interviewer reactions | | |
| Interviewee reactions | | |
| Type of information | | |
| Strategies used | | |

**Figure 7.1** Grid for Activity 7.4

# The difference between planned and spontaneous exploration

In both types of exploration, information is collected and greater depth of understanding is achieved, but the process is different because the roles of leader and follower are reversed. In the real world of patient care, this distinction in the types of exploration may not be obvious because there is give and take between a nurse and patient. The roles of leader and follower are continuously shifting.

Whether leading or following, nurses use similar skills and techniques, although the type and frequency of skills used may be different. For example, more questioning techniques are employed in planned exploration than in spontaneous exploration. Planned exploration, such as the formal interview, often follows a prescribed format, even if the sequence is altered; spontaneous exploration has no set format. Planned exploration aims to solicit standard information, while spontaneous exploration is more a search for meaning and for a patient–nurse relationship in which more information and feelings can be shared. The differences are highlighted in Table 7.1.

The summary of Activity 7.4 is most likely to show that the second interview (with no questions used) created more anxiety. The interviewer in these circumstances often feels uncomfortable and sometimes even selfish. Nevertheless, the type of information obtained when no questions are asked is often more personal, focused and meaningful in getting to know the interviewee. Asking no questions usually results in increased reciprocal sharing during the interview, and this eventually leads the interviewer to a greater understanding of the interviewee on a personal level. The first interview usually collects a lot of facts about the interviewee but does not really uncover subjective opinions and ideas. The first interview usually covers more breadth, while the second one covers more depth.

Questions tend to focus on collecting information and are associated with formal interviews. Exploratory statements tend to focus more on reciprocal sharing of ideas, opinions, beliefs and feelings and reflect a conversational style of interacting. Each type of exploration yields different types of information; how information is collected affects what information is gleaned.

## TABLE 7.1  Planned versus spontaneous exploration

| PLANNED EXPLORATION | SPONTANEOUS EXPLORATION |
| --- | --- |
| Directive | Responsive |
| Nurse-led | Patient-led |
| Prescribed format (usually) | No prescribed format |
| Information solicited | Meaning sought |
| Topic areas determined by the nurse | Topic areas introduced by the patient |
| More questioning techniques (probes) used | More exploratory statements (prompts) used |

# THE SKILLS OF EXPLORATION

As demonstrated in Activity 7.4, exploration can be accomplished with or without using questions. This section divides the skills of exploration into two major categories: prompting and probing. Prompting skills are exploration techniques that are statements; probing skills are exploration techniques that are questions.

# Prompting skills

Verbal prompts are a means of instigating further interaction and serve to help patients elaborate and expand on partially expressed ideas. Prompting skills include:

- minimal encouragement
- one-word/phrase accents
- gentle commands
- open-ended statements
- finishing the sentence
- self-disclosure.

## Minimal encouragement

Minimal encouragement is expressed by verbal responses such as 'uh huh', 'mm hum' and 'yes'. Often, they are utterances that are not really classified as words, yet convey messages such as 'I'm with you', 'I'm following what you are saying' and 'I want to hear more'. They are signals that acknowledge the patient's verbalisation and encourage further elaboration. Visualise a person on the telephone who keeps repeating 'yes' and 'uh huh'. Although you cannot hear the person on the other end of the line, you can ascertain that the person is encouraging the other person to carry on the conversation. A person talking on the telephone uses minimal encouragement extensively because non-verbal messages are limited. In face-to-face communication, minimal encouragement reinforces attentive listening but is not really a substitute for it. Attentive and active listening (see Ch 5) is, in itself, an effective prompt because it conveys messages similar to those of minimal encouragement.

Sometimes minimal encouragement is used without conscious awareness, even when active listening is absent. If this is the case, the verbal and non-verbal messages are incongruent. Because of this incongruence, minimal encouragement, without attentive listening, probably would not prompt further interaction. Try it in a conversation. Keep uttering 'uh huh' while not really attending and listening to the other person. Eventually, the person speaking to you either gives up or says, 'Hey, you're not listening to me!'.

Minimal encouragement works best when patients are willing and able to continue the interaction. When patients are having difficulty verbalising their experiences, more explicit prompting and probing techniques need to be employed.

## One-word/phrase accents

One-word/phrase accents are the repetition of key words or phrases and are an effective way to both extend and focus the interaction. The choice of which word or phrase to repeat is important because it determines the direction of the exploration; it becomes the focus. It is best to repeat words or phrases that are judged to be the most central or critical. The following example illustrates the uses of accents:

Patient: *My son won't be visiting me while I'm here in hospital.*

Nurse: *Won't be visiting?*

Patient: *Yes, he says he can't stand the sights and smells of the hospital.*

Notice how the accent encourages the patient to expand the initial comment. Nurses effectively use the accent to explore what they perceive to be the most significant part of the patient's statement. Had the nurse repeated the words 'your son?', the interaction may have taken a different direction. In this regard, one-word/phrase accents are controlled by the nurse, although they are always in response to what the patient has said. If a patient does not elaborate, a nurse should follow the patient's lead and end the discussion.

## Gentle commands

Gentle commands are explicit requests for information or elaboration. Although specific topics are often introduced with gentle commands, they are open-ended because they allow the patient to determine the direction and flow of the response. Examples of gentle commands include:

- 'Tell me about your family.'
- 'Can you describe that in more detail?'
- 'Tell me more.'
- 'Let's talk about that further.'
- 'Tell me what it's like for you to be in hospital.'
- 'Go on, say what's on your mind.'

In response to the first example, 'Tell me about your family', patients can choose whatever they wish to share about their family. One patient could say how many children they have, while another may focus on relationships with their extended family. The gentle command is directive in one sense, yet allows the patient to control the direction in another sense.

Gentle commands should always be said in a way that allows patients to maintain a sense of control; they should not be demands. Although the idea of commanding patients to tell the nurse something sounds a bit harsh, the qualifier 'gentle' must not be forgotten. 'Gentle' means that the command is stated as an interested request for more information rather than an order to speak. The qualifying phrase 'Can you?' is often placed before the command for this reason. 'Can you tell me about your family?' sounds less harsh than 'Tell me about your family'. Technically, the addition of 'Can you?' turns the statement into a closed question, and a patient can simply respond 'yes' or 'no' without any further elaboration. In general, this does not happen because the underlying message that the nurse wants to hear more than a simple 'yes' or 'no' is generally understood by most patients.

The gentleness of the command is conveyed primarily through non-verbal messages. Practise a few of the examples cited, using a variety of vocal tones and facial expressions, and include the qualifier 'Can you?' at the beginning of the statement. Note that the words can sound harsh if said in a controlling, demanding manner. Nevertheless, if gentleness is put into the tone and facial expression, such commands are quite effective in exploring patients' experiences.

## Open-ended statements

Open-ended statements provide a broad introduction to topics for discussion and are sometimes referred to as 'indirect questions'. They indicate to a patient that the nurse would like to hear more about something and provide an open invitation for the patient to speak about a topic. Examples of open-ended statements include:

- 'So, this is the first time you are having surgery.'
- 'I wonder how it is being sick when you've been so healthy all of your life.'
- 'I hear from your family that you are quite the athlete.'
- 'You've been giving yourself insulin injections for a few years now.'

It is clear from these examples that the nurse making the statement is interested in hearing more about the topic that is introduced. Open-ended statements are invitations to patients to say more, if they choose to accept the invitation. In this way, open-ended statements are similar to gentle commands because they allow the patient to determine the direction and depth of the interaction. Open-ended statements are often a good way to begin an interaction because they introduce a topic but still allow the interaction to take various directions. While they introduce a topic, they do not control the direction of the conversation.

## Finishing the sentence

This exploration technique is similar to open-ended statements. Instead of completing a sentence, the nurse begins it, then trails off with an expectation that the patient will finish the sentence. Examples of finishing the sentence include:

- 'So you're most worried about …'
- 'And when you are in pain you usually …'
- 'Today has been …'
- 'What you really would like to know is …'

To be effective, finishing the sentence relies heavily on an inquisitive, anticipatory facial expression that lets the patient know that the nurse has not had a lapse in memory or become preoccupied with other thoughts or activities. The non-verbal message, conveyed through facial expression and body posture, communicates that the nurse is waiting for the patient to complete the sentence.

## Self-disclosure

Sometimes the most effective way to encourage patients to explore their experiences with nurses is for nurses to share their own thoughts. Through self-disclosure, nurses open an area for exploration by stating their own reactions, feelings or thoughts. Self-disclosure must always be honest. There is little point in nurses fabricating information about themselves in an attempt to make patients open up. Self-disclosure is not the same as giving an opinion or a valuative judgment. Examples of self-disclosure as an exploration technique include:

- 'If I were in your place, I'd be angry.'
- 'I don't handle pain all that well.'
- 'If it were me I'd be wondering what was wrong.'

Self-disclosure lets the patient know that the nurse is not afraid to be open. When used in the context of exploration, it serves as a trigger for the patient to expand and elaborate because it creates a climate of safety.

It works well as an exploration technique with patients who seem reluctant to reveal themselves. While self-disclosure is utilised here as a means of encouraging exploration, a complete discussion of it can be found in Chapter 8.

# Probing skills

Probing skills are the techniques associated with asking questions. Carefully worded and well-timed questions frequently provide the backbone of effective exploration and interviewing. Questions come in different varieties, yielding different responses and taking the interaction in different directions, depending on the type used. Both planned and spontaneous explorations combine the various types of questions. There are two major types of probing skills: open-ended questions and closed questions. Closed questions have two subtypes, which are particularly relevant to exploration within the nursing context: focused and multiple-choice questions.

## Open-ended questions

Open-ended questions are those that require more than a one-word response (such as 'yes' or 'no'), thereby encouraging more elaboration in the answer. Examples of open-ended questions include:

- 'How well did the medication control your pain during the night?'
- 'What concerns you most about the surgery?'
- 'What types of food do you enjoy eating?'
- 'What happened when you visited the outpatient department?'

Open-ended questions begin with interrogative words such as who, what, when, where, why and how. Not all questions beginning with these words are open-ended. For example, 'Where do you live?' is a closed question, while 'Where do you see yourself in five years' time?' is an open-ended question. Questions that are open-ended often yield more information than closed questions because their replies include more detailed expansion and elaboration. Additionally, open-ended questions allow more flexibility in response than closed questions. In answering open-ended questions, patients can highlight what is most relevant to their experience and therefore retain a sense of control in the interaction. Nevertheless, an open-ended question, no matter how well-stated, can pressure patients to disclose personal matters before they feel trusting enough to share their inner experiences. Because open-ended questions often probe more deeply than closed ones, nurses need to be mindful about the level of trust established before delving too deeply into the patient's experience.

## Closed questions

Closed questions are those that are usually answered with a simple 'yes', 'no' or other one-word response. They control the direction of the conversation and limit the amount of information that is shared or obtained. If closed questions are overused, an interaction begins to resemble an interrogation and can result in a patient feeling put on the spot because, short of refusing to answer or lying, the patient often feels obliged to answer direct questions posed by a nurse. Examples of closed questions include:

- 'Have you been in hospital before?'
- 'Do you wear eye glasses?'
- 'Is your wife coming to visit you tonight?'
- 'Do you have any children?'
- 'When did you last have something to eat?'

## *Focused, closed questions*

At times it is necessary for nurses to ask closed questions that are focused and directed at obtaining information about a specific clinical situation. These questions are based on the nurse's clinical knowledge and experience. Without them, important and even vital information may be missed. Examples of focused, closed questions include:

- 'Are you feeling nauseous?' (to a patient recovering from anaesthesia)
- 'Do you ever feel dizzy when you get out of bed quickly?' (to a patient whose blood pressure is low)
- 'Is your mouth dry?' (to a patient taking medication that produces a dry mouth as a side effect).

Each of these examples is a closed, focused question that is appropriate under the circumstances. The trigger for these closed questions is the nurse's awareness and understanding of what is pertinent to explore in a given clinical situation. Patients may not recognise the significance of their clinical symptoms and therefore feel reassured by such questions. An open-ended question may not yield the information needed or reveal progress in a particular direction.

## *Multiple-choice questions*

Multiple-choice questions are another form of specific, closed questioning that is based on the nurse's understanding of a particular clinical phenomenon. In multiple-choice questions, the nurse provides options to the patient in an attempt to obtain an answer to the question, 'Which of these is correct?' A good example is when a nurse tries to obtain a complete description of a patient's pain. An open-ended question such as 'How does the pain feel?' or even 'How would you describe the pain?' is often met with responses such as 'It feels like pain; it hurts' or 'I don't know, pain just feels like pain'. A multiple-choice question is helpful under such circumstances. In posing a multiple-choice question, the nurse asks, 'Is the pain burning, grabbing, crushing, pinpoint, dull or sharp?' This type of questioning about pain yields specific information about the nature of the patient's pain. In the example provided, the nurse uses knowledge of the various types of pain to focus and direct the exploration.

### ACTIVITY 7.5  Converting probes into prompts

**Process**

Questions (probes) are often overused as a means of exploration. This activity challenges participants to turn closed questions into exploratory statements (prompts). Table 7.2 demonstrates how this is accomplished.

1. Make a list of closed questions pertinent to the nursing context. Divide a piece of paper into three columns and place the closed questions down the left column.

2. Convert each of these questions into an exploratory statement by first making the closed question into an open-ended one. Place these in the middle column of the page.

3. Now convert the open-ended question into an exploratory statement or a prompt. Place these in the right-hand column.

**Discussion**

1. Which of your closed questions were easy to convert to exploratory statements? Which were difficult? Were there any you found impossible to convert?

2. Review each of the exploratory statements and discuss how making a statement instead of asking a question would alter the interaction between a nurse and a patient.

3. Would you obtain different information from an exploratory statement? If so, is the information obtained more relevant?

4. Which of the exploratory statements seem appropriate to the topic being discussed? Do any seem inappropriate or foolish?

5. Can you imagine yourself using the exploratory statements? Why? Why not?

| | TABLE 7.2 Converting probes into prompts | |
|---|---|---|
| **CLOSED QUESTION** | **OPEN-ENDED QUESTION** | **EXPLORATORY STATEMENT (PROMPT)** |
| Are you feeling all right? | How are you feeling? | Tell me how you are feeling. |
| Will it help to make you more comfortable if I rearrange your pillows? | What would help you to be more comfortable in the bed? | Perhaps if I rearrange your pillow, you'll be more comfortable. |
| Did that medication help to relieve your pain? | How did that medication help in relieving your pain? | You had your pain medication 30 minutes ago, I see. |
| Do you want your sponge now? | When would you like your sponge? | You can have your sponge now or later. |
| Would it help if I stayed with you a while? | How would you feel if I stayed with you a while? | Perhaps if I stayed with you a while, it would help. |

## Open-ended versus closed questions

As a general rule, using open-ended questions is more effective as an exploration technique than using closed questions because responses to open-ended questions are more elaborate and encourage expansion of ideas. They also allow the patient to direct the interaction and therefore a nurse who asks an open-ended question is likely to hear what is most significant to the patient at the time.

Does this mean that closed questions should be avoided? Not necessarily, because closed questions have a legitimate place in the context of patient–nurse interaction. The choice between open-ended and closed questions depends on what information is being sought, who is seeking it, who is being asked, in which context and to what end. In making the decision to use one type or the other, nurses must consider their relationship with the patient as well as the need for specific information. For example, when a nurse wants to know whether a patient can tolerate aspirin, they might begin by asking, 'Have you ever used aspirin?' Then, if the answer is affirmative, questions such as 'How much?', 'How often?', 'For what reason?' and 'What effects were noted?' may follow. Asking open-ended questions such as 'How do you experience aspirin?' or 'What do you think about aspirin?' are nonsensical and inappropriate to the content being explored and the information required.

On the other hand, a question such as 'How was your first pregnancy?' is appropriate in exploring an experience as personal and unique as pregnancy. Nevertheless, questions such as 'How do you feel about being pregnant?' probe too deeply if the patient and nurse have not yet established a trusting relationship. Questions need to probe at a depth that is appropriate to the level of trust between the patient and the nurse.

The decision about which type of question to use should be based on an understanding of each type of questioning. Table 7.3 compares the two types of question and provides useful guidelines for the selection.

If the open-ended type is selected as more suitable, the next choice is which open-ended question is best, given the circumstances. In most instances, questions

## TABLE 7.3 Comparison of open-ended and closed questions

| OPEN-ENDED QUESTIONS | CLOSED QUESTIONS |
| --- | --- |
| Yield information and facilitate elaboration | Yield information and limit elaboration |
| Allow a patient to determine the direction of the interactions | Focus a patient in one direction |
| May not be useful when specific information is required | Are useful in obtaining specific information |
| Probe subjective experiences and may threaten a patient if trust is not established | Maintain interpersonal safety by keeping the interaction on a less-personal level |

## SCENARIO

Nurse: *Have you ever had surgery before?* [Closed]

Patient: *Yes, once before.*

Nurse: *What happened that you needed surgery?* [Open]

Patient: *I had my appendix removed when I was 10 years old.*

Nurse: *Were you in hospital?* [Closed]

Patient: *Yes.*

Nurse: *How was that hospitalisation?* [Open]

Patient: *Fine, the nurses were great, my mum was with me the whole time and I don't remember being in any pain.*

Nurse: *So, you have good memories of that?* [Closed]

Patient: *Yes.*

Nurse: *What do you expect will happen this time in hospital?* [Open]

Patient: *Well, I am a lot older, so my mum won't be here the whole time. I'm a bit worried about the pain.*

Nurse: *What worries you most?* [Open]

Patient: *That nobody will be able to help me with the pain ... I'm a bit of a baby.*

Nurse: *You will have a patient-controlled device so you can have pain medication when you need it, and the nurses are here to make sure you are not in pain. You do realise that.* [Closed]

Patient: *Yes, I guess ... but I don't know what you will do to help.*

beginning with 'who', 'what', 'where' and 'when' yield factual, objective data, while questions beginning with 'how' yield more personal, subjective information. For example, 'What surgery did you have in 1998?' will yield a factual answer such as 'I had my appendix removed'. If this is followed by a question such as 'And how was that surgery?', exploration of the patient's subjective experience of the surgery is achieved. This general guideline is not a hard-and-fast rule. For example, 'What were your feelings about the surgery?' is a question that probes on a personal level. The focus of the question is as important as its type.

The most effective exploration will include a combination of both open and closed questions, as illustrated in the following interaction.

Notice how, in this interview, the nurse moves between closed and open-ended questioning and each question is appropriate to the content and the purpose of the interview. During the interaction, the nurse gathers objective data (previous experience with surgery) as well as subjective data (the patient's personal experience of the surgery). Open and closed questions are not inherently good or bad because their 'goodness' or 'badness' depends on what information is being sought, and for what reason.

## Pitfalls of using probing skills

Despite the fact that questions are neither good nor bad within themselves, there are some common pitfalls in using questioning, including some types of question that are best avoided altogether. Common pitfalls include overuse of questions, continuous multiple questions, the 'why' question and the leading question.

### Overuse of questions

The most common pitfall in probing is the overuse of questions. Asking too many questions during an interaction can interrupt and confuse the patient. Overuse of questions runs the risk of continually shifting the focus of the interaction. Additionally, it has the potential to convey the message that the nurse is in an overbearing position of authority. In order to be effective, questions need to be mixed with exploratory, prompting statements.

### Continuous multiple questions

Another pitfall in questioning is using multiple questions, asked in succession, without allowing time for a reply from the patient. For example, 'How did you sleep last night? Did the sleeping tablet help? Was there too much noise?' While this manner of questioning sounds a bit ridiculous, it does occur in patient–nurse interactions. Asking multiple questions in succession is counterproductive to the exploration process. If a question is asked, the nurse needs to ensure that enough time is allowed for the patient to respond before proceeding.

### The 'why' question

The 'why' question is a tricky one because often in the nursing context the answer to why needs to be sought. 'Why does Mr Ahmad experience so much pain, even after maximum pain relief is administered?' 'Why is Ms Wu having so much difficulty breastfeeding her baby?' Although it is important to uncover the reasons for such occurrences, asking the question 'why?' directly of patients can have a negative impact, and may not be the most effective way to find the answer. This is partly due to the fact that the question 'why?' often creates anxiety and a defensive reaction. It implies that patients have to justify and explain their actions and feelings, or that something is not right about their actions and feelings.

Imagine you are about to administer a medication to a patient and another nurse approaches you and asks, 'Why are you giving that medication now?'. Your internal reaction may range from, 'What's it to you?' to 'Oh no, maybe I've made a mistake!'. Perhaps your colleague just wants to know if the patient receiving the medication is still experiencing pain. Somehow, your reaction to the 'why' question does not acknowledge such a well-intentioned motive on your colleague's part. Instead, you become defensive or anxious.

The reaction to a 'why' question is often defensive because the question has a way of sounding like a negative evaluation. This may be due to experiences in childhood, such as when Mum asked, 'Why did you spill the milk on the floor?' as she stands there, hands on hips, looking and sounding quite cross. It quickly becomes apparent to the child that Mum is not the least bit interested in why the milk was spilt. (Does she want an explanation about gravitational force?) The message conveyed by the 'why' question in this instance is, 'Don't do it again; I get cross when milk is spilt'. This possible socialisation as to the interpretation of the 'why' question, and the potential defensiveness produced by it, are reasons for avoiding its use in patient–nurse interactions.

Frequently, the 'why' question is asked in an attempt to explore feelings; for example, 'Why do you feel sad, Kate?'. The use of the 'why' question in this instance assumes that Kate knows why she feels sad and that these feelings have a rational basis. Patients often do not know why they feel a certain way but may think they need to justify or rationally explain their feelings when asked 'why?'. Again, the reaction may be a defensive one – a justification of feelings. In general, it is best to avoid the 'why' question altogether. It is often counterproductive to exploration because of its potential to close off further interaction.

## *The leading question*

Another type of question to avoid is the 'leading' question. Leading questions are not exploratory but rhetorical because they have an implied answer and are often designed to confirm what nurses think they already know. Examples of leading questions include:

- 'You're all right, aren't you?'
- 'Why don't you just cooperate with us?'
- 'Are you really going to ring the doctor at this hour of the night?'
- 'Is your anger really justified?'

## ACTIVITY 7.6 Alternatives to 'why'

### Process

The following patient statements have the potential to elicit a 'why' question from nurses. Read each and record an alternative to 'why'.

1. Patient (who has been on renal dialysis for a long time and is awaiting a renal transplant): 'I want to stop dialysis.'

2. Patient (who is awaiting results of diagnostic tests): 'I had a really bad night's sleep because I'm so worried.'

3. Patient (who is a recently arrived resident of a nursing home): 'How would you like being stuck in here? I hate this place and just want to die.'

4. Patient (who has recently undergone coronary artery bypass surgery): 'I really thought I was going to die this morning.'

5. Patient (who has been told she should have a hysterectomy): 'I can't possibly spare the time to have this operation.'

### Discussion

1. Did you find you were tempted to ask 'why?' in response to each statement?

2. Review your alternatives to the 'why' question. Are any of them 'why?' in disguise (e.g. 'How come?' or 'What makes you feel that way?').

3. What type of exploratory response did you develop? Are any of the responses exploratory statements?

4. Compare your responses with those of other participants. How much variety exists between the responses?

5. Try to use some of your responses with other participants playing the role of the patient. Ask the person who is playing the patient to describe the effects of each response.

- 'What's making you so hard to get along with?'
- 'You really don't want any more medication, do you?'

Leading questions are not really questions at all. They are statements in disguise, 'dressed up' to look like questions. Like the 'why' question, they have a tendency to put the other person on the defensive because they usually contain a value judgment. It is far better to make a statement than to pretend to want an answer to a question that does not really have one. Review the previous examples of leading questions, turn them into statements and note the difference.

## ACTIVITY 7.7 Recognising types of questions  335

**Process**

Classify each question according to its type, using the following key:

    A  closed question

    B  open-ended question

    C  leading question

    D  disguised 'why' question.

1. What makes you feel scared?
2. How are you feeling today?
3. What is your doctor's name?
4. Do you really enjoy drinking heavily?
5. When does your pain get worse?
6. Are you interested in seeing a volunteer from Alcoholics Anonymous?
7. What are your reasons for refusing your medication?
8. What kind of nurse do you think I am?
9. You really don't want any more pain medication, do you?
10. What did the doctor say?
11. Did that medication help with the nausea?
12. How do you like your breakfast tray to be arranged?
13. How did you go with physiotherapy today?
14. What makes you say that?
15. How old are your children?
16. How was the visit with your family last night?
17. Did you sleep well after having the sleeping tablet?
18. When are you going to stop bothering the other patients?
19. Are you worried about having sex after your heart surgery?
20. Don't you think you had better try to stick to your diet this time?
21. How do you usually manage your diabetic diet?
22. Are you still hurting your baby by smoking while you are pregnant?
23. What would help you to be more comfortable?

(Note: The answers to this activity can be found at the end of this chapter.)

# FOCUSED EXPLORATION

The skills of exploration can be employed effectively in the process of focusing an interaction between a patient and a nurse. The process of focused exploration deepens the nurse's general understanding of the patient's experience by concentrating on a specific aspect. This process of focusing is sometimes referred to as 'funnelling' because of the way in which it continues to narrow the topic being explored. Any of the various exploration skills identified can be employed in the process of focusing. The following interaction, from a postpartum maternity ward, is an illustration of focusing.

## SCENARIO

Nurse: *How are you today?* [Open-ended question]

Patient: *Okay, I guess.*

Nurse: *You guess?* [One-word accent]

Patient: *I didn't sleep very well last night.*

Nurse: Couldn't *sleep?* [One-word/phrase accent]

Patient: *No, I kept worrying about my baby.*

Nurse: *What, in particular, was worrying you?* [Open-ended question]

Patient: *The paediatrician was here last night to examine him and he noticed his high-pitched cry.*

Nurse: *And?* [Minimal encouragement]

Patient: *Well, the doctor said it was probably nothing to worry about because it was most likely due to some swelling in my son's brain as a result of the labour. I was in second stage for a long time, you know.*

Nurse: *Yes, it might clear up in a few days. I have seen babies with that cry before and it was due to temporary swelling that went away after a few days. But it doesn't really stop the worry just because you know it might be nothing.* [Open-ended statement]

Patient: *What is most worrying is that the doctor said it could be a sign of brain damage.*

Nurse: *And that's what has you most worried?* [One-word/phrase accent]

Patient: *Yes. I kept asking the doctor what else besides temporary swelling could be causing the cry. Now I'm sorry I asked. I might have been better off not knowing. There's nothing I can do now but worry and wait.*

Notice how the nurse in this interaction begins broadly then keeps focusing and narrowing the conversation. This is accomplished through using a variety of exploration skills. The nurse chose to focus on what she perceived to be the most significant aspect of the patient's messages. The focusing process serves to highlight and elaborate on a particular topic.

---

### ACTIVITY 7.8  Developing exploratory responses (II)

**Process**

1. Refer to your responses in Activity 7.1: 'Developing exploratory responses (I)'. Label each of your responses according to the skills outlined in this chapter. You may have used more than one type of exploratory response.

2. Determine if you have a tendency to use one type of exploratory response in preference to the other types.

3. If you tend to ask closed questions, make these open-ended.

4. Do any of your questions begin with 'why'? If so, find an alternative.

5. Turn your exploratory questions into exploratory statements. What possible effects would these changes have on the interaction with the patient in the situation?

---

# NURSES' CONTROL IN EXPLORATION

Previously in this chapter, planned exploration was differentiated from spontaneous exploration. In planned exploration, the nurse leads and takes charge of the direction and focus of an interaction. In spontaneous exploration, the nurse follows the patient's lead, usually through clarifying and probing patient cues. The same skills are used in both types of exploration, although not to the same extent. For example, closed questions may be more prevalent when the nurse is leading, and one-word/phrase accents may be more prevalent when the nurse is following.

At the heart of the difference between spontaneous and planned exploration is the notion of who is in control. Control in the context of patient–nurse interaction refers to who dominates in determining the flow of information exchange. When the patient is in control, they dominate. The reverse is true when the nurse controls the interaction. Ideally, a balance is achieved when both the patient and the nurse share control of interactions.

In order for this ideal balance to occur, nurses need to be alert to the cues of patients and to be able to follow the patient's lead. Likewise, nurses will at times control the interaction when they are obtaining specific information. Self-aware nurses who reflect on their interactions will notice whether they tend to be controlling in their interactions.

## ACTIVITY 7.9  Patient interview  335

### Process

1.  Each participant is to obtain a blank nursing history form from a healthcare agency. Review the form and determine the most appropriate way to explore each area with a patient.

2.  Form groups of three and designate one person as A, another as B and the third as C.

3.  A conducts a nursing history interview, with B acting in the role of a patient. C acts as an observer. A informs B about the setting and the circumstances of the patient interview. C records the types of exploratory skills used by A during the interview by keeping a record of the name of each skill used.

4.  C now interviews A, who plays the role of a patient. B is now the observer. Continue as per the instructions in step 3.

5.  B now interviews person C, who plays the role of a patient. A is now the observer. Continue as per instructions in step 3.

### Discussion

1.  What types of exploratory skills were used during the interviews? Were some types used more frequently than others?

2.  Were there areas of the nursing history that lent themselves to using a certain skill more than other areas? If so, what were these areas? Which skills seemed most appropriate for these areas?

3.  How did it feel when you were in the role of the patient? Did you think you had enough opportunity to tell your story? Did you think the nurse got to know you as a person during the interview?

4.  When you were the nurse, what was easy to explore? What was difficult? Were there any areas you thought were not covered adequately? How well did you come to understand the patient during the interview? What would you change in the interview if you had the opportunity?

5.  What generalisations can be made from the activity in terms of conducting interviews between patients and nurses?

# SUMMARY

The process of exploration is one of the most important aspects of patient–nurse interaction because it not only provides the means by which information is obtained but demonstrates the nurse's active regard for understanding the patient's experience. During planned exploration, nurses focus on what is most significant for them to know about patients. During spontaneous exploration, nurses focus on what is most significant to the patient at the time. Both types of exploration require the use of effective questioning (probes) and exploratory statements (prompts). When used in conjunction with other interpersonal skills, exploration helps to shape effective and facilitative patient–nurse interactions and leads to greater understanding.

# REFERENCES

Brandes, K., Linn, A.J., Smit, E.G., et al., 2015. Patients' reports of barriers to expressing concerns during cancer consultations. Patient Educ. Couns. 98, 317–322.

Chan, E.A., 2014. Cue-responding during simulated routine nursing care: a mixed method study. Nurse Educ. Today 34, 1057–1061.

de Leeuw, J., Prins, J.B., Uitterhoeve, R., et al., 2014. Nurse-patient communication in follow-up consultations after head and neck cancer treatment. Cancer Nurs. 37 (2), E1–E9.

Finset, A., Heyn, L., Ruland, C., 2013. Patterns in clinician responses to patient emotion in cancer care. Patient Educ. Couns. 93, 80–85.

Griep, E.C.M., Noordman, J., Vandulmen, S., 2016. Practice nurses mental health provide space to patients to discuss unpleasant emotions. J. Psychiatr. Ment. Health Nurs. 23, 77–85.

Grimsbø, G.H., Ruland, C.M., Finset, A., 2012. Cancer patients' expressions of emotional cues and concerns and oncology nurses' responses, in an online patient–nurse communication service. Patient Educ. Couns. 88, 36–43.

Sheldon, L.K., Hilaire, D., Berry, D.L., 2011. Provider verbal responses to patient distress cues during ambulatory oncology visits. Oncol. Nurs. Forum 38 (3), 369–375.

Zimmermann, C., Del Piccolo, L., Finset, A., 2007. Cues and concerns by patients in medical consultations: a literature review. Psychol. Bull. 133, 438–463.

# ANSWERS TO ACTIVITIES

## Activity 7.3: cues and inferences

1   Cue – Answered interview questions completely.
2   Inference – Uninterested in the interview.
3   Cue – Changed the topic when asked about her family.
4   Inference – An open person.
5   Cue – Sleeping quietly.
6   Cue – Shallow, rapid respirations.
7   Inference – Doesn't understand prescribed medications.
8   Cue – Keeps asking questions about diagnostic tests.
9   Cue – No eye contact during the interview.
10  Cue – Speech is pressured.
11  Cue – Puzzled expression on his face when I asked him about the surgery.
12  Inference – Doesn't know what to expect.
13  Cue – No visible signs of distress.

## Activity 7.7: recognising types of questions

KEY:
A    closed question
B    open-ended question

C    leading question

D    a disguised 'why' question

1    D – What makes you feel scared?

2    B – How are you feeling today?

3    A – What is your doctor's name?

4    C – Do you really enjoy drinking heavily?

5    B – When does your pain get worse?

6    A – Are you interested in seeing a volunteer from Alcoholics Anonymous?

7    D – What are your reasons for refusing your medication?

8    C – What kind of nurse do you think I am?

9    C – You really don't want any more pain medication, do you?

10   B – What did the doctor say?

11   A – Did that medication help with the nausea?

12   B – How do you like your breakfast tray to be arranged?

13   B – How did you go with physiotherapy today?

14   D – What makes you say that?

15   A – How old are your children?

16   B – How was the visit with your family last night?

17   A – Did you sleep well after having the sleeping tablet?

18   C – When are you going to stop bothering the other patients?

19   A – Are you worried about having sex after your heart surgery?

20   C – Don't you think you had better try to stick to your diet this time?

21   B – How do you usually manage your diabetic diet?

22   C – Are you still hurting your baby by smoking while you are pregnant?

23   B – What would help you to be more comfortable?

# 8

# Intervening: comforting, supporting and enabling

## CHAPTER OVERVIEW

- Nurses need to take action beyond listening, exploring and understanding.
- These actions are psychosocial in nature because they are enacted through the patient–nurse relationship.
- These psychosocial actions are grouped into three major areas: comforting, supporting and enabling.
- The primary comforting action is the skill of reassuring patients.
- Supporting actions promote patients' use of resources.
- Enabling actions are aimed at encouraging patients to actively participate in their own care, primarily through sharing information and providing explanations to patients.
- Challenging and self-disclosure are two further examples of enabling actions.

Visit the Evolve site for video content to support the themes and skills explored in this chapter: http://evolve.elsevier.com/AU/Stein-Parbury/patient/

# INTRODUCTION

The material in the previous chapters has laid a theoretical foundation and a practical framework for establishing effective patient–nurse relationships. Thus far, this book has alluded to how nurses take direct action in helping patients, but active intervention has not been fully explained. In fact, moving too quickly into action has been shown to be inappropriate in the absence of a relationship based on understanding. Focusing prematurely on action, intervention and outcome has the potential to stifle a nurse's understanding and appreciation of a patient's current experience.

There is inherent danger in taking action without first understanding a patient's unique orientation to the world. Interventions cannot be applied in a context-free manner, selected from a list of options like one selects a recipe from a cookbook. Such non-specific, potentially hit-and-miss approaches can actually do more harm than good. For example, enabling patients to participate in their care by sharing information is most effective if nurses first determine how much information a patient wants and can use.

This suggestion, to initially curtail direct intervention, may prove frustrating to some nurses because a felt need to do something often overrides the need to understand the patient's experience from the patient's perspective. Time is a precious commodity in nursing practice, and the time spent in coming to understand patients' experiences may be perceived as a luxury. Nevertheless, the time and effort expended in coming to understand the patient's frame of reference are well spent because actions, which direct and influence patients, are then based on such understandings.

# PSYCHOSOCIAL ACTIONS THAT COMFORT, SUPPORT AND ENABLE

Often nursing actions are aimed at physical care and treatment of a disease (e.g. administering medication to provide physical relief from pain), and technical competence is perceived by patients as caring (see Ch 2). But nursing actions are also psychosocial in nature. Psychosocial actions are aimed at promoting psychological ease and relief of distress (e.g. through explanations that orient patients to what is happening around them). While physical and psychosocial actions are inextricably linked in nursing practice, this chapter focuses on psychosocial nursing actions that promote health and healing in patients and are accomplished through the patient–nurse relationship.

## Indications of the need for psychosocial action

When listening and understanding, nurses are guided by patients. When taking psychosocial action, nurses assume a more active role in guiding patients. This does not mean that a nurse takes charge and control of a patient's life but intervenes in a way that encourages the patient to assume as much control as possible. For example, when an understanding is reached that a patient is facing a decision, the nurse takes action to help the patient make the decision rather than taking over and making the decision for the patient. Actions that are psychosocial in nature are liberating, not restrictive, and they always work from within the patient's experience.

Taking action is based on indications that it is needed. The following list includes examples of patient situations that indicate a need to intervene directly. Psychosocial action may be required when patients are either:

- in need of more information
- emotionally distressed (e.g. feeling overwhelmed)
- facing a health-related decision
- learning new skills
- lacking in available resources
- inadequately using existing resources, or
- experiencing difficulties in coping, adjusting and adapting.

## Patient outcomes

Psychosocial nursing actions of comforting, supporting and enabling are focused on outcomes and resources. When nurses employ these actions, they do so with the deliberate intention of producing positive changes or reinforcing adaptive ones in patients. While the desired outcome may not always be directly observable and measurable, action is taken for a focused purpose. Some examples of desired outcomes include helping patients to:

- adjust and adapt to changes in living imposed by illness
- maintain self-esteem
- find meaning in illness
- feel secure and in control
- contain and control emotional distress within manageable limits
- make decisions about healthcare
- access and use helpful resources.

Outcomes are based on the indication of a need for action. For example, the indication that a patient is emotionally distressed calls for an outcome of containing and controlling that distress within manageable limits. Not only is it important for nurses to relate desired outcome to patient need but, more importantly, nurses must work with patients in determining needs and outcomes from the patients' perspective.

## Patient resources

Psychosocial nursing actions are most effective when nurses work with patients' natural resources, their capabilities and means for coming to terms with health-related and illness-related issues. Some actions work with a patient's existing resources, while others focus on identifying, developing and using new or unused resources. It is important for nurses to understand the patient's resources. Examples of resources include: the patient's knowledge, will, desire, strength and courage; family members and friends; other patients; self-help groups; and health services and providers. Possible resources are endless for some patients, and quite limited for others. Essential to using a patient's resources is the recognition and acknowledgement that nurses themselves are but one, usually temporary, resource in helping patients. Nurses must look to longer term resources, basing their outlook on the belief that patients are themselves resourceful and capable.

Often there are times when patients are vulnerable and uncertain (see Ch 9) and are in need of responses from nurses that provide comfort and reassurance to enable them to actively participate in their care.

# COMFORTING

Comforting is associated with relief from distress and pain, easing anxiety and rising above and beyond problems (Kolcaba 2017). To be comfortable is associated with being relaxed, contented, and free from pain and anxiety. Providing comfort to patients was considered by Nightingale (1859) to be a primary goal in nursing care, as comfort is a central aspect of healing. Many years later Morse (1992) urged nurses to reconsider the claim that caring is the essence of nursing (see Ch 1) and refocus nursing to the concept of comfort. She argued that caring focuses on what the nurse does, while comfort focuses on the patient. Caring is process-oriented and is the motivation for nursing actions. Comfort is outcome-oriented and is the aim of nursing actions. Caring is *why* nurses act; comforting is *how* they act.

Morse's argument is compelling in the sense that it offers nurses a focus of care that can be described through practices that comfort patients. Caring is more nebulous in the sense that it offers little in the way of clear guidelines for clinical performance, especially for beginning nurses. Because comfort focuses on outcomes rather than process, it offers a framework for nursing action. Comfort represents what patients want and need and what nurses want to provide, as it increases job satisfaction (Boudiab & Kolcaba 2015).

While providing comfort is mostly associated with physical care, such as pain relief and end-of-life care, it is now recognised that comforting goes beyond these circumstances (Oliveira 2013; Pinto et al 2016). Comforting also eases patient anxiety, assists in tolerating uncertainty and enhances general wellbeing. Comforting also involves providing reassurance and emotional, informational and social support.

When nurses' responses are comforting they express a sense of concern for the patient, demonstrated through being unhurried, making eye contact and using a soothing tone of voice. Research has demonstrated that patients are in a state of comfort when they feel secure in the knowledge that nurses are competent, and assistance is available. In addition, patients are comforted by information.

Perhaps most importantly, patients are comforted when they feel valued and can establish connected relationships with nurses (Williams et al 2011).

All the skills in this chapter could be subsumed under the umbrella of the comforting strategies that have been explicated through research; this reinforces the centrality of comforting in nursing. Nevertheless, for the purpose of simplicity and clarity, reassurance is the main skill that is fully developed as a comforting action. Supporting is another comforting action, which is described in a separate section. Other skills, such as informing and challenging, are developed under the umbrella of enabling patients to participate in care.

# Reassuring patients

Reassuring patients is a common nursing activity, often cited as a planned, purposeful intervention in nursing care. But how is reassurance actually offered and provided by nurses? Under what circumstances is it indicated? How can reassurance be engaging and not dismissive of patients? Unless the answers to these questions are clearly thought through and understood, there is a danger that reassurance will be oversimplified as nothing more than a natural human response. They are not really natural but are culturally conditioned. Sometimes cultural conditioning will result in a reassuring action that is not focused on the patient but protective of the nurse. This is false reassurance.

## False reassurance

In everyday social situations, reassurance is frequently offered in the form of trite, trivial clichés and platitudes, repeated so often that they have lost their meaning. Ready-made comments such as 'Everything will work out', 'Don't worry' and 'It will be all right' are uttered in an almost automatic, stereotypical manner. These types of 'reassuring' response were presented in Chapter 6 as examples of false reassurance. They do little to ease discomfort in the person being offered them. When reassurance is offered in this way, the effect is often opposite to its intention.

In saying to patients 'Everything will be all right', nurses may believe that patients will be comforted; however, patients often feel dismissed by such an expression. Not only have nurses failed to meet patients in their world but they have also actually denied its existence or diminished its importance.

False reassurance distances patients from nurses and may be used by nurses to distance themselves from unpleasant or difficult aspects of nursing. Telling a patient not to worry may make the nurse feel better but, as a general rule, unless the patient receives concrete reassuring evidence, this alone does little to comfort a patient who is concerned and distressed.

Unless they are careful and thoughtful, nurses may inadvertently find themselves slipping into this automatic mode of falsely reassuring patients. Because years of socialisation are difficult to change, it is likely that a platitude or cliché will 'slip out' before a nurse realises it. The realisation that such responses are not truly reassuring, and even potentially alienating, to patients may produce a sense of failure in the nurse if this happens.

Nevertheless, a nurse who inadvertently utters a trite cliché can recover by following the cliché with a comment that indicates awareness and sensitivity. Here are some examples of how to recover:

- *'Everything will be all right*, but my saying so won't necessarily make it so.'
- *'Don't worry*. That's easy for me to say, isn't it?'
- *'Things have a way of working out*, but that thought may not help you to feel any better.'
- *'Some good will come out of all of this*. That doesn't really help you, though, does it?'

Recovering comments, such as these, demonstrate the nurse's awareness and usually result in the interaction proceeding rather than generating feelings of alienation and rejection in the patient. After recovering, the nurse is now free to proceed with a more realistic reassuring response.

## Comforting reassurance

If effective reassurance is not about presenting such falsely reassuring responses, then what does it involve? To reassure is to restore confidence and to promote a sense of safety, control, hope and certainty. Reassurance calms the anxious, abates the uneasiness of the worried and decreases concern in the uncertain. Reassurance is concrete and directly related to a patient's situation, rather than global and non-specific as clichés are. Realistic reassurance is novel, imaginative, unique and, most importantly, specific to the patient.

The desired outcome in providing reassurance is a restored sense of confidence and feelings of safety within a patient. To reassure literally means to assure again. In this sense, reassurance is restorative. By supporting their inherent power and ability, effective reassurance enables patients to face situations with equanimity. Reassurance may not 'make everything all right' (sometimes this is not possible), but a patient who is reassured can face experiences with confidence, hope and courage.

Like the previous analysis of caring and comforting, reassuring is what the *nurse* does (i.e. it is nurse-focused), and coping is the desired patient outcome. Nevertheless, providing reassurance does not guarantee that a patient will feel more certain and confident and therefore cope better. This lack of guarantee, however, should not stifle attempts to reassure patients.

## Patients' need for reassurance

As with all intervening skills, recognising a patient's need for reassurance and an understanding of their experience in relation to this need precede action. Nurses must understand and appreciate the concrete, specific nature of a patient's worry. The following scenario serves as an illustration of the importance of assessing a patient's need for reassurance.

## SCENARIO

Jacob is scheduled for an above-the-knee amputation of his right leg. He has diabetes, which has been difficult to control and manage. Prior to surgery he expresses concern by making statements such as 'I don't know how this is all going to turn out' and 'It's a bit of a worry'. The nurse caring for him avoids saying 'Oh, don't worry, everything will be all right', appreciating the futility and potential harm of such a statement. Instead, the nurse explores what, specifically, is worrying Jacob. Perhaps he fears pain postoperatively; he could be worried about how he will manage to get around after the surgery; perhaps he is concerned about loss of income (he is self-employed) during and after hospitalisation; perhaps he fears not being able to return to his usual occupation. Perhaps ... perhaps ... the list is almost endless.

Unless the nurse responding to him understands what exactly is worrying him, any attempts to reassure him may be misguided. Through the use of exploration and understanding skills, the nurse comes to know that the fear of postoperative pain is worrying him most.

Now that the specific focus of his concern is identified, the nurse can reassure Jacob, with specific information, about how much pain he can expect and, more importantly, what will be done to alleviate and control his pain.

In nursing practice there are everyday patient situations that indicate the need for reassurance. Awareness of these general situations, however, does not replace the necessity of exploring and understanding each patient's experience in relation to the need for reassurance.

The need for reassurance arises out of situations in which patients are apprehensive, doubtful, uncertain, worried, anxious and full of misgivings or lacking confidence. In nursing practice there are myriad circumstances that result in patients experiencing such feelings and perceptions. Some examples include:

- an unclear/unknown medical diagnosis
- facing unfamiliar situations
- an ambiguous future
- painful procedures.

The common theme in situations indicating a need for reassurance is uncertainty. The need for reassurance arises out of situations that are unfamiliar, unknown, unsettling, threatening and confusing. Patients facing such situations often experience a loss of control and need to have their confidence restored. They are in need of something on which, or someone on whom, they can rely to decrease their uncertainty. The intention in reassurance is then to decrease uncertainty and restore a sense of control.

## ACTIVITY 8.1 Situations requiring reassurance

**Process**

1. Working individually, record a patient situation that you have experienced or can imagine that indicates the patient's need for reassurance. Ask yourself: 'What made me think the patient needed reassurance?' Describe the situation as fully as possible.

2. Form groups of five to six and distribute the recorded situations randomly among the participants.

3. Have each participant review the situation and write a key word or phrase from the recorded situation that indicates the need for reassurance. Make a list of patient cues from the recorded situation that expressed the need for reassurance.

4. Record all key words and phrases, including those that are repetitive, on a sheet of paper visible to all participants.

5. On a separate sheet of paper, visible to all participants, record the identified patient cues.

**Discussion**

1. What themes are expressed in the key words and phrases?

2. How much variation is there in the list of patient cues?

3. What generalisations can be made about patient situations that indicate a need for reassurance?

## Patient cues indicating uncertainty

Because of their uniqueness, patients will express uncertainty in a variety of ways. Return to the list of patient cues indicating a need for reassurance, developed in Activity 8.1. Some examples of patient cues indicating feelings of uncertainty, and therefore the potential need for reassurance, include:

- openly stating fears and anxieties
- asking numerous questions
- continuous activity
- becoming quiet and withdrawn
- crying
- making numerous requests and demands.

A perceptive nurse will notice such cues, place them within the context of the patient's current situation, integrate them with an understanding of this patient's experience and explore and validate the presence of uncertainty and need for reassurance. A general discussion of how to explore patient cues is found in Chapter 7. Having established the presence of a need for reassurance, nurses can now proceed to provide it in a variety of ways.

Nurses reassure patients in myriad ways, not just through verbal responses. They provide reassurance to patients through their presence and manner, as well as through reassuring actions and verbal responses.

### ACTIVITY 8.2 Ways nurses reassure patients

**Process**

1. Recall a time in your life when you were filled with uncertainty about something that was happening, or about to happen, to you.

2. Reflect on the situation and circumstances surrounding it.

3. What, if anything, would have allayed or did allay your uncertainty? Describe, on a piece of paper, how you were/might have been reassured.

4. Form groups of five to six and discuss both the described situations and the ways of reassuring.

5. List the identified ways of reassuring.

6. Compare each small group's list, developed in step 5.

7. Prepare a list that combines each small group's list.

**Discussion**

1. Of the identified ways of reassuring, which are appropriate within the nursing context?

2. How might a nurse reassure patients?

3. What hinders nurses in their attempts to reassure patients? What helps?

## Reassuring presence of the nurse

Patients are reassured by the knowledge that a nurse will be there, as the presence of another human being is reassuring in itself, especially during times of disquiet. Being present involves more than simply a physical presence; it involves the emotional presence of a nurse who is fully attending and listening. When the nurse is fully present, patients are comforted and reassured (Kostovich 2012). Patients experience a reassuring presence as 'being with me' and 'being there for me'. Accessibility of a nurse is the key factor in a patient's sense of feeling reassured. Chapter 5 describes this presence with specific reference to the comforting presence of a nurse whose entire focus is on the patient.

In addition, patients are reassured in knowing that the nurse will remain present and will not abandon them, no matter how difficult, painful or overwhelming circumstances are for them. This vigilant, constant and reliable presence promotes confidence within patients, thus providing reassurance.

## Reassuring manner of the nurse

When a nurse conveys, primarily through non-verbal means, calmness and confidence, patients are reassured. This highlights the need for self-understanding (see Ch 3) because nurses may unconsciously (non-verbal behaviour is usually out of conscious awareness) communicate a sense of uneasiness to the patient. A nurse's uneasiness may or may not have reference to the immediate patient, but it will compound the worry of an already worried patient. A nurse who appears unsure or uncertain can contribute to a patient's uneasiness and uncertainty.

A nurse's reassuring presence and manner maintain meaningful human contact between a patient and a nurse. Other non-verbal forms of communication, including touching, holding hands, massaging and ministering, are examples of physically comforting, reassuring acts.

## Reassuring actions

In addition to the reassuring presence and manner of nurses, a number of actions reassure patients. Example include:

- positive affirmation
- concrete and specific feedback
- explanations and factual information.

These skills are considered facilitative because they encourage patients to reinterpret their situations in light of different or new information. They are especially helpful when a patient's current interpretation of a situation is threatening – for example, a new mother who believes her 'blue' feelings after birth are a sign she is 'losing her mind' (see 'Illness representation' in Ch 9).

### *Positive affirmation*

A positive affirmation is a pledge, promise or guarantee made with the intention of reassuring a patient. Examples include:

- 'The pain medication that we will give you routinely after your surgery is quite effective. I think you'll find it really helps.'
- 'This wound is going to heal nicely because you are a fit, healthy person.'
- 'I will visit your family every two weeks. Most families find this sufficient, but if you need to contact me in between visits you can reach me on this number.'

Notice how making a positive affirmation is similar to sharing information. While sharing information is related to positive affirmation, it is not exactly the same. A positive affirmation usually contains an interpretation, which the patient is asked to accept without analysis. Information may be added to strengthen a positive affirmation, but information itself does not provide an interpretation.

Positive affirmations are similar to false reassurance, although they should not be empty promises or false guarantees. The difference between a false reassurance and a positive affirmation is the nurse's focus. When a cliché or platitude is focused on protecting the nurse and hiding distress, it is not reassuring. When it is focused on the patient, such a comment, genuinely and spontaneously stated, can result in comfort and reassurance.

## Concrete and specific feedback

Feedback about how a nurse perceives a situation can be reassuring to patients. In order to be helpful in providing reassurance, feedback needs to be concrete and specific to the patient. Simply saying to a patient 'I think you are progressing just fine' is not concrete enough to fully reassure the patient. Examples of helpful feedback include:

- 'I can tell you're getting a little stronger each day because yesterday you could only walk to the edge of the bed. Today you made it to the shower on your own.'
- 'You've been through a lot with your father's illness. It's no wonder you're feeling a bit drained.'
- 'Last month you weren't sure what you were going to do about the tumour; this month, I see a different person.'

Like positive affirmation, feedback provides the patient with a new interpretation of the situation. This interpretation is based on the nurse's view of the situation, which is usually informed and knowledgeable. It is based on the nurse's view, but helpful feedback is not a judgment, an evaluation or an analysis of the patient's situation.

For feedback to be truly reassuring, it is essential that the nurse establishes first that the patient wants it and can use it. In addition, feedback that focuses on a patient's strengths and resources is more helpful than feedback that highlights weaknesses and shortcomings.

## Providing explanations and factual information

Sharing information, especially about what is usual/expected under the circumstances is reassuring to patients, particularly to those patients whose interpretation is based on faulty or misguided information. For example, a patient who is nil by mouth, and receiving intravenous fluids, may fear they will literally 'starve to death' due to lack of understanding. Explanations provide patients with an opportunity to re-evaluate their situation in light of new, more valid information. Providing factual information restores a patient's sense of control over situations and reduces their uncertainty.

### ACTIVITY 8.3 Reassuring interventions

**Process**

1. Return to Activity 8.1, 'Situations requiring reassurance', and randomly redistribute the recorded patient situations to each participant.

2. Each participant reviews the patient situation and records how they would provide reassurance under the circumstances.

*cont.*

*Activity 8.3 continued*

3. The recorded situations, along with the suggested way to reassure the patient, are again randomly distributed to all participants.

4. Each situation and suggestion for reassurance is then read aloud by the participants. The types of reassurance suggested are recorded on a tally sheet, under the broad headings provided in the text.

**Discussion**

1. Which methods of providing reassurance were most preferred? Discuss the possible reasons for this.

2. Which methods of providing reassurance are easy to employ? Which are more difficult? Discuss reasons for this.

# SUPPORTING PATIENTS

To support is to provide a means of holding up something to prevent it from falling apart. Foundations support houses; beams support ceilings – their enduring presence provides the means to keep a structure intact and prevent its collapse.

In supporting patients, nurses 'stand in the wings' awaiting a call for assistance. Being supportive is an essential quality of nurses and it is needed whenever nurses relate to patients. The foundation skills of listening and understanding are the primary means of conveying a supportive attitude. Their use demonstrates that the nurse is available, accepting and encouraging. Nurses also express their support by upholding an inherent belief in patients' capabilities and resources and through maintaining a sense of hope. In this regard, support encompasses a variety of skills because it is predominantly an attitude of being with and for the patient.

## Types of support

Providing support occurs within an interpersonal process that involves: emotional support, often expressed as comfort; instrumental support, which involves providing direct assistance; and informational support in the form of explanations and education (Tay et al 2013; Thoits 2011). Nurses provide support to patients in a variety of ways. First, there is informational support. Sharing information with patients is supportive because information assists patients in coming to terms with their health status, making decisions about healthcare and understanding what is usual and expected for a given situation. Another type of support comes in the form of direct aid and assistance. This type of support is the concrete, often observable, 'lending a helping hand'. Helping a hospitalised patient out of bed is a clear example of this type of support. Another type of support is providing positive affirmation and encouragement to patients. This type of support is emotional in nature, and an example of it is the proverbial 'pat on the back'. It involves standing by and offering encouragement to a patient. The last type is the most common usage of the term 'support'. Emotional support has been linked with positive health outcomes such as quality of life and recovery from illness and self-care (Graven & Grant 2013; Koetsenruijter et al 2016; Sharply et al 2015).

From the preceding description of the types of support, it is apparent that nurses provide support to patients in varied ways. An effective relationship with a patient provides support. Nevertheless, nurses must also bear in mind that they are but one, often temporary, source of support for patients. Patients also rely on their social network as a source of support (Ch 9). Patients often rely on their family and friends to provide emotional support, while they depend on nurses and other healthcare providers to provide informational support (Arora et al 2007). In addition to informational support, patients also feel supported when: they are treated as an individual, as opposed to a number; when care is not rushed or mechanical; and when there is continuity with healthcare providers (Drageset et al 2016).

# Mobilising patient resources

Another way for nurses to provide support for patients is through direct intervention to mobilise 'other' sources of support. The following scenario is an illustration of how nurses mobilise support for patients.

## SCENARIO

Emily is in hospital following the stillbirth of a baby girl at full term. The pregnancy, her first, was planned, and both she and her husband eagerly anticipated the birth. The loss and disappointment following the stillbirth were, as expected, devastating for Emily. The nurses found her to be remote, non-communicative and inaccessible, although her emotional pain was visible to them. They understood Emily's sadness but were especially concerned by her lack of responsiveness when interacting. Although every effort was made to interact with Emily, the nurses began to feel helpless because they could not 'connect' with her. They recognised that their concern was greater than usual and assessed the need for active intervention.

Of all the nurses caring for Emily, Sue had established the most meaningful relationship with her. Although mostly unresponsive, Emily spoke more with Sue than any of the other nurses. Through exploration, Sue learnt that Emily's husband, Jake, had refused to discuss the death of their daughter with her. Jake's attitude and approach was one of maintaining a 'stiff upper lip'. He saw no reason to 'cry over spilt milk' and dwell on the negative; he just wanted their lives to return to normal as soon as possible. Sue noticed that, when Emily discussed Jake's reaction, she became a bit more communicative and animated. More than anything, Emily wanted to talk to Jake about her feelings of despair and sadness. In this situation, one of Emily's supports, Jake, was not available to

*cont.*

*Scenario continued*

her. What she needed, more than anything, was to be able to talk to Jake about what had happened. Sue decided to intervene to mobilise this support for Emily.

The next time Jake came to visit, Sue made the effort to spend time with them both. Up to this point, the nurses had left the two of them alone during visiting time, out of respect for their need for privacy. During the interaction with Emily and Jake, Sue encouraged Jake to discuss his reactions to what had happened. When he said there was no reason to cry and feel sorry for himself, Sue suggested that, although he himself may not wish to cry, perhaps his approach was preventing Emily from expressing how she felt. At this point, Emily began to cry. Jake appeared a bit surprised but made an effort to console her. Sue left the room, with Emily and Jake in an embrace. The next day Emily's general appearance and demeanour had changed. Although still quite sad, she was more talkative and open. Clearly, she felt better as a result of receiving support from her husband.

This story illustrates, quite clearly, the importance of nurses perceiving support as more than something they supply directly. Through mobilising support for Emily, rather than focusing exclusively on the patient–nurse relationship, Sue provided an intervention that was helpful and effective.

# ENABLING PATIENTS

Enabling patients involves nursing care that is focused on recognising and supporting patients' capacities to have control over their lives through active participation (Hudon et al 2011). Patient participation varies from involving patients in care by considering their viewpoints to having patients acting as equal partners in decisions about their care (see Ch 1). Partnership implies a working association between two people, which is usually based on a contract. As such, both partners are knowledgeable about the work of the partnership.

Involving patients in care, on the other hand, is more one-way, with the nurses being more knowledgeable, yet taking into consideration their patient's point of view. Whether at the level of partnership or involvement, there is overwhelming evidence that there must be an interpersonal relationship between a patient and nurse in order for patient participation to occur (Angel & Frederiksen 2015; Hudon et al 2011; Kolovos et al 2015; Mavis et al 2015; Snyder & Engström 2016; Thórarinsdóttir & Kristjánsson 2014; Tobiano et al 2016a). Involving patients in participating in their own care is contingent on having a trusting, connected relationship in which the nurse comes to know the patient and what they need and want.

The relationship enables participation to be negotiated between patients and nurses. This negotiation process is essential because patients vary in their desire and capacity to participate (Papastavrou et al 2016; Tobiano et al 2015a, 2015b).

Not all patients either want to or are able to participate in their own healthcare. The extent to which they do depends on congruence between their desire to participate and the extent to which nurses interact with them to promote such participation, as the nurse's behaviour can inhibit or stimulate participation (Papastavrou et al 2016; Larsson et al 2011). In order to promote participation, nurses must relinquish control and power (Angel & Frederiksen 2015; Mavis et al 2015; Tobiano et al 2015a) because patients who want to participate often feel powerless within the healthcare system (Sheridan et al 2012) (see *Research highlight*).

---

## RESEARCH HIGHLIGHT Patients' perception of participating in nursing care

*Tobiano, G., Bucknall, T., Marshall, A., et al., 2016b. Patients' perceptions of participation in nursing care on medical wards. Scand. J. Caring Sci. 30, 260–270.*

### Background

The quality and safety of nursing care is enhanced when patients are active participants in their care. Nurses and patients may hold different views about participation. Therefore, it is important to understand how patients view their participation in nursing care.

### Purpose of the study

The aim of this study was to explore hospitalised patients' perceptions of participation in nursing care, including aspects that both facilitated and inhibited participation.

### Method

Interviews with patients were conducted, as one aspect of a larger ethnographic study, to explore their views on participation in nursing care while in hospital. Interview data were collected from 20 patients from a variety of hospital settings. Data were transcribed and analysed interpretively, in an ongoing manner, in order to develop themes.

### Key findings

Four themes emerged from the analysis. The first was that patients valued an opportunity to participate in their nursing care and felt motivated to do so. The next theme related to their pursuit in seeking knowledge about what was occurring in their care, done primarily through asking questions. The third theme indicated that they monitored their own care in an effort to attend to their own safety. The final theme demonstrated how they recognised the inherent power imbalance between them and the nurses; as a result, they complied with care and treated the nurses with kindness and respect.

### Implications for nursing practice

Nurses need to recognise that patients positively regard their input into nursing care. Nonetheless, they also recognise that they need to be compliant with that care, so their

*cont.*

The major theme in the literature on patient participation is that patients need information in order to participate in their care. Therefore, having patients participate in their care is contingent on them having knowledge about that care. Herein lies one of the major challenges to participation. Sharing information with patients is an important skill in meeting this challenge.

## Sharing information

The skill of sharing information encompasses a range of actions – from providing explanations, to giving instructions, to imparting knowledge, to formal teaching. When explaining to a patient the reasons for an extended delay in a scheduled procedure, the nurse is sharing information. When engaged in informing patients what they can expect to happen postoperatively, the nurse is sharing information. When teaching a patient how to care for a colostomy, the nurse is sharing information.

What nurses perceive as ordinary and everyday in the routine of healthcare delivery can seem foreign to patients. Patients may have little previous knowledge and experience to draw on in trying to understand this sometimes strange, often frightening, world of healthcare. Clearly, nurses are in a prime position to help patients make sense of the environment and their experiences in it through sharing information.

Nurses play a key role in keeping patients informed, not only because of their sustained, continual presence but also because of their close proximity to the patient's specific experience. When sharing information, a nurse operates from within the patient's experience. It is the nurse who comes to know how much adjustment a patient must make in order to follow a prescribed therapeutic diet. It is the nurse who appreciates the demands being placed on a new mother who has recently arrived in the country and is isolated from her usual support systems. Empathy and understanding of a patient's experience enable nurses to share information that is specific to the patient and to appreciate what the patient wants to know in relation to health status and care.

Sharing information is more than merely providing information, or imparting knowledge. In sharing, there is concern with how the information is received, understood and used. It is a two-way process. Providing information involves merely supplying information to patients and is a one-way process. In this sense, books, pamphlets and videos provide information to patients. Sharing information, on the other hand, is interactive. By connecting the patient's experience with the need for information the nurse is able to consider how the information is received and treat the patient as an active participant, not as a passive recipient.

As with all the skills of intervening, sharing information is grounded in an understanding of the patient. To some patients, remaining fully informed, down to the level of minute detail of their care, is extremely important to their sense of wellbeing. Other patients prefer not to know every detail and feel best when told only the bare essentials. Nevertheless, some information (e.g. orienting information about the routine of the clinical setting) is necessary, regardless of the patient's frame of reference and expressed desire to know.

## Effects of sharing information

Having meaningful information about their health status and care helps patients gain a sense of control over sometimes confusing or disturbing events. Providing meaningful information helps them to feel safe. Frequently, information is shared when a patient is prepared for an anticipated health event. For example, knowing what can be expected following abdominal surgery assists patients in coming to terms with the usual postoperative course of events. Accurate information can do much to alleviate unnecessary anxiety stemming from false beliefs, misconceptions and even fantasies. Patients facing decisions in relation to healthcare are able to determine the best course of action when they are fully informed. Explanations alleviate the anxiety of guessing what will happen next.

## A nursing perspective on sharing information

Nurses are sometimes reluctant to embark on sharing information with patients because the information to be shared is perceived as exclusively medical in nature. While it is inappropriate for nurses to assume the role of doctor in presenting initial information about a medical diagnosis, nurses frequently serve as the interpreters of such information. Patients often rely on nurses to provide them with needed information because nurses are more accessible than doctors. Simply referring them to the appropriate doctor is often not enough. Nurses can assist patients to obtain relevant medical information by helping them to develop questions to ask the doctor. In this sense, nurses act as guides for patients.

Nevertheless, there is more to sharing information than helping patients to obtain and understand input that is medical in nature. Patients also need assistance in understanding how their health status, including their medical diagnosis (when present and known), will affect their day-to-day living. They need to learn how to adjust and adapt to the demands that are placed on them by alterations in health status. When nurses share information about these aspects of health, they are functioning within a nursing perspective. By focusing on these aspects, nurses concern themselves more with patients' responses to their health status, rather than just their health status per se.

Examples of a nursing perspective on sharing information include helping patients to:

- make sense of what is happening to them
- learn new skills in caring for themselves
- make adjustments and adaptations in relation to the demands placed on them by alterations in health status.

In short, nurses are in a position to share information about patients' daily living in relation to health status.

## Sharing information versus giving advice

It is easy to confuse giving advice with sharing information (this was mentioned briefly in Ch 6). In sharing information, nurses offer a range of alternatives to patients. In giving advice, nurses present solutions to patients. There are times when patients expect advice and place nurses in the role of knowledgeable expert. Before assuming this role, however, nurses need to be clear that certain risks are inherent in advising.

## SCENARIO

Sarah has been visiting the local early childhood centre regularly since her first son, Connor, was born 11 months ago. During a recent visit she related that she is becoming increasingly distressed because Connor is still waking during the night to breastfeed. Although Connor feeds quickly during the night and settles back to sleep quite easily, Sarah is distressed by her continual nights of broken sleep.

Eleanor, the registered nurse in the centre, has been working with mothers and babies for 12 years. Sarah asks Eleanor for advice about what to do because she is becoming desperate for an unbroken night's sleep. Eleanor begins by explaining that Connor is of sufficient weight and age to go through the night without a feed. She then proceeds to explain that Sarah has various options. She could let Connor cry until he returns to sleep; she could use the 'controlled crying method' to get him back to sleep without a feed; Sarah's husband could tend to Connor in the middle of the night; or she could continue to feed him, knowing that some day waking during the night will cease. Eleanor then continues, explaining how other mothers she knows have dealt with similar circumstances. Finally, she shares her own experiences learnt through caring for her own three children.

After presenting the options, Eleanor explains to Sarah that only she can decide what is best for herself, Connor and the family. She finishes by stating that there are numerous theories about how to care for babies, and a variety of possible approaches, but it really comes down to what Sarah can live with. She then explores each of the options with Sarah to determine what Sarah would like to try.

When functioning within the nursing perspective, nurses share information in an attempt to help patients adjust and adapt to their daily living. By advising patients about what is 'best' to do, nurses assume they are experts about each patient's life. Clearly, patients are the most qualified experts when it comes to managing their lives. The risks of playing the expert when it involves another person's life are apparent – the advice can be unsuitable, unacceptable, inappropriate or even dangerous.

It is better to present alternatives, through sharing information, and enable the patient to determine which course of action might be best. The following scenario highlights the process of presenting alternatives versus giving solutions.

Obviously, Eleanor could have advised Sarah about what she should do rather than share information and let Sarah decide. In doing so, however, she would have run the risk of suggesting a solution that is unacceptable or unworkable for Sarah. Even if the advice is acceptable, it may not work, so Sarah would be left with no other options. Under these circumstances, Sarah probably would not ask Eleanor again and may even blame her for the failure of her recommendation. Most importantly, by giving advice, Eleanor becomes responsible for the outcome. Sarah could be left with feelings of inadequacy as a result. These are the risks of presenting solutions, rather than alternatives.

Giving advice is not the same as presenting factual, clinical information to patients, or explaining the potential consequences of certain health-related behaviours. Advice offers solutions when patients are facing situations that they can potentially manage. Instructing a patient to cough and breathe deeply following surgery, in order to help prevent pulmonary complications, is an example of presenting information and instructions, although this could be construed as advice. There are times when nurses effectively offer advice to patients, but this should be undertaken with full awareness of the risks involved.

## Approaches to sharing information

Sharing information begins with the nurse's recognition of the patient's need for it. While it could be said that all patients need certain information in order to cope with changes in health status, the specific need within each patient may be variable. Recognition and appreciation of a patient's unique requirements for information stem from the nurse's understanding.

While a patient's unique experiences provide a useful starting point for using any intervening skill, there are some general situations that indicate a specific need for information. These include:

- facing new and unfamiliar situations
- coping with demands of altered health status
- developing new skills
- being misinformed
- requesting information and explanations
- expressing the need for reassurance and informational support.

## Readiness to learn

Timing is crucial when sharing information, and this is best expressed as capturing a patient's readiness to learn. If information is shared before a patient is ready, it may 'fall on deaf ears' or, worse, create undue anxiety. When it occurs too late, sharing information fails to achieve its desired outcome.

Capturing a patient's readiness to learn is a sophisticated process. The degree of sensitivity to patient cues required for this level of practice is developed through experience and involvement with numerous patient experiences. To beginning nurses, the concept of the 'right time' to share information may seem vague and elusive. Nevertheless, an acceptance and recognition that there is a right time to 'strike while the iron is hot' enables beginning nurses to make the effort to observe and notice patient cues that indicate readiness.

A good example occurs in teaching patients to care for a colostomy – a complex, sometimes overwhelming, task for most patients. Because patients must first come to terms with the reality of a colostomy, they will not be ready to learn the details of caring for it themselves until this happens. Cues indicating readiness include looking at the colostomy in more than just a fleeting manner, not reacting with disgust when looking at it and asking questions of the nurse who is changing the colostomy bag. This is but one example of the importance of noticing when the patient seems ready to learn.

Obviously, capturing a patient's readiness means that nurses must be flexible enough to change their immediate plans in order to accommodate this readiness.

## Beginning to share information

Once the need for information is established, and the readiness to receive the information is noted, it is best to begin sharing information by establishing what the patient wants to know. Often patients will ask questions without prompting or probing, but it may be necessary for the nurse to use exploration skills (see Ch 7) to establish what the patient wants to know first. Questions that are useful include:

- 'What questions are on your mind?'
- 'What would you like to know?'
- 'Where would you like me to begin explaining this?'

Through exploring what patients want to know, the nurse is requesting and encouraging the patient to ask the questions. It is important that these questions are answered at the depth and level at which they are asked. A simple question need not be met with a complicated, involved answer. Likewise, a complex question should not be brushed aside with a superficial answer. It is often a good idea to paraphrase (Ch 6) the patient's question prior to attempting to answer it.

After answering a patient's question, the nurse needs to check that the response satisfied the question. This is accomplished by following the response with another question such as 'Does that answer your question?'. The nurse may be surprised when the patient answers 'No'. Under this circumstance, it is obvious that the nurse needs to develop another response, or have the patient pose the question again, using different words.

From this point, the nurse now can move into further, more focused exploration of what the patient already understands. A person who has experienced repeated hospitalisations may understand a great deal about ward routine. This exploration provides a good opportunity to correct any misinformation or misperceptions. The nurse can also use the patient's current level of understanding as a springboard for elaboration. Notice how beginning in this manner encourages the patient to direct the flow of information. It also provides an opportunity for the nurse to further assess the patient's readiness to receive information.

## Limiting the amount of information shared

When nurses are expanding into sharing new information, they need to appreciate that there are limits to how much information can be absorbed at one time. Too much information presented at one time can overload a patient's information-processing capacity. Presenting detailed, complex information all at once can create more confusion within the patient. A general guideline is to present no more than three new items at one time.

## Using appropriate language

Another important facet of sharing information is to use language that matches the patient's age, experience and cultural background. Nurses sometimes become so accustomed to the jargon of healthcare that they fail to appreciate that patients do not understand some of the language used. Terms such as 'IVs', 'nil by mouth', 'obs' and even 'bedrest' can create confusion in patients. For example, some patients think 'bedrest' literally means to have a rest in bed and liken it to an afternoon nap, thinking this is sufficient to maintain bedrest. Not only should standard medical and nursing terms and jargon be fully explained to patients, but also their use should be kept to a minimum, if not avoided altogether.

## Tailoring information to the patient

Of even greater importance when sharing information is the need to tailor explanations to individual patients. Cultural variations (see Ch 4), especially as they relate to how health and illness is perceived and understood (see 'Illness representation' in Ch 9) need to be taken into account (Glattacker et al 2012). It is equally important to work from the patient's background and experience. For example, an engineer can easily relate the functioning of the heart to already acquired knowledge of closed systems that work on pressure, pumps, one-way valves and electrical conduction. Knowing a patient's background is necessary for this guideline to be enacted.

## The need for reinforcement

It is often helpful to reinforce explanations and information verbally shared with prepared pamphlets, diagrams, models and spontaneously written notes. Using an alternative means of expression, such as one or more of these, provides helpful reinforcement for patients. Summarising (see Ch 6) the shared information is another helpful means of reinforcing. Often patients' anxiety levels interfere with their ability to absorb information; reinforcing will help them retain it.

Additionally, there may be a need to reiterate information. Repetition provides reinforcement, although the need to repeat information may prove frustrating to the nurse. A patient may need to hear it more than once in order to incorporate the information, and put it to some use.

## Checking a patient's understanding

Sharing information is more than imparting knowledge, so the nurse sharing the information needs to periodically check that the patient understands the information. It is better to check frequently throughout an information-sharing interaction than to wait until it draws to a close. The skills of exploration (see Ch 7) are employed for this purpose.

## Expressing understanding when sharing information

When nurses are sharing information, they need to be sensitive to the impact of the information on the patient. For the patient, there may be surprises and challenges contained in the information. Observing patient cues that indicate their reactions, reflecting observed feelings and expressing empathy are all helpful skills to employ for this purpose. In the absence of patient cues, it may be necessary for nurses to explore patients' reactions to the information that is shared.

## A final word on sharing information

Before embarking on sharing information, nurses must be reasonably confident with their own level of knowledge about a patient's situation. This is not to say that nurses should 'know everything' there is to know about all patient situations, but there is little point in trying to share information when the basics of the situation are not understood. If this is the case, a cursory assessment of the patient's need for information could be undertaken, but there are limits (e.g. a patient's misunderstanding might not be immediately corrected if the nurse lacks knowledge).

There are likely to be situations in which a patient's request for information is beyond what a nurse currently understands and knows. There is no real harm in nurses admitting that they do not know, as long as they are willing to find out for the patient or refer the patient to an appropriate resource. When referral to another person (e.g. the patient's doctor) is the most appropriate course of action, nurses can assist patients in framing questions to ask of this person.

**ACTIVITY 8.4  Sharing information**   **336**

**Process**

1. Working in groups of five to six, develop a list of patient situations that indicate that the patient needs more information.

2. Each group member now writes a brief scenario, based on one of the situations from the developed list. Include patient cues indicating a need for information.

3. Distribute the scenarios to each of the group members. Members are to take the scenario away from the session and gather the information required to fully inform the patient described in the scenario.

4. At the next class gathering, participants form groups of three. Identify one member of the group as the patient, one as the nurse who will share information and the third person as an observer.

5. For each scenario, have the nurses share information with the patients. The observer uses the 'Guide for sharing information' (see the appendix, page 336).

**Discussion**

1. What was easy about sharing information? What was hard?

2. What were some of the difficulties experienced in sharing information? Refer to questions on the observer guides that were answered 'no'.

3. How did the nurses assess the patients' current level of knowledge?

4. How did the nurses determine the patients' comprehension of the information?

5. What kind of wording and language was used in sharing the information?

# Challenging

When challenging, nurses urge patients to reconsider their current perspectives and assist them to develop new perspectives. A challenge encourages patients to evaluate their views, feelings and interpretations of a situation. This can be achieved by directly presenting a different interpretation, or by exploring alternative perspectives with the patient. Either way, a successful challenge enables patients to reframe their experiences in a new light and therefore participate in care with this new view.

Challenging is a skill that is high in terms of influencing patients. This is because the nurse is asking patients to call into question their experiences and to develop new perspectives on their experience. Challenging often forces patients to call on new or unused resources.

## The nature of challenging

Effective challenging is beneficial because it encourages patients to look at their situations in new and different ways. This reframing and reinterpretation may prove unsettling at first, and patients may experience anxiety as a result. For this reason, nurses are often uncomfortable with the notion of challenging a patient because it seems unsupportive to cast doubt on the patient's current perspective. Perhaps this is due to a lack of understanding of the nature and helpfulness of a challenge.

Challenging is not the same as disagreeing with or rejecting the patient's perspective, although it does rely on the nurse's judgment that another perspective may be more productive. For example, a patient may believe that having a myocardial infarction results automatically in permanent disability and dramatic alteration to previous functioning. An interpretation such as this can lead to feelings of depression and even despair. Such a patient is at risk of becoming a 'cardiac cripple'. By challenging this perspective, the nurse enables the patient to develop a more realistic view of the situation post-infarction.

When challenging, it is important to focus on the patient's strengths and resources, not just weaknesses and failures. In this regard, challenging is employed with an attitude of respect for the patient's inherent capabilities.

## The conditions needed for effective challenging

As with all the psychosocial action skills, challenging is preceded by acknowledging the reality of the patient's current experience (see Ch 6). Nurses 'earn the right' (Egan 2014) to challenge by first demonstrating understanding of a patient's viewpoints and experiences. In this sense, understanding is a prerequisite to challenging.

Before embarking on challenging skills, a nurse must also consider the strength of the relationship with the patient. If little rapport, trust and understanding has developed, it is likely that a challenge will be ineffective. In fact, without trust, challenging may be counterproductive to further developing the relationship. Patients will accept a challenge from a nurse who has demonstrated interest, accessibility, reliability and understanding. Challenging is more likely to be effective in longer term relationships.

Other aspects to consider before embarking on a challenge relate to the vulnerability and fragility of the patient. Nurses must be reasonably certain that the patient being challenged has the strength, resilience and resources to develop and accept a new perspective. Minimally, the patient needs to be able to acknowledge that alternative views are possible.

## The need to challenge

The need to challenge stems from the existence of patients' perspectives that are unproductive, unsatisfying, poorly informed, unacceptable and/or unnecessarily painful or distressing to them. The importance of that final phrase, *to the patient*, cannot be stressed enough. It is important that challenges are not presented as negative judgments that give the impression that patients 'should not' think or feel the way they do. Although nurses rely on a judgment that a new perspective may be needed, they must operate from within the patient's value system in order to be most effective. A nurse cannot decide, without consultation, that a patient's perspective needs to be altered.

## Tentativeness of the challenge

Challenges are best presented in a tentative manner but not so tentative that nurses lack assertiveness in the process. A nurse wishing to challenge a patient can begin by suggesting there may be another way of looking at the situation. This is an effective way to determine the patient's readiness to accept alternative perspectives.

## Approaches to challenging

The ability to be assertive (see Chs 3 and 10) is necessary when challenging. Some examples of assertive challenging responses include:

- 'I see your situation in a different light from you.'
- 'I'm concerned that if you continue along these lines, you will just wither away.'
- 'You say you are doing everything to help yourself, but I can see some more things that you could do.'

When patients indicate, often through subtle cues, that their current view is unproductive or difficult to maintain, nurses can proceed not only by sharing information but also by exploring consequences and sharing their own experiences.

### *Exploring consequences*

Another way to begin the challenge is to explore the consequences of a patient's present perspective. While this approach relies on effectively using exploring skills (see Ch 7), it is a focused exploration into the possible effects of the patient's current perspective and delves into the potential risks and benefits of that perspective.

A nurse may be tempted to take the idea of consequences one step further and actually point them out to patients. This approach should be used sparingly (Ivey et al 2013) because of its potential to degenerate into a judgmental, coercive activity that preaches warnings and punishment. Nurses need to be cautious about admonishing patients because this can translate to 'blaming the victim'. If this happens, patients may form the impression that the nurse doesn't want to understand.

### *Sharing own experiences*

Self-disclosing is a skill whereby nurses share their own thoughts, feelings, perceptions, interpretations and experiences in the interest of helping the patient. Self-disclosure helps nurses to make an interpersonal connection with the patient, as this displays the nurse's humanity. One of the most frequent ways that self-disclosure is effective occurs when a nurse has experienced a situation that is similar to the patient's. For example, a nurse who has had the experience of a family member with cancer may share this experience with the family of a patient who is diagnosed with cancer. Under circumstances such as these, nurses share their experiences, not only to demonstrate to the patient a personal understanding of the situation but also to present an alternative perspective.

Self-disclosure also serves as a way to reassure patients that nurses are real people with real lives. Being open enough to share their own stories with patients demonstrates that nurses trust patients as much as they want patients to trust them. The genuineness and personal involvement that is demonstrated by self-disclosure has the potential to draw the nurse and the patient closer. But it also may frighten some patients who do not desire this degree of intimacy, or who prefer nurses to remain distant.

This notion of sharing one's self with patients does challenge some notions of 'professionalism'. At times, professionalism is equated with distance, detachment and non-involvement with patients. This notion of professionalism is explored fully in Chapter 2. Self-disclosure raises questions about how much information about themselves nurses should share with patients.

In deciding how much of one's self to share with patients, there will almost certainly be differences that are based on the personality of each nurse. Like all people, some nurses are more willing to share personal experiences than others. Irrespective of personality, a general rule of thumb can be applied in deciding how much of oneself to share. The general rule stems from the nature of the relationship between the patient and the nurse. Although this relationship involves give and take and, at times, is quite intimate, the nurse must remain oriented towards the patient. When self-disclosure is used to benefit the nurse, the orientation has shifted onto the nurse.

## Pitfalls of self-disclosure

Self-disclosure does not mean that nurses should ask patients to bear some of the burden of their own personal difficulties and problems. This is one of the potential pitfalls of self-disclosure. Self-disclosing has the potential to shift the focus from the patient to the nurse and, as a result, the nurse dominates the interaction with discussions about themselves. In this case, the self-disclosure runs the risk of burdening the patient with the nurse's personal story. Obviously, if this happens, questions are raised about how helpful this might be for the patient. It takes awareness to recognise when this is happening, and an aware nurse will shift the focus back onto the patient, perhaps by employing an exploration skill.

When sharing their own experiences with patients, nurses need to be careful not to use the self-disclosure as a subtle way of rejecting a patient's experience in favour of their own. Nor should self-disclosure be used in a competitive manner of 'let's see who has the best/worst story to tell'. Before disclosing themselves to patients, nurses should pass the disclosure through the following proverbial gate: 'Am I sharing this in order to benefit the patient or our relationship?' If the answer is 'yes', the gate opens for self-disclosure.

## Patients' requests for personal information

The discussion about self-disclosure also raises the question of how nurses should respond when patients request information that is personal in nature. In this regard, the patient prompts the self-disclosure. Clearly, the decision about how much nurses share of themselves is a personal one, but there are also professional reasons to disclose or not to disclose. First, the context must be considered. In an inpatient mental health setting, for example, there may be sound reasons for nurses to avoid too much disclosure of personal details about their lives. Other aspects of the context that should be considered include:

- the possible reasons the patient requests the information
- the degree of personal depth in the request
- the potential consequences of answering or not answering the question.

Nurses are encouraged to reflect and explore how much or how little information about themselves they are willing to share with patients.

---

### ACTIVITY 8.5  Self-disclosure

**Process**

1. As a large group, discuss the following:

   **a.** How much personal information about themselves should nurses share with patients?

   **b.** Is there anything of a personal nature that nurses should not share with patients? If so, what?

   **c.** Discuss the reasons for the answers to each of these questions.

**Discussion**

1. How much disagreement was there between participants in answering questions 1a–c?

2. Were there areas of agreement about what should and should not be shared with patients? What are they?

3. How do you account for the agreement and disagreement in the questions posed?

---

# SUMMARY

The skills presented in this chapter focus on psychosocial actions of comfort, supporting and enabling. Nurses employ the skills of comforting in order to reassure patients. Effective reassurance releases patient anxiety so that energy can be used for dealing with the health event at hand. Effective support offers assistance and aid, again freeing the patient's energy to cope. Enabling patients to participate in care by sharing information and challenging helps them to reframe their perspectives on their situation. All of these skills involve taking direct action to positively influence patients and, more importantly, free energy to cope with health events.

The power necessary for nurses to influence patients in these ways is not automatic; a nurse who has taken the time to fully understand a patient earns it. Taking action is most effective when it works from within the patient's experience; therefore, the continual need to listen, explore and understand has been emphasised throughout the chapter. Nurses are most effective when they use psychosocial actions with the view that patients are capable and resourceful. With this view, the skills in this chapter are used to mobilise, utilise and reinforce patients' capabilities and resources.

# REFERENCES

Angel, S., Frederiksen, K.N., 2015. Challenges in achieving patient participation: a review of how patient participation is addressed in empirical studies. Int. J. Nurs. Stud. 52, 1525–1538.

Arora, N.K., Finney Rutten, L.J., Bakos, A.D., et al., 2007. Perceived helpfulness and impact of social support provided by family, friends, and health care providers to women newly diagnosed with breast cancer. Psychooncology 16, 474–486.

Boudiab, L.D., Kolcaba, K., 2015. Comfort theory: unraveling the complexities of veterans' health care needs. Adv. Nurs. Sci. 38 (4), 270–278.

Drageset, S., Lindstrøm, T.C., Giske, T., 2016. Women's experiences of social support during the first year following primary breast cancer surgery. Scand. J. Caring Sci. 30, 340–348.

Egan, G., 2014. The Skilled Helper, tenth ed. Brooks Cole, Belmont CA.

Glattacker, M., Heyduck, K., Meffert, C., 2012. Illness beliefs, treatment beliefs and information needs as starting points for patient information – evaluation of an intervention for patients with chronic back pain. Patient Educ. Couns. 86, 378–389.

Graven, L.J., Grant, J., 2013. The impact of social support on depressive symptoms in individuals with heart failure update and review. J. Cardiovasc. Nurs. 28 (5), 429–443.

Hudon, C., St-Cyr Tribble, D., Bravo, G., 2011. Enablement in health care context: a concept analysis. J. Eval. Clin. Pract. 17, 143–149.

Ivey, A.E., Ivey, M., Zalaquett, C.R., 2013. Intentional Interviewing and Counseling: Facilitating Client Development, seventh ed. Brooks/Cole, Belmont, CA.

Koetsenruijter, J., van Eikelenboom, N., van Lieshout, J., et al., 2016. Social support and self-management capabilities in diabetes patients. Patient Educ. Couns. 99, 638–643.

Kolcaba, K., 2017. Comfort. In: Peterson, S.A., Bredow, T.S. (Eds.), Middle Range Theories: Application to Nursing Research and Practice. Wolters Kluwer, Philadelphia PA, pp. 196–211.

Kolovos, P., Kaitelidou, D., Lemonidou, C., et al., 2015. Patient participation in hospital care: Nursing staffs' point of view. Int. J. Nurs. Pract. 21, 258–268.

Kostovich, C.T., 2012. Development and psychometric assessment of the presence of nursing scalc. Nurs. Sci. Q. 25 (2), 167–175.

Larsson, I.E., Sahlsten, M.J.M., Segesten, K., et al., 2011. Patients' perceptions of barriers for participation in nursing care. Scand. J. Caring Sci. 25, 575–582.

Mavis, B., Rovner, M.H., Jorgenson, S., et al., 2015. Patient participation in clinical encounters: a systematic review to identify self-report measures. Health Expect. 18, 1827–1843.

Morse, J.M., 1992. Comfort: the refocusing of nursing care. Clin. Nurs. Res. 1 (1), 91–106.

Nightingale, F., 1859 (1992). Notes on Nursing: What It Is and What It Is Not. Reprinted. Lippincott, Philadelphia, PA, originally published by Harrison & Son, London.

Oliveira, I., 2013. Comfort measures: a concept analysis. Res. Theory Nurs. Pract. 27 (2), 95–114.

Papastavrou, E., Efstathiou, G., Tsangari, H., et al., 2016. Patients' decisional control over care: a cross-national comparison from both the patients' and nurses' points of view. Scand. J. Caring Sci. 30, 26–36.

Pinto, S., Caldeira, S., Carlos Martins, J.C., 2016. A systematic literature review toward the characterization of comfort. Holist. Nurs. Pract. 30 (1), 14–24.

Sharply, C., Hussain, R., Wark, S., et al., 2015. The influence of social support on psychological distress in older persons: an examination of interaction processes in Australia. Psychol. Rep. 117, 883–896.

Sheridan, N.F., Kenealy, T.W., Kidd, J.D., 2012. Patients' engagement in primary care: powerlessness and compounding jeopardy: a qualitative study. Health Expect. 18, 32–43.

Snyder, H., Engström, J., 2016. The antecedents, forms and consequences of patient involvement: a narrative review of the literature. Int. J. Nurs. Stud. 53, 351–378.

Tay, L., Tan, K., Diener, E., et al., 2013. Social relations, health behaviors, and health outcomes: a survey and synthesis. Appl. Psychol. Health Well Being 5 (1), 28–78.

Thoits, P.A., 2011. Mechanisms linking social ties and support to physical and mental health. J. Health Soc. Behav. 52 (2), 145–161.

Thórarinsdóttir, K., Kristjánsson, K., 2014. Patients' perspectives on person-centred participation in healthcare: a framework analysis. Nurs. Ethics 21 (2), 129–147.

Tobiano, G., Bucknall, T., Marshall, A., et al., 2015a. Patient participation in nursing care on medical wards: an integrative review. Int. J. Nurs. Stud. 52, 1107–1120.

Tobiano, G., Bucknall, T., Marshall, A., et al., 2015b. Nurses' views of patient participation in nursing care. J. Adv. Nurs. 71 (12), 2741–2752.

Tobiano, G., Marshall, A., Bucknall, T., et al., 2016a. Activities patients and nurses undertake to promote patient participation. J. Nurs. Scholarsh. 48 (4), 362–370.

Tobiano, G., Bucknall, T., Marshall, A., et al., 2016b. Patients' perceptions of participation in nursing care on medical wards. Scand. J. Caring Sci. 30, 260–270.

Williams, A.M., Pienaar, C., Toye, C., et al., 2011. Further psychometric testing of an instrument to measure emotional care in hospital. J. Clin. Nurs. 20, 3427–3482.

# PART

# 3

# SKILLS IN CONTEXT

In Part 2 various skills and concepts of interacting with patients were presented without direct reference to situational variables that affect the use of these skills. The skills of interacting were placed in the context of the relationship that develops between a nurse and a patient. While the various patients' stories in these chapters have served as illustrations in using the skills, no attempt has been made so far to place the skills into specific nursing care contexts.

Part 3 places interpersonal skills in context by addressing transitions through health and illness and how people cope with these transitions in order to successfully navigate through them (see Ch 9). In addition, there is information regarding how nurses can assist in these transitions. Chapter 10 includes a discussion of difficult encounters that may challenge nurses in their therapeutic endeavours and includes a discussion of conflict and the need for assertiveness in its resolution. Dealing with patient anger and possible aggression is also included in this discussion. Particular challenges that may be faced when communicating with older people are then considered, incorporating a discussion of how to interact with a person who is cognitively impaired.

The final chapter (Ch 11) explores healthcare environments, with a particular emphasis on those with cultures that support interpersonal nursing care and promote quality and safety. The importance of interprofessional collaboration and peer support are emphasised as critical factors in building a supportive workplace. Strategies for self-care are included as a means of dealing with the inherent occupational stress in nursing.

# Transitions through health and illness

## CHAPTER OVERVIEW

- Nurses need to know how to assist people who are in the process of transitioning through health and illness.
- How people make efforts to cope with such transitions is important for nurses to understand.
- Coping efforts often reflect how people conceptualise illness, called 'illness representation'.
- There is a relationship between coping efforts and illness representation.
- Resilience, a sense of coherence and social support, are resources that assist with coping.
- Common themes in the experience of illness include uncertainty, vulnerability, loss/grief and hope.

# INTRODUCTION

Nurses relate to people in a variety of contexts, and for the most part these people will be in the throes of significant life events such as the transition from health to illness. These transitions, whether major or minor, often create interruptions and disruptions in the lives of the people experiencing them. Understanding the particular ways in which people experience illness enables nurses to help people navigate their transition because nurses can use this understanding to individualise their care for each person. Individualising care involves recognising personal responses to illness and a patient's own particular journey in healthcare transitions.

People experiencing a transition often feel uncertain and vulnerable, especially as they meet the demands and cope with the changes that often occur as a consequence. Nurses are in a prime position to ease the path of transition by decreasing uncertainty and vulnerability and by assisting people to cope with changes brought about by illness.

A clear understanding of coping and illness enables nurses to appreciate the variety of ways that people may respond. Nurses can adapt their interpersonal approach to how a particular patient is responding in order to assist that person through their transition. However, the emphasis is not simply to understand how patients are coping but to use this understanding in making interpersonal connections. Forming helpful relationships remains at the heart of nursing care.

# TRANSITIONS AND COPING

People who are cared for by nurses are often experiencing life transitions. They may be adults moving from being independent to being permanently or temporarily dependent on others for their survival. It may be a family coming to grips with a catastrophic illness or a terminal diagnosis of one of its members. Others may be awaiting a medical diagnosis after experiencing symptoms of illness. For others again, it will be dealing with the challenges of chronic illness, often exacerbated by bouts of acute illness and the continual need for readjustment. All of these circumstances involve transition – a movement from one way of being to another. The process of transition is important for nurses to understand, not only because of its pervasiveness in healthcare but also because nurses are in a position to help facilitate a transition (e.g. by assisting patients to learn new skills in their healthcare). Credited with the development of the nursing theory of transitions, Meleis (2010) claims that it is a concept central to nursing.

In its simplest definition, transition is a passage from one place to another. In this regard, transition refers to relocation; in healthcare settings, such passages are often far-reaching. Transitions through health and illness are often transformative in the sense that lives are altered. A health transition is the passage from one life stage, condition or health status to another (Meleis 2010). Through such transitions, people often redefine their sense of self and redevelop self-agency in response to disruptive life events' (Kralik et al 2006). Distress, anxiety, loss and grief may also mark health transitions, as people cope with life alterations such as being unwell, getting well again, becoming disabled and approaching death.

In the process of facilitating a transition with patients, nurses' efforts are aimed at understanding the patient's experience of illness. Understanding the illness requires knowledge of the patient's physical condition, medical diagnosis and treatment; this is 'case knowledge', described in Chapter 1. Nevertheless, understanding illness is more than simply knowing about diseases; it entails knowing something about the person who experiences illness. This is knowledge of how the person is responding to the disease, also discussed in Chapter 1 as 'patient and person knowledge'.

In nursing practice, the focus is on the relationship between illness and disease (Benner 1984) – that is, the personal, subjective experiences of patients. Disease is a medical diagnosis that explains symptoms of an illness. Illness is the experience of disease – in other words, how disease affects a person's life. Illness is also the whole personal experience of a disease – the 'story' of the patient. 'Illness is the human experience of loss or dysfunction whereas disease is the manifestation of aberration at a cellular, tissue or organ level' (Benner & Wrubel 1989, p. 8). Illness is the human response to disease; however, there can be illness in the absence of disease. Similarly, a person can have a disease, yet not experience illness.

The experience of illness is not inherently negative in nature. Transitions, even one from health to chronic illness, are neither positive nor negative; often they are both. This is because transitions bring with them opportunities for positive growth (Meleis 2010). Consider the following scenario.

## SCENARIO

When Ted had a myocardial infarction (heart attack) at the age of 52, he was not surprised. Many years earlier he had witnessed his father suffer numerous myocardial infarctions that eventually left him debilitated and ultimately resulted in his death. Ted knew there was a strong possibility that he also might experience a fate similar to his father. Because of his family history, Ted had quit smoking and reduced both his cholesterol intake and his weight, 10 years prior to his infarction. Ted received early warning signals in the form of angina three years prior to his infarction, and the diagnosis of coronary artery disease was confirmed at that time. When Ted had the diagnosis confirmed, he began an exercise program and visited a cardiologist regularly. None of these measures prevented his ultimate heart attack; however, Ted knew that his efforts had helped to decrease both the severity and the effects of the infarction.

One aspect of Ted's life had not been altered in his efforts to reduce his risk of progressive coronary artery disease. It was his job. His work as an information technology expert in a large multinational company was stressful, and recent events in the industry had placed more demands than ever on Ted. When he had the heart attack, Ted realised that it was time to consider altering his

*cont.*

current work activities. Just how he would or could do so was not immediately apparent, but the recognition that something had to be done to either reduce his work-related stress or cope with it in different ways became clear in Ted's mind as he lay on a bed in the coronary care unit.

Ted underwent coronary artery bypass surgery within weeks of his infarction. His recovery from a medical and surgical viewpoint was uneventful, but the experience dramatically altered Ted's life. When he returned to work six weeks after the surgery, he did so on a part-time basis. No longer would he spend endless hours at work. Ted also altered his attitude towards work. No longer would he react with anger and frustration at what he perceived to be improper decision making at upper management levels. He successfully changed both his attitude and his reactions to work-related demands. While still functioning effectively on the job, he successfully altered his perception of his work environment and his response to it.

After two more years as an information technology manager, Ted was offered and accepted a newly created position in his company. This position was more relaxed and enabled him to have more flexibility and control over his work environment. After three years in this position, Ted decided to take a lucrative early retirement package when it was offered.

Prior to his illness, the idea of retirement had frightened Ted because he could not imagine what he would do with his time if he was not at work. His illness changed all that. He took up more leisure activities in an effort to relax and keep physically fit. When his final days at work approached, Ted was ready and able to leave it all behind, eagerly anticipating his new life as a retired worker. Many years later, he remains content in his retirement, relaxed and able to enjoy the slower pace of life that it brings. Ted sometimes reflects back on his illness and wonders what might have happened had he not seized the opportunity to slow down and enjoy life. He remains grateful that his heart attack caused him to reconsider his lifestyle and take action to alter what had become unhealthy work practices.

The scenario illustrates how a transition to illness can serve as a catalyst for learning and change. Ted met the challenges presented by his illness by seizing the opportunity in a positive way, achieving a sense of wellbeing with a life now redefined. Transition is not simply change but rather the process that people go through to incorporate the change or disruption into their lives (Kralik et al 2006). Success in transition is considered to occur when feelings of distress are relieved and the person feels a sense of mastery of the event that brought about changes in their life.

In facilitating successful transitions, it is important that nurses have a basic understanding of how people make sense of life changes and make efforts to cope. Coping is concerned with efforts to manage demands for adjustment and adaptation and the emotions that they generate (Lazarus 2006). Efforts to cope are psychological mechanisms that manage stress and anxiety in both positive and negative ways.

# Coping efforts

The link between coping and transitions is premised on the notion that transitions mean change, and this engenders demands for adjustment. When helping to facilitate a smooth transition, nurses need to understand how the patient is attempting to cope with such demands. Coping is defined as 'constantly changing cognitive and behavioural efforts to manage specific external and/or internal demands that are appraised as taxing or exceeding the resources of the person' (Lazarus & Folkman 1984, p. 141). Coping efforts include all attempts that are made in response to these demands. Attempts to cope range from denying the significance of an event to mastering new skills in order to meet the demands of the situation. Coping efforts may be focused on reducing the anxiety, mastering the situation, minimising its significance or simply tolerating it.

People make efforts to cope in two identifiable ways. They can attempt to change the situation and meet its challenges by developing capabilities such as self-care so that it doesn't continue to be so stressful, or they can attempt to change the way the stressful situation affects them, thus altering their response to it. The first of these attempts is known as 'problem-focused' or active coping because they address problems directly. The second is known as 'emotion-focused' or passive coping because they regulate emotional responses. Active coping focuses on the problem at hand by solving the problem and developing new skills. Passive coping focuses on the emotional response to the problem at hand (e.g. by pushing the problem to one side and thinking about something else) (Lazarus & Folkman 1984). These two types of coping are illustrated in Fig. 9.1.

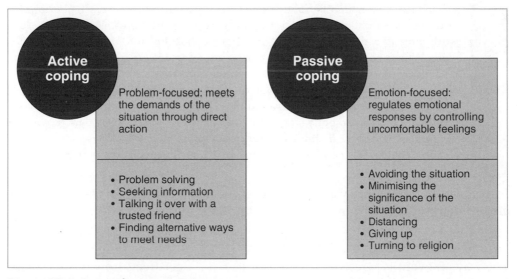

**Figure 9.1** Active and passive coping

## Denial

Coping efforts that are aimed at avoiding the situation are often considered to be a form of denial. Denial is frequently used as a means of emotion-focused coping and is effective in containing anxiety within manageable limits. Denial can take many forms, ranging from denial of feelings about an illness to denial of the existence of a disease, even when it has been diagnosed and explained to a patient. It is an effective way for patients to manage the perceived consequences of an illness. Denial is often used whenever these consequences are dire for the patient, for example, when life goals are under threat.

There is often an automatic tendency by nurses to judge denial as negative, making statements such as 'This patient is in denial', and therefore not cooperating with care or accepting what nurses view as the reality of their situation. As a result, nurses might confront and challenge denial because they perceive denial as an ineffective way of coping with an illness. Before challenging denial, nurses need to understand and appreciate the benefits of it.

Denial serves as a buffer for a disturbing and disruptive reality by allowing a temporary respite from this reality. Because patients will let reality (*their* reality) seep into their awareness at a rate that is manageable for them, the degree of denial is in keeping with this rate. This rate may be different from the nurse's desired rate. Whenever nurses are tempted to challenge a patient's denial, it is essential that the patient's readiness to accept the challenge be assessed. The nurse wishing to challenge denial must ask, 'Is this for the *patient*, or for *me*?'

More importantly, rather than perceiving denial as a negative response, it is useful for nurses to consider that the patient is in an early stage of acceptance. Consider the following scenario.

### SCENARIO

When Lisa, a young mother of two small children, noticed a change in her bowel patterns she sought help from her general practitioner. After preliminary diagnostic work indicated disease she was admitted to hospital for further diagnostic work. When she was diagnosed by a specialist doctor with an aggressive form of cancer, she told a nurse that she was feeling optimistic about treatment, stating that 'maybe I am just in denial'. The nurse responded by saying 'Not really. If you were in denial you would have not sought any help at all. I would say that you are in an early stage of acceptance because it takes time to come to grips with a cancer diagnosis'. After a thoughtful moment, Lisa responded by saying, 'That's really comforting. Thank you. I hadn't thought about it that way'.

In this scenario the nurse was able to not only pass judgment on the patient but also to demonstrate a comforting understanding of her perception.

## Cognitive appraisal

The way an event is perceived in terms of its relevance affects how it is handled. In order to cope effectively, people must be able to construct an interpretation of an event so that meaningful action can be taken. The perception of the event, referred to as 'cognitive appraisal' (Lazarus & Folkman 1984), affects coping efforts. Cognitive appraisal relates to how an event is evaluated in terms of its perceived outcome in relation to personal life goals and values and an assessment of coping skills to achieve this outcome. The appraisal influences the person's coping response.

Coping efforts that are aimed at keeping anxiety under control (passive or emotion-focused coping) are effective in situations that are perceived as futile (i.e. when there is considered to be a lack of control over the outcome). These types of coping efforts are usually focused on maintaining emotional control. When the outcome is perceived as overwhelming or disruptive to major life goals and there is little that can be done to alter the outcome, then temporary denial or avoidance may be the most effective alternative.

When people believe they can influence the outcome of an event through some effort, they are likely to take active measures to meet the challenges and demands of the event (active or problem-focused coping). Most people use a combination of both types of coping efforts. People must be able to keep emotional responses within manageable limits by using avoidance mechanisms (emotion-focused coping) while simultaneously altering, adjusting and adapting to the demands placed on them by stressful events (problem-focused coping) (Lazarus & Folkman 1984).

People need to be able to employ both types of coping effort. Passive coping efforts assist in maintaining emotional equilibrium by diffusing emotional responses and keeping anxiety under control. Active coping efforts enable people to change and grow through stressful experiences. Although it is a somewhat paradoxical concept, people simultaneously maintain equilibrium and grow throughout life and its transitions. According to Lazarus (2006) there are dangers in treating the two types of coping as separate and competing, as they often complement each other and combine to form the complete coping process.

Lazarus (2006) has warned that an emphasis on the two types of coping, while necessary, may be inadequate because the types refer to only part of the coping process – the cognitive or thought processes. He urges an equal emphasis on the personal meaning of events, especially in relation to the emotions that are engendered when facing life stresses. For nurses to appreciate how a patient is coping, they must also understand meanings that the patient attaches to illness (i.e. their own perception of the event and their feelings about it).

# Coping effectiveness

Like transitions, coping methods are not inherently good or bad, and nurses need to view patients' coping efforts within the overall context of the situation (e.g. the effects of coping on significant people in the patient's life). An evaluation of the effectiveness of coping efforts relies on the use of a variety of criteria, expressed in the following questions:

- Does the coping effort help to keep anxiety and distress within control?
- What are the long-term effects of the coping efforts?
- Does the coping effort help to maintain a sense of self-esteem?

- Is the coping effort helping to maintain interpersonal connections?
- Is there flexibility in the thinking about and the approach to the situation?

Effective coping is a sophisticated juggling act that simultaneously maintains self-esteem and internal equilibrium, sustains interpersonal relationships, assists in securing adequate and relevant information and promotes autonomy and freedom and flexibility of approach. These factors are important to take into account when nurses are considering the effectiveness of coping efforts.

Some people have a characteristic style of coping that is not effective for the health situation at hand. For example, when symptoms are experienced yet no definitive diagnosis can be made, or is delayed through extensive testing, patients with the tendency to attack situations head-on may not cope effectively because they are essentially trying to come to grips with an unknown. As long as there is an effort made to determine the cause of symptoms, patients in this situation may be better off temporarily forgetting or denying the possibilities. Focusing on 'what-if' scenarios could lead to increased distress and anxiety.

Consider the following scenario.

## SCENARIO

Leanne was 43 years old when she was diagnosed with a brain tumour. Her symptoms during the three years prior to diagnosis had been annoying, puzzling and, at times, alarming to her. But, despite these symptoms, she did not see herself as ill. It was her gradual loss of hearing in her left ear and the subsequent referral to a neurologist that finally resulted in tests that confirmed the presence of the tumour. Initially, she was shocked and frightened but relieved when a biopsy showed that the tumour was benign.

Nevertheless, she was informed that she would need to undergo a lengthy and complicated surgical procedure to remove the tumour. She began to prepare herself for this. She was accustomed to leading an active and involved life, filled with a job she enjoyed, friends and family and extensive travel. From what the surgeon explained, Leanne realised that her life would change dramatically in the immediate months following the surgery. Although the long-term prospects for full recovery were hopeful, Leanne realised that there were no guarantees. She understood the implications of her surgery and knew her future was filled with uncertainty.

Leanne's friends and family were amazed by the way she was facing the situation. Naturally, she had periods of distress, anxiety, sadness and even anger. But most of the time she thought about and discussed her impending surgery with an informed awareness of what it would entail. She understood and accepted that her recovery would take time and require effort to relearn some daily functions that she previously took for granted.

In the weeks leading up to the surgery, however, Leanne found that she focused less and less on what was about to happen. Instead, she busied herself by sewing fancy nightgowns so she would at least 'look nice' while in hospital. There was really no more for her to do but wait and try not to dwell on her worries.

Leanne's story illustrates how a combination of efforts is used to cope with an illness. Initially, she focused on 'attacking' the problem by having all the necessary tests and gathering information that would help her to understand the surgery. Once plans for surgery were under way, she coped with the waiting period by focusing her energies elsewhere. Worrying seemed of little value to Leanne at this time, so she coped by 'not thinking too much' about the surgery.

Experienced nurses who are involved with people dealing with major life transitions that are disruptive and sometimes shattering cannot help but be struck by the strength of the human capacity to cope. Some people seem to have limitless capacity to psychologically weather the storm of serious illness, while others become overwhelmed and incapacitated by minor inconveniences. The difference is not necessarily related to the seriousness and extent of an illness but to how the person perceives the situation and uses resources in the dynamic process of coping.

# Coping resources

Coping resources are personal assets that increase the likelihood of effectiveness as people adjust and adapt to health transitions; as such, they provide protection against distress. Referred to as protective factors, they help people to cope with life challenges. Three such resources are of particular relevance in relation to the process of coping with illness. Those selected for review here are resilience, a sense of coherence and social support. Not only can nurses learn to recognise these particular resources, they can also use an understanding of them when facilitating the process of transition through health and illness.

Promoting the positive aspects of coping and focusing on patients' strengths, and enhancing a sense of coherence rather than focusing on problems (e.g. dire medical diagnoses), is in accord with a nursing perspective of healthcare (Gottlieb 2014); nurses need to work with patients' strengths and resources, not just deficits. With an emphasis on health, nurses assist patients in dealing with the whole of a health event, not simply managing a disease. They do so as people who are skilled in the practice of comforting, supporting and enabling (see Ch 8).

## Resilience

People who are resilient have the ability to 'bounce back' in the face of adversity and remain optimistic in the face of threats to their wellbeing (Garcia-Dia et al 2013). Resilient people are capable of being injured and they do bend under stress, but they are equally capable of subsequent rebound and recovery. They adapt and adjust in order to overcome adversity; in fact, resilient people often thrive and flourish in the face of adversity (Aburn et al 2016).

Resilience is characterised by a strong sense of self-esteem and self-reliance, high flexibility and adaptability and an optimistic outlook that includes a sense of humour about oneself and life in general, which is accompanied by positive, caring, strong social connections and support (Garcia-Dia et al 2013). Resilient people possess a strong sense of self, and they are able to find meaning and purpose in life. Once considered a personality characteristic that moderates the negative effects of stress, resilience is now recognised as a dynamic process that is learnt and therefore modifiable (Aburn et al 2016).

As a process, resilience is a response to stress in which a person directs energy to minimise the impact of stressful events through novel approaches to problem solving and reframing their perceptions. When faced with negative circumstances, resilient people use positive emotions and are likely to construct positive meaning in negative events. They are able to manage adversity through positive adaptation and maintain functioning at an optimal level.

Resilience is associated with positive health outcomes, such as wellbeing and physical health (Eicher et al 2015), and lower mortality rates when compared with non-resilient people (Elliott et al 2014). It is for these reasons that nurses should make an effort to build resilience in patients, for example, by assisting them in reframing negative perceptions and constructing positive meaning in health events (see Ch 8).

Resilience is the direct opposite to the concept of vulnerability. When people feel vulnerable they feel inadequate to meet the demands of a situation. Resilient people feel adequate and are resourceful. Consider the following scenario.

## SCENARIO

Jacinta wouldn't rest until she had an answer that made sense to her about what she felt in her breasts. Dissatisfied with what the doctors were telling her about her symptoms, she persisted in seeing more medical specialists. She didn't believe there was 'nothing wrong'. She told herself and her friends, 'Just because the tests have come back negative doesn't mean I'm fine. I know there's something wrong and I'm not going to settle until somebody does something'. Jacinta knew she could not afford to take any chances. Her family, especially her three children, needed her.

She was not at all surprised by the diagnosis of cancer when a specialist finally agreed to do a breast biopsy. While the diagnosis and subsequent mastectomy were extremely distressing, at least some action was being taken. She felt strong because she knew what she was fighting. And fight she did. Through every course of radiotherapy and chemotherapy, Jacinta remained incredibly optimistic. She reassured her friends and family members when they expressed worry or fear. In fact, Jacinta's fortitude was an inspiration to everybody. When secondary sites of the cancer were found, she was a bit disheartened but not discouraged. She courageously endured three years of cancer therapy and never lost the beaming smile on her face. Her major frustration was a low level of energy and the need to curtail her usual activities. Sleeping during the day was not her style, but she adjusted to the change of pace in her life. Her friends and family members stepped in to assist with her daily responsibilities of caring for her children.

Despite ongoing treatment, the cancer gradually invaded all of Jacinta's body. When it became clear that no more active treatment was indicated, some of her friends and family members fell apart. Nevertheless, Jacinta didn't. She

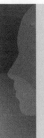

remained an inspiration to all. Her cheerfulness was unending. Even though her 'fight' with the cancer was over, she did not feel or act defeated. She enjoyed every day that she had with her family. Jacinta was thankful for and cherished every moment until the end of her life. When she died peacefully and in comfort in her home, her friends and family members were grief-stricken. But they also knew that Jacinta and her phenomenal strength and human spirit had enriched their lives.

Jacinta showed remarkable resilience throughout her illness. Her ability to remain optimistic in the face of adversity, along with her equanimity and responsiveness to others, are demonstrations of the characteristics of resilience.

## Sense of coherence

Aaron Antonovsky (1987) developed a theory about how people stay healthy in order to counteract the tendency in healthcare to focus on why people get sick. In doing so, he emphasised the resources that people use to successfully cope with the stresses of life. These resources combine and converge to form what Antonovsky refers to as a sense of coherence. A sense of coherence (Antonovsky 1987, 1996) is marked by three attributes: an ability to understand and make sense of situations that happen in life (*comprehensibility*); an abiding trust that things will work out because there are resources available to meet the demands of life's various situations (*manageability*); and the motivation to invest time and effort in life's challenges (*meaningfulness*).

People who have a strong sense of coherence perceive life's challenges as having some structure and clarity as opposed to the perception that life is a series of random events. This is what is meant by comprehensibility. Manageability, the second attribute, is the extent to which a person perceives that resources to cope successfully are available and adequate. The final characteristic, meaningfulness, is the extent to which a person believes it is worth putting time and effort into coping with life stresses. Comprehensibility is the cognitive or thinking aspect of coherence, manageability is the behavioural or action aspect and meaningfulness is the motivational or feeling aspect. All three – thoughts, behaviours and feelings – come together to form a sense of coherence.

A strong sense of coherence is likely to diffuse the negative effects of stressful situations and promote health in two ways. First, a sense of coherence diffuses the negative effects of stress through a perceptual process of accenting the positive because optimism has been shown to be related to a sense of coherence (Gustavsson-Lilius 2012). This is referred to colloquially as 'seeing the world through rose-coloured glasses'. In addition to its effect on perception, a sense of coherence results in coping that involves problem solving (active coping) rather than avoidance (often associated with emotion-focused coping). Not only does the disposition towards coherence result in effective coping, it also positively influences health status in general (Geulayov et al 2015).

A sense of coherence creates an orientation towards life's challenges that averts tension and assists in managing life stress and transitions. Such a disposition contributes to a sense of wellbeing (Grevenstein et al 2016) and health-related quality of life (Chumbler et al 2013; Vogel et al 2012). In addition, a strong sense of coherence is associated with lower mortality from any cause (Geulayov et al 2015), alleviating distress in cancer (Gustavsson-Lilius et al 2012) and better self-management in chronic illness (Chumbler et al 2013; Silarova et al 2014; Stein-Parbury et al 2012).

While initially considered by Antonovsky as stable by the age of 30 years, a sense of coherence has been shown to change in response to life events (Bergman et al 2011) and strengthens in old age (Silverstein & Heap 2015). Therefore, it is not a static disposition but a dynamic process that is open to change through life experiences and interactions with others. This holds promise as the disposition of coherence can be enhanced through helpful interventions – for example, by assisting people to 'restructure' the meaning of illness, framing it in a positive light and developing coping strategies in illness. The way that nurses care for patients has the potential to promote a sense of coherence in patients (Kvåle & Synnes 2013). For example, providing explanations helps patients to comprehend their circumstances; validating their worth as a person helps them to find meaning; and supporting their self-care helps them with managing their health (see *Research highlight*).

## RESEARCH HIGHLIGHT How nurses promote a sense of coherence in patients

*Kvåle, K., Synnes, O., 2013. Understanding cancer patient's reflections on good nursing care in light of Antonovsky's theory. European Journal of Oncology Nursing 17, 814–819.*

### Background

Cancer patients who have a strong sense of coherence experience less distress, depression and anxiety than those with a weaker sense of coherence. As sense of coherence is not static, it is important that nurses understand what type of care enhances a patient's sense of coherence.

### Purpose of the study

The aim of this study was to explore cancer patients' perceptions of good nursing care. This analysis of the data was based on Antonovsky's theory of the factors that support health and wellbeing.

### Method

Twenty patients who were hospitalised for cancer were interviewed in order to ascertain their perceptions of how nurses cared for them. The data from the interviews were initially analysed from a phenomenological perspective. This was a reanalysis based on how nursing care related to their sense of coherence.

### Key findings

In making sense of their situation (comprehensibility) patients wanted nurses who could explain what was happening – for example, discussing the side effects of medications. Having information helped them to feel in control. Patients expressed that they preferred to talk with nurses about their normal life rather than focusing on the negative emotions aroused by their illness. This helped them find meaning that life was worth living for and investing energy into despite an uncertain future (meaningfulness). Finding meaning in their daily life helped them to feel less overwhelmed by their situation (manageability).

### Implications for nursing practice

It is important that nurses are able to explain aspects of a patient's illness and its treatment. Nurses need to appreciate the importance of talking to patients about what is important in their lives and not just the experience of their illness.

## Social support

Both resilience and a sense of coherence have a common thread – the presence of a social network that provides support to the person. Social support involves connection with and mutual obligation to other people; people who experience social support feel cared for, loved and esteemed (Tay et al 2013; Thoits 2011). Social support is based on the assumption that people need to have supportive relationships with other people in order to manage the demands of daily living and cope with life transitions. These relationships serve to fulfil social needs for affection, approval, belonging, security and identity.

In Chapter 8 the concept of nurses as providers of support was explored, but emphasis was placed on the importance of nursing care that mobilises other sources of support for patients. In this chapter, social support refers to these other sources that come from close associates such as family and friends. If these usual sources cannot provide needed support, people look to other sources of support such as healthcare professionals.

Support from other people in the form of aid, assistance, personal affirmation and information is necessary when stressful events such as transitions in health and illness are experienced. While support from other people does not necessarily alter the demands of a situation, it does lessen its consequences. Appropriate support aids provide further capability for meeting demands and counteracts feelings of helplessness and hopelessness.

Social support helps people to: evaluate their situation realistically; challenge and alter their existing perspectives; maintain their self-esteem by reinforcing a belief that they are able to manage; and establish emotional balance by absorbing the impact of strong feelings. Other people's involvement can also serve as a temporary distraction from distress. Cultural and religious rituals, beliefs and practices, largely social in nature, can also provide support during stressful events.

As a result of supportive social networks, people experience a sense of competence, empowerment and wellbeing; they feel validated. There is a robust evidence of a positive correlation between being strongly connected through a social network and physical and mental health (Deindl et al 2016; Heinze et al 2015; Tay et al 2013; Thoits 2011; Vogel et al 2012), and reduced mortality (Becofsky et al 2015; Idler et al 2012). In addition, social support is positively related to health and recovery from illness (Graven & Grant 2013; Sharply et al 2015), as well as self-care in chronic illness (Cornwall & Waite 2012; Koetsenruijter et al 2016). The evidence of this connection is so strong that social relationships should be considered as important as other lifestyle interventions (e.g. exercise and diet) in health promotion and recovery from illness (Becofsky et al 2015).

How do social relationships influence health and recovery from illness? There are numerous ways in which support from other people buffers stress and assists with coping. The first is that having people around who are caring, concerned and understanding boosts a person's self-esteem and sense of security and belonging, as well as providing emotional support. In addition, other people often provide tangible and practical aid such as providing transport to medical appointments or encouraging shared, regular exercise. Another way that other people provide support is by helping to perceive and appraise a situation (i.e. looking at the world through different eyes). Whether by providing information or offering a different perspective, other people often help with seeing a situation in a new and different light (Thoits 2011). All of these instances of social support have a positive effect on coping and being healthy.

To be effective in stressful situations, support from other people must be available, usable and suitable to the context. A hospitalised patient's relative who cannot cope with the sights and sounds of a hospital will be of little value in the situation. In this sense, the effectiveness of the support needs to be evaluated in light of the current context. A supportive person who lives in another state or country may not be able to provide support, regardless of how helpful this person may be. That is, social support must always be considered specifically within a context. And in the case of a person without a network, nurses can become an integral feature of support.

The concept of social support is sometimes presented as all positive, expressed through catch phrases such as 'your friends are your best medicine'. Nevertheless, this is a simplistic notion of social connections because people in a social network can place demands on each other as well as offer assistance. Friends and family can create stress as well as alleviate it. Also, support that is offered must match what is needed (Thoits 2011). There is no use in a friend offering help that actually hinders – for example, by offering advice or information that is neither wanted nor useful.

Therefore, social support is a complex, multidimensional concept that is not well understood despite an abundance of research (Cornwall & Waite 2012). One aspect is that social support encompasses an acknowledgment of the importance of social relationships. Other aspects include descriptions of social networks and the interrelationships between the people in that network (e.g. an extended family). In addition, there are functional aspects of social relationships, the perceived availability of support and actual support that is received. Because of its complexity, social support has many definitions. At their most basic level, social connections between people are part of a healthy life.

# FACILITATING TRANSITIONS IN ILLNESS

In coping with an illness, patients call upon needed resources. Nurses are potential resources if they are involved, interested and concerned. But nurses can only be resources when they have taken the time to understand the situation from the patient's perspective.

Nurses help patients cope with illness by assisting them in many ways; they can help patients to contain uncomfortable feelings, generate a sense of hope and redefine the situation in solvable terms. Perhaps most significant is the way in which nurses assist patients in maintaining or regaining their self-esteem.

Throughout an illness, patients must be able to maintain a sense of self-esteem and their capability for meeting the demands of the situation. Illness often threatens this sense – for example, when there is loss of physical functioning or an alteration in body image. Acknowledging and understanding patients' experiences is one of the most effective ways that nurses can help maintain a patient's self-esteem.

Whenever people become ill, there is a personal assessment of the meaning of the illness. Benner and Wrubel (1989, p. 9) express this by stating that, 'Every illness has a story – plans are threatened, relationships are disturbed and symptoms become laden with meaning depending on what else is happening in the person's life'. They go on to say that, 'When illness strikes, the illness and possible ways to cope with it are understood in light of personal background meanings, the situation and ongoing concerns in the patient's life' (Benner & Wrubel 1989, p. 88).

While it might be easier for nurses to consider a patient's responses in light of what they know about the clinical condition of the patient, they also need to understand how the patient perceives and interprets the meaning of the illness in relation to its impact on their life. The impact and meaning of an event will influence whether or not the event will create anxiety and distress. Some patients view admission to hospital for routine surgery as a minor inconvenience. But a mother of small children who is unable to arrange adequate childcare in her absence may view the same event as a major inconvenience and disruption to her daily life.

Often there is a perception of threat or danger in illness, especially when it begins or exacerbates: threat that the person's life may no longer be the same; threat that there may be an inability to proceed with life as anticipated and planned; and threat in the sense that the body once relied on to perform and work effectively is no longer able to do so. This sense of threat is often accompanied by anxiety and fear, and if these feelings become too strong or pose too much of a disruption, they are met with efforts to keep them under control.

Of primary importance in coping with illness is the ability to maintain emotional balance. Patients must be able to keep distressing feelings within manageable limits in order to cope with other demands of illness. If feelings of anxiety and fear become overwhelming, patients become disorganised or almost paralysed. Passive coping efforts such as minimising, denying, rationalising and ignoring are all examples of how feelings of anxiety are kept in check.

In Chapters 6 and 7 there are references to the importance of recognising when patients are trying to control their emotions and appreciating the importance of not focusing on feelings during these times. The reasons for this are reinforced in this section, and nurses who understand the importance of timing their responses will be able to refrain from discussing feelings with patients who are coping by containing and controlling their emotional responses.

# Illness representation

How patients perceive an illness (i.e. how they make sense of it) involves a complex cognitive and emotional process that results in creating a mental representation of the illness (Leventhal et al 2003). Referred to as the 'lay view' or 'common sense' model of illness, this representation is based on the sources of information that are available to people in order to make sense of and manage an illness event (Petrie & Weinman 2012). The sources include: previous experiences and cultural understandings; information from other people including authoritative sources such as healthcare professionals; and current perception of and previous experience with the illness.

The illness representation includes five cognitive dimensions: cause, consequences, identity (of the symptoms), timeline and cure/controllability. The dimension of *cause* refers to biological factors such as a virus, as well as psychological ones such as overwork or mental attitude. In this regard, causes can be seen as internal and/or external to the person. The next dimension, *consequences*, relates to the impact of the illness on the person in relation to overall quality of life, as well as functional capacity. *Identity* refers to the recognition and experience of the symptoms of illness, and *timeline* involves beliefs about the course of an illness (e.g. whether it is perceived as short-term or chronic). The *cure/controllability* dimension includes the perception of the effectiveness of coping behaviours (e.g. the belief that taking medication, as an active coping effort, will cure an illness). Taken together, these five dimensions capture how a person makes sense of an illness as a whole.

The original work on illness representation included these five dimensions, which are cognitive in nature. More recently, the role of emotional reaction (i.e. how a person feels about the illness) has been recognised as equally important (Kucukarslan 2012). Illness representation is not only what people think but also how they feel about what is happening to their health. For example, the diagnosis of an 'incurable' cancer may have different emotional meaning to a 96-year-old person who feels satisfied that they have lived a good life than it would to a 26-year-old person who has small children. The emotional stakes and impact are different in each of these situations.

There is evidence that illness perceptions not only affect the way people cope but also are associated with healthcare outcomes, such as functioning, healthcare utilisation, adherence to treatment and mortality, across a range of illnesses (Petrie & Weinman 2012). In relation to medication adherence, all dimensions of illness perceptions, with the exception of coherence, have an impact for better or worse (Kucukarslan 2012). There are poorer clinical outcomes when an illness is perceived as chronic, with serious consequences and poor control (Glattacker et al 2012). In a meta-analysis of studies, Dempster et al (2015) concluded that views about the consequences of an illness and emotional perceptions were the aspects of illness representation that had the strongest relationship with distress in a range of illnesses.

In patients with cancer, passive coping responses were employed when they perceived their illness to be long-lasting, emotionally burdensome and having negative consequences (Hopman & Rijken 2015). In patients with chronic kidney disease, having greater knowledge, along with a poor perception of control, was associated with treatment adherence (Vélez-Vélez & Bosche 2016). In patients with chronic pain, illness representation contributed significantly to depression and anxiety more than the intensity of actual pain (Costa et al 2016).

Each of the dimensions of illness representation also affects how people cope with a health event. Consider the following scenario.

## SCENARIO

The discovery of a lump on her breast during a routine visit to her general practitioner took Julia by complete surprise. At the age of 39 she felt fit, well and quite happy with her life. Her two sons, aged eight and 10, were doing well with school and friendships. She was happily married to a loving man and enjoyed an active social and community life. She adored her part-time work as an interior designer, a job in which she not only found enormous professional satisfaction but also one that had brought her public accolades and honours from peers. Having just learnt that she had been nominated for an international industry award for innovative design, the news of the lump in her breast that same day brought her right down to the ground.

When a biopsy revealed that the lump was cancerous, Julia faced the resultant surgical removal of the lump and radiotherapy with the optimistic and cheerful outlook that pervaded the rest of her life. She did not dwell on thoughts of 'why me?' and accepted the illness as happenstance for her; she did not 'blame herself' for the illness, nor did she dwell on what she might have done to contribute to it. She was mindful of the frequency with which she heard of more and more women experiencing breast cancer and considered that she was just one of the unlucky many.

This did not stop her from taking every action she could to restore her health and wellbeing. She altered her diet dramatically based on the advice of a naturopath; she began practising yoga regularly in an effort to learn to more effectively relax and meditate. Her close and supportive network of friends, family and work colleagues were involved and included in all of her efforts.

*cont.*

*Scenario continued*

Because of her outgoing nature, she met many women who had experienced breast cancer and was eager to hear of their experiences, whether good or bad.

In addition to her changes in lifestyle, Julia remained diligent in her regular health checks and yearly mammograms. After five years, a mammogram revealed 'suspicious' changes in the breast that initially had the cancer, and Julia was once again confronted with the fear of ongoing cancer and the need to have further treatment. Complete removal of her breast was indicated, and she faced the surgery with her usual level of optimism, albeit with an ongoing, nagging fear of cancer spreading throughout her body.

The results of the biopsy of the removed breast and further exhaustive testing revealed there was no need for ongoing concern. Her surgeon was most reassuring that the cancer had been removed from her body. However, he did recommend referral to an oncologist. Until this point in time, the medical practitioners caring for her shared Julia's optimism about her future health. While she willingly accepted the advice of her surgeon to see an oncologist, she was filled with anxiety because doing so somehow made her a 'real' cancer patient.

She easily formed a good working relationship with the oncologist, as she had with her other doctors. She was willing to heed any advice that she was offered. However, the oncologist was not as directive as her GP and surgeon had been. Instead, she presented Julia with a set of statistics and options, offering little in the way of advice. The oncologist assured Julia that there were no signs of cancer in her body at present but did inform her that there was a five per cent chance that her cancer would recur because there could be 'rogue' cancer cells present in her body even in the absence of any current medical evidence to indicate this was so. The oncologist informed Julia that chemotherapy was an option to eliminate the shadow of doubt, based on the five per cent probability. However, she stressed that the decision to undergo chemotherapy was entirely Julia's decision and would not offer advice either way.

Suddenly, what seemed fairly straightforward in relation to treatment became murky and ambiguous. Chemotherapy had numerous side effects that Julia found distasteful, especially the loss of her hair. Her family and friends were reluctant to say what they thought she should do, and she did not place them in the position of doing so by asking. She knew that she alone would have to make the decision.

After a few weeks of serious contemplation and much soul-searching, Julia decided to undergo the chemotherapy. She based her decision on the fact that she had a young family to raise and that she was still young herself. More importantly, she reconciled that living with even a small chance of cancer recurrence could become too burdensome mentally and she preferred to relieve her anxieties by undergoing the treatment. She came to terms with the hair loss and purchased a stylish wig to get her through what seemed to be the most troublesome aspect of the therapy.

She underwent the chemotherapy with a positive attitude, secure in the knowledge that it would relieve a large degree of her worries. It was temporary pain for long-term gain. She was extra cautious in her self-care, taking even more time for herself and her health than was her usual nature.

One year following the chemotherapy, Julia was feeling herself again. Her body had been through much and would never be the same in appearance. She mentally accepted that she would always be considered a 'cancer patient'. Yet she was able to move forward with her life. Receiving the international design award had helped to boost her spirits, but she realised that what mattered most in life was her health and the love of her family and friends. She was proud of her achievement and at ease with her body. She experienced a renewed sense of her life values.

Julia's story reveals how an illness representation affects a person's response to a transition in health. She perceived that the cause was external to her and just a matter of chance. Nonetheless, she did take measures to control its consequences through changes in her lifestyle that improved her overall quality of life. Prior to her illness, she was more likely to place the needs of others ahead of her own. As a result of the illness, she was able to match concern about her own wellbeing with her concern for others. While she accepted that she would continue to be a 'cancer patient', she did not perceive her illness as chronic. The measures she took to seek and accept medical treatment were based on her belief that the cancer could be contained, if not controlled. Her abiding belief in the treatment that she chose enabled her to progress with her life in a reassured manner. In summary, her representation of her illness affected how she coped with it.

## Working with a patient's illness representation

While the theory of how people come to understand an illness is relevant, nurses must also have the skills of working with a patient's illness representation. Any approach to be of assistance will only be effective if the patient's understanding of their health condition and its cognitive appraisal is taken into account. For example, patients who feel responsible for causing their illness will need understanding and support with feelings of guilt and remorse. Patients who perceive that the consequences of their illness are life-threatening will need assistance in understanding if this is really the case; they may need factual information if there is every chance that they will recover. If their condition is chronic they will need help in making any necessary adjustments to their lifestyle. Having a sense of how long an illness is likely to last will enable them to make life plans. When, from a biomedical perspective, there is little possibility of recovery, nurses need to comfort and support patients in their struggle to come to terms with their condition. Finally, nurses need to understand how a patient feels about their illness and express empathy for these feelings. Therefore, nurses need to adapt each of the skills presented in this book to their patient's perceptions of their health condition.

# THEMES IN ILLNESS

Nurses come into contact with patients who are facing a variety of situations. For example:

- A disease is suspected yet unknown or unclear, and the patient feels unwell but no identifiable cause is known.
- The patient's condition is one in which full recovery is anticipated, although the patient may be ill and incapacitated for a period of time.
- Although recovery is likely, the patient experiences complications that delay recovery and create the possibility of a long-term illness.
- The patient's condition is one that is likely to proceed on a progressive downhill course, leaving the patient increasingly incapacitated and ill.
- The patient develops a chronic condition that is usually characterised by periods of illness and periods of wellness.
- There is a life-threatening condition that brings uncertainty both immediately and in the future.
- The patient's condition is one in which death is likely to occur in the near future.

Each of these situations represents a different set of circumstances, and each patient facing the situation will experience it differently. Nevertheless, there are commonalities that specifically relate to how nurses approach patients who are experiencing these situations. These commonalities are uncertainty, vulnerability, distress, loss and grief and hope.

## Uncertainty

Whenever there is an alteration to a patient's health status, they are dealing with uncertainty. What is wrong? Will recovery occur? What type of medical intervention will be required? Can the demands of such intervention be met? Will there be a permanent alteration to lifestyle? Will there be pain and suffering? Uncertainty in illness is the inability to interpret the meaning and to predict the outcomes of a health-related event (Mishel 2013). Therefore, there is no way to understand what is happening and develop a mental representation of the illness.

Uncertainty is experienced as confusion, ambiguity and fear of the unknown. It is accompanied by insufficient information and cues to structure the experience (Cypress 2016). It is the opposite of feeling confident of the way forward and in control. A high level of uncertainty results in emotional distress and anxiety (Hansen et al 2012), especially if coping resources are inadequate to resolve the ambiguity or manage emotions. Mishel (2013) considers uncertainty to be the greatest single psychological stress when adults experience an acute illness.

In understanding the experience of illness, nurses are often sensitive to the uncertainty that is part of the experience. There may be clinical uncertainty in establishing a diagnosis of an illness, or there may be functional uncertainty in understanding what will happen after a diagnosis occurs. Perhaps the widespread existence of uncertainty in the illness experience is the reason that nurses so frequently offer false reassurance by directing patients not to worry (see Ch 6).

Factors thought to contribute to and influence the level of uncertainty in illness include severity of illness, specificity of diagnosis, cognitive capacity of the patient, resources to aid in the interpretation, degree of social support and trust and confidence in healthcare providers. Of these possible contributors to uncertainty in illness, the lack of useful and relevant information (e.g. a specific diagnosis) is associated with increasing uncertainty (Hansen et al 2012). Therefore, the availability of healthcare professionals providing relevant information has been shown to decrease uncertainty. This information should include explanations about how the healthcare system is organised and how it operates. Nurses are seen by patients as credible authorities in health and illness, therefore patients will turn to them for information to reduce uncertainty (Ch 8).

Furthermore, support from family and friends eases the anxiety that accompanies uncertainty (Mishel 2013). These people help find meaning in an illness event in relation to a person's life. This makes mobilising social support (Ch 8) particularly relevant in reducing uncertainty.

Like other aspects of transitions in illness, uncertainty can be perceived as both a threat and an opportunity. Patients who perceive uncertainty as a threat are likely to use emotion-focused coping (passive); those who see uncertainty as an opportunity will use problem-focused coping (Mishel 2013). Passive coping efforts – such as not thinking too much about the possibilities of illness, especially when a diagnosis is unknown or ambiguous – are effective in reducing anxiety and distress. Active measures such as seeking further information or re-evaluating life goals address the uncertainty directly. Nurses need to appreciate and support both types of efforts, as both are effective means of coping.

# Vulnerability

'Vulnerability' is a term used in epidemiology to describe groups of people who are 'at risk' of certain health problems. For example, type 2 diabetes is associated with risk factors such as obesity and a sedentary lifestyle. Although useful as an objective measure in population studies that identify 'at risk' groups of people, vulnerability as it is discussed in the context of this chapter refers to the subjective state of vulnerability as individual people experience it.

In this sense, vulnerability refers to the subjective experience in which people make the interpretation that the demands of a situation exceed their personal capabilities for meeting these demands. Vulnerability is experienced as feeling unprotected or in need of protection (Sarvimäki & Stenbock-Hult 2016). Most people will experience a sense of vulnerability; it is considered part of the human condition (Gastmans 2013). However, the vulnerability experienced by people who are ill and in need of healthcare exceeds this fundamental level of vulnerability (Gjengedal et al 2013). For example, in serious or critical illness, the sense of vulnerability is heightened because patients in these circumstances are highly dependent on healthcare providers and are therefore unable to meet their own basic needs for survival. Responding to vulnerability is considered to be the essence of care (Gastmans 2013). This is first done through understanding the patient's perspective – that is, 'knowing the patient' (see Ch 1).

Coming into contact with nurses can compound a patient's vulnerability. The very fact that they perceive their situation as one that requires using healthcare resources (e.g. nurses) indicates that they evaluate their own capabilities for dealing with the situation as inadequate. The potential dependence resulting from the need for healthcare may further increase feelings of vulnerability. On the other hand, the fact that patients have mobilised healthcare resources may indicate a sense of competence and resilience. They may still perceive themselves as capable of handling the situation but recognise the need for professional assistance.

Professional healthcare practices may actually increase a patient's sense of vulnerability. For example, when patients are not involved in decisions that affect them, they are denied choice and influence, therefore increasing their sense of vulnerability. Providing information and explanations reduces a patient's sense of vulnerability (Hansen et al 2012) and enables them to be involved in decisions that directly affect them (Ch 8).

# Loss and grief

Losses are often experienced during illness. There may be loss of ability to function, loss of ability to achieve life goals, loss of hope, loss of contact and connection with significant people or loss of flexibility and freedom to determine life goals. Coping with loss is a process of letting go of what was lost, often accompanied by feelings of sadness, anxiety and sometimes guilt. Patients who are facing or experiencing loss are frequently consumed by this process and therefore are unable to focus their thoughts.

Most often, there is emotional pain as patients come to grips with a loss. There is a tendency to focus on the deprivation created by the loss. Patients whose loss is acute often feel immersed in the experience. When this natural process of healing is allowed to happen, what often follows is a new sense of gain in meeting the demands of the illness.

Grief is a natural reaction to loss. Grief is defined as 'an involuntary, spontaneous, and multi-dimensional internal state of distress catalyzed by a real or perceived loss of someone or something valued or cherished' (Bagbe Darian 2014). It, too, is a process of letting go, mourning, reflecting, reliving memories and eventually summoning resources to proceed with life, despite the fact that it may never be the same. Through the experience of grief, people learn to 'let go' and adjust, and eventually adapt to changed life conditions. Grief is a process of closing a chapter of life and gathering energy to begin the next chapter. While there may be energy to begin new phases of life, unveiling the closed chapter is still possible. But this is done as a way of recollecting how it was, of choosing to remember, rather than remaining in the acute pain of loss and grief.

Current understanding of grief and loss have been influenced by the seminal work of Elisabeth Kübler-Ross (1969). Against what was considered taboo at the time, she talked openly with patients who were dying about their experiences and observed an identifiable pattern in their thoughts and feelings. She developed a theory about loss and grief that was based on these observations and in 1969 published her ground-breaking work in a book titled *On death and dying*, which is still available today. Her work revolutionised thinking about death and grief and has influenced millions of people worldwide. Its relevance is no longer considered exclusive to the experience of death but to that of any significant loss.

Kübler-Ross' theory was based on the notion that people pass through stages in their grieving. The five stages are:

- denial – characterised by a sense of numbness, shock and disbelief
- anger – in which people experience frustration, even rage, and ask, 'why me?'
- bargaining – trying to negotiate the inevitable, often through bargaining with a 'higher power'
- depression – feeling sad and guilty over what is happening
- acceptance – coming to peace and finding a way forward, often with a sense of hope.

While this theory of the grieving process enabled an understanding, it is not without its pitfalls and criticisms. First, the use of the term 'stages' is problematic because this implies a linear process, much like the stages of growth and development. Rather than being sequential, people can pass through the stages in any order and may not experience all of the stages. Although Kübler-Ross never intended the stages to be viewed in this way, there is a tendency to apply the theory in this manner. Second, she was also clear that the stages were not a fixed road map but should be used as a guide for understanding the grieving process (Kübler-Ross & Kessler 2007).

A nurse who understands and appreciates that grieving is a natural process of healing is able to facilitate its spontaneous progression. Through understanding, nurses are able to accept patients' expression of feelings, as well as their reliving and reflecting as an expected and usual progression towards healing. The process of reflection is often associated with a search for meaning.

It is better for nurses to come to grips, on a personal and professional level, with the reality of the pain of loss. Accepting that loss is an aspect of nursing that cannot be denied or avoided minimises the risk of treating it as something that can be intellectually 'problem solved'. In dealing with patients who are experiencing or facing loss, nurses must be able to assist them with reviving memories of what has been lost. Nurses must be comfortable in allowing patients' feelings to emerge and be expressed. When the experience of loss is shared with and understood by nurses, patients feel consoled and nurtured.

# Hope

Throughout interactions with patients in transition, it is also important that nurses maintain a sense of hope that the successful passage through the illness can occur.

Hope is an emotion considered to be a vital resource in coping and counteracts feelings of despair (Duggleby et al 2012; Lazarus 1999). Hope is characterised by a sense of possibility and creates the anticipation of a positive outcome, even when life goals have been altered and there is a redefined future (Fitzgerald Miller 2007). Hope is engendered through a sense of belonging and affiliation with other people (i.e. it is a relational process). It is promoted through the presence of other people who demonstrate acceptance, tolerance and understanding.

During an illness, no matter how serious or minor, a sense of hope must be promoted and maintained. Nurses who demonstrate confidence in patients' capabilities to cope with and manage the situation promote hope. In addition, helping people to find meaning in illness promotes a sense of hope (Fitzgerald Miller 2007).

In the absence of hope, patients often give up, perceiving that their efforts to cope are in vain. This frequently occurs for brief periods during recuperation from a long-term illness or when illness is chronic. If it becomes pervasive, patients may fail to put any effort into recovering or adjusting.

While it is important that nurses maintain a sense of hope, this should not take the form of presenting false reassurance, minimising the significance of patients' distress or promoting a false sense of wellbeing through deception. At times, nurses may think that deceiving patients is in the patient's best interest. Conversely, deceit signals a lack of respect for the patient's abilities to cope and undermines any trust the patient may be feeling in the nurse. While it may be tempting to offer false hope, such actions are usually counterproductive to establishing an effective relationship and successful transition.

# SUCCESSFUL TRANSITION

Despite the vulnerability, uncertainty and distress that accompanies illness, people are often able to make a smooth transition. Consider and contrast the following two scenarios.

## SCENARIO

Tran was returning home from work one rainy evening when she was involved in a low-speed, head-on collision close to her home. Awaiting her arrival at home were her five children, ranging in age from three to 12 years, and her husband. The accident left Tran's legs severely damaged. There was a chance that one of her legs would need to be amputated. Her family, friends and neighbours were shocked and devastated by the news of Tran's condition.

But Tran's outlook was positive right from the beginning of what was to become a long journey back to functioning. She was grateful to be alive and thankful that she had not sustained injuries to her brain or other internal organs. Although her physical pain was great, especially in the early days after the accident, she remained pleasant and cheerful. Even during the time when amputation of her leg was being considered, Tran maintained that if it eventuated she could find 'other ways of getting around', despite the fact that she may do so 'with only one leg'.

Friends who visited her in hospital in the early days found her attitude uplifting and remarked that they left her bedside feeling better because Tran herself was in such good spirits. Some thought that it was only a matter of time before Tran would plunge into despair, sadness and anxiety about what was happening to her. But this was not to happen, for Tran's outlook remained positive throughout the immediate and long-term recovery periods.

As soon as she was able, Tran contacted the driver of the other vehicle involved in the collision. She expressed her concern and reassured this young man, who was not physically injured in the accident, that it was just an unfortunate incident for which no one could be blamed. Tran's family and friends rallied around and took care of her family's household needs while she was in hospital. The day she was able to get out of bed and into a wheelchair, Tran began visiting the other patients who were on the hospital ward. She spent the remaining six weeks of her acute hospitalisation visiting other patients, bringing encouragement and showing genuine interest in each of them.

Tran's hardiness and the way she approached her situation impressed the nurses who cared for her. She remained optimistic, pleasant and understanding, even when she was suffering excruciating pain. Fortunately, Tran's leg did not require amputation, but she did undergo a long period of rehabilitation during which time she learnt to walk again. Throughout the entire recovery period, Tran demonstrated an ability to cope, had available resources for her assistance and was able to maintain a realistic and positive view of the situation.

## SCENARIO

Joanne and Harold had been married for 50 years when Harold suffered a heart attack. The heart attack was minor from a medical viewpoint, and physical recovery was expected. Harold's hospitalisation and convalescence were following the usual pattern of recuperation, without complications. The nurses in the coronary care unit recognised that although Harold was progressing towards recovery, Joanne remained extremely anxious. Each time she visited Harold she asked the same questions over and over again. Her questions centred on the theme of Harold's recovery, and she expressed fears that he was not going to be 'all right'. She kept focusing on a fear that Harold might die.

No matter how many times the nurses attempted to reassure Joanne through offering factual, encouraging information about Harold's continued improvement, she remained visibly anxious. In fact, her anxiety seemed to be escalating as Harold recovered. With each visit she appeared more distraught. One day as she was leaving the hospital, Joanne's anxiety mounted to near panic. She

*cont.*

*Scenario continued*

began to cry uncontrollably and reached a state where her behaviour became disorganised. She was making random attempts to cope with the situation and her verbalisation reflected that she was having difficulty keeping her thoughts on one track. Joanne needed immediate attention.

Victor, one of the nurses caring for Harold, took Joanne to a quiet area of the ward. He listened to Joanne in an effort to understand what was happening. It took some time to piece together the story that Joanne relayed, but Victor learnt that Joanne and Harold had both been survivors of a train crash that occurred many years ago when they were young. They lived through the ordeal but lost family and friends in the accident. The event brought them closer together, bonding them in a common experience that would remain significant for the rest of their lives.

Joanne believed the nurses were just telling her everything was all right because they didn't want to worry her. She hadn't been sleeping or eating well since Harold was admitted because 'they always did these things together'. Harold and Joanne's only son was out of town on a business trip that had been delayed because of Harold's illness but could not be postponed any longer. Many of Joanne and Harold's friends had either died or moved away after retirement.

Joanne's perception of the situation was that Harold would die, despite what she was hearing from the nursing and medical staff. Her major way of coping previously was to talk things over with Harold, an avenue that was not available to her under the circumstances. Her representation of illness as fatal, her lack of adequate and usable coping skills and the absence of available social supports disrupted her ability to make a smooth transition in Harold's illness.

# SUMMARY

Whether it is temporary or long-term, an illness places coping demands and challenges on people, requiring the use of physical, personal and social resources. Through their interactions and relationships, nurses assist patients in meeting the challenges and demands of illness. Appreciating and understanding the nature of the illness experience – the narrative in the person's life – enables nurses to provide such assistance. Understanding such narratives is a central aspect of nursing care.

When forming relationships with patients, nurses must consider how the health status of the patient affects the relationship and their interactions. This chapter has explored patients' health status from the viewpoint of transitions and themes in illness. The many considerations that illness brings to the relationships between patients and nurses create a context for these relationships.

While these considerations may seem to complicate the process of learning how to interact effectively with patients, they also add richness to the experience. While nurses are interacting with patients, they come to appreciate and know the complexity and abundance of human experiences of illness.

# REFERENCES

Aburn, G., Gott, M., Hoare, K., 2016. What is resilience? An integrative review of the empirical literature. J. Adv. Nurs. 72 (5), 980–1000.

Antonovsky, A., 1987. Unraveling the Mystery of Health: How People Manage Stress and Stay Well. Jossey-Bass, San Francisco, CA.

Antonovsky, A., 1996. The sense of coherence: an historical and future perspective. Isr. J. Med. Sci. 32, 170–178.

Bagbe Darian, C.D.Y., 2014. A new mourning: synthesizing an interactive model of adaptive grieving dynamics. Illn. Crises Loss 22 (3), 195–235.

Becofsky, K.M., Shook, R.P., Sui, X., et al., 2015. Influence of the source of social support and size of social network on all-cause mortality. Mayo Clin. Proc. 90 (7), 895–902.

Benner, P., 1984. From Novice to Expert: Excellence and Power in Clinical Nursing Practice. Addison-Wesley, Menlo Park, CA.

Benner, P., Wrubel, J., 1989. The Primacy of Caring: Stress and Coping in Health and Illness. Addison-Wesley, Menlo Park, CA.

Bergman, E., Malm, D., Berterö, C., et al., 2011. Does one's sense of coherence change after an acute myocardial infarction? A two-year longitudinal study in Sweden. Nurs. Health Sci. 13, 156–163.

Chumbler, N.R., Kroenke, K., Outcalt, S., et al., 2013. Association between sense of coherence and health-related quality of life among primary care patients with chronic musculoskeletal pain. Health Qual. Life Outcomes 11 (1).

Cornwall, E.Y., Waite, L.J., 2012. Social network resources and management of hypertension. J. Health Soc. Behav. 53 (2), 215–231.

Costa, C.V., Vala, S., Sobral, M., 2016. Illness perceptions are the main predictors of depression and anxiety symptoms in patients with chronic pain. Psychol. Health Med. 21 (4), 483–495.

Cypress, B.S., 2016. Understanding uncertainty among critically ill patients in the intensive care unit using Mishel's theory of uncertainty of illness. Dimens. Crit. Care Nurs. 35 (1), 42–49.

Deindl, C., Brandt, M., Hank, K., 2016. Social networks, social cohesion, and later-life health. Soc. Indic. Res. 126, 1175–1187.

Dempster, M., Howell, D., McCorry, N.K., 2015. Illness perceptions and coping in physical health conditions: a meta-analysis. J. Psychosom. Res. 79, 506–513.

Duggleby, W., Hicks, D., Nekolaichuk, C., et al., 2012. Hope, older adults, and chronic illness: a metasynthesis of qualitative research. J. Adv. Nurs. 68 (6), 1211–1223.

Eicher, M., Matzka, M., Dubey, C., et al., 2015. Resilience in adult cancer care: an integrative literature review. Oncol. Nurs. Forum 42 (1), e3–e16.

Elliott, A.M., Burton, C.D., Hannaford, P.C., 2014. Resilience does matter: evidence from 10-year cohort record linkage study. BMJ Open 4, e003917. doi:10.1136/bmjopen-2013003917.

Fitzgerald Miller, J., 2007. Hope: a construct central to nursing. Nurs. Forum 42 (1), 12–19.

Garcia-Dia, M.J., DiNapoli, J.M., Garcia-Ona, L., et al., 2013. Concept analysis: resilience. Arch. Psychiatr. Nurs. 27, 264–270.

Gastmans, C., 2013. Dignity-enhancing nursing care: a foundational ethical framework. Nurs. Ethics 20 (2), 142–149.

Geulayov, G., Drory, Y., Novikov, I., et al., 2015. Sense of coherence and 22-year all-cause mortality in adult men. J. Psychosom. Res. 78, 377–383.

Gjengedal, E., Ekra, E.M., Hol, H., et al., 2013. Vulnerability in health care – reflections on encounters in everyday practice. Nurs. Philos. 14, 127–138.

Glattacker, M., Heyduck, K., Meffert, C., 2012. Illness beliefs, treatment beliefs and information as starting points for patient information – evaluation of an intervention for patients with chronic back pain. Patient Educ. Couns. 86, 378–389.

Gottlieb, L.N., 2014. Strengths-based nursing. Am. J. Nurs. 114 (8), 24–32.

Graven, L.J., Grant, J., 2013. The impact of social support on depressive symptoms in individuals with heart failure: update and review. J. Cardiovasc. Nurs. 28 (5), 429–443.

Grevenstein, D., Aguilar-Raab, C., Sweitzer, J., et al., 2016. Through the tunnel: why sense of coherence covers and exceeds resilience, optimism, and self-compassion. Pers. Individ. Dif. 98, 208–217.

Gustavsson-Lilius, M., Julkunen, J., Keskivaara, P., et al., 2012. Predictors of distress in cancer patients and their partners: the role of optimism in the sense of coherence construct. Psychol. Health 27 (2), 178–195.

Hansen, B.S., Rørtveit, K., Leiknes, I., et al., 2012. Patient experiences of uncertainty – a synthesis to guide nursing practice and research. J. Nurs. Manag. 20 (2), 266–277.

Heinze, J.E., Kruger, D.J., Reischl, T.M., et al., 2015. Relationships among disease, social support, and perceived health: a lifespan approach. Am. J. Community Psychol. 56, 268–279.

Hopman, P., Rijken, M., 2015. Illness perceptions of cancer patients: relationships with illness characteristics and coping. Psychooncology 24, 11–18.

Idler, E.L., Boulifard, D.A., Contrada, R.J., 2012. Mending broken hearts: marriage and survival following cardiac surgery. J. Health Soc. Behav. 53 (1), 33–49.

Koetsenruijter, J., van Eikelenboom, N., van Lieshout, J., et al., 2016. Social support and self-management capabilities in diabetes patients. Patient Educ. Couns. 99, 638–643.

Kralik, D., Visentin, K., van Loon, A., 2006. Transition: a literature review. J. Adv. Nurs. 55, 320–329.

Kübler-Ross, E., 1969. On Death and Dying. Macmillan, New York, NY.

Kübler-Ross, E., Kessler, D., 2007. On Grief and Grieving: Finding the Meaning of Grief Through Five Stages of Loss. Scribner, New York, NY.

Kucukarslan, S.N., 2012. A review of published studies of patients' illness perceptions and medication adherence: lessons learned and future directions. Res. Social Adm. Pharm. 8, 371–382.

Kvåle, K., Synnes, O., 2013. Understanding cancer patients' reflections on good nursing care in light of Antonovsky's theory. Eur. J. Oncol. Nurs. 17, 814–819.

Lazarus, R.S., 1999. Hope: an emotion and a vital coping resource against despair. Soc. Res. (New York) 66 (2), 653–678.

Lazarus, R.S., 2006. Emotions and interpersonal relationships: toward a person-centered conceptualization of emotions and coping. J. Pers. 74 (1), 9–46.

Lazarus, R.S., Folkman, S., 1984. Stress, Appraisal and Coping. Springer Verlag, New York.

Leventhal, H., Brissette, I., Leventhal, E.A., 2003. The common-sense model of self-regulation and illness. In: Cameron, L., Leventhal, H. (Eds.), The Self-Regulation of Health and Illness Behavior. Routledge, London, pp. 42–65.

Meleis, A.I., 2010. Transitions Theory: Middle Range and Situation Specific Theories in Nursing Research and Practice. Springer, New York, NY.

Mishel, M.H., 2013. Theories of uncertainty in illness. In: Smith, M.J., Liehr, P.R. (Eds.), Middle Range Theory for Nursing, 3rd ed. Springer, New York, pp. 53–86.

Petrie, K.J., Weinman, J., 2012. Patients' perceptions of their illness: the dynamo of volition in health care. Curr. Dir. Psychol. Sci. 21 (1), 60–65.

Sarvimäki, A., Stenbock-Hult, B., 2016. The meaning of vulnerability to older persons. Nurs. Ethics 23 (4), 372–383.

Sharply, C., Hussain, R., Wark, S., et al., 2015. The influence of social support on psychological distress in older persons: an examination of interaction processes in Australia. Psychol. Rep. 117, 883–896.

Silarova, B., Nagyova, I., Jaroslav Rosenberger, J., et al., 2014. Sense of coherence as a predictor of health-related behaviours among patients with coronary heart disease. Eur. J. Cardiovasc. Nurs. 13 (4), 345–356.

Silverstein, M., Heap, J., 2015. Sense of coherence changes with aging over the second half of life. Adv. Life Course Res. 23, 98–107.

Stein-Parbury, J., Gallagher, R., Chenoweth, L., et al., 2012. Factors associated with good self-management in older adults with a schizophrenic disorder compared with older adults with physical illnesses. J. Psychiatr. Ment. Health Nurs. 19, 149–153.

Tay, L., Tan, K., Diener, E., et al., 2013. Social relations, health behaviors, and health outcomes: a survey and synthesis. Appl. Psychol. Health Well Being 5 (1), 28–78.

Thoits, P.A., 2011. Mechanisms linking social ties and support to physical and mental health. J. Health Soc. Behav. 52 (2), 145–161.

Vélez-Vélez, E., Bosche, R.J., 2016. Illness perception, coping and adherence to treatment among patients with chronic kidney disease. J. Adv. Nurs. 72 (4), 849–863.

Vogel, I., Miksch, A., Goetz, K., et al., 2012. The impact of perceived social support and sense of coherence on health-related quality of life in multimorbid primary care patients. Chronic Illn. 8 (4), 296–307.

# 10

# Challenging interpersonal encounters

## CHAPTER OVERVIEW

- Nurses are sometimes challenged in their interpersonal encounters with patients.

- Patients may become so distressed that they act out in anger towards nurses.

- There may be conflict associated with a patient's anger towards a nurse, and this can escalate into physical aggression. Nurses need to be able to successfully negotiate when conflict occurs.

- Nurses can preserve relationships with patients by using assertive communication skills and conflict resolution techniques.

- In addition to conflict, nurses are sometimes challenged when caring for older people who experience problems related to sensory losses or cognitive impairment.

Visit the Evolve site for video content to support the themes and skills explored in this chapter: http://evolve.elsevier.com/AU/Stein-Parbury/patient/

# INTRODUCTION

There are times when therapeutic relationships may prove difficult to establish, challenging nurses in their interpersonal efforts to relate in a helpful manner. There are fundamental skills, such as those reviewed in previous chapters, that help nurses meet the challenges of difficult encounters with patients. But some encounters require the use of more advanced skills. For example, all nurses should be able to respond to a patient's anger in a helpful way; they need basic skills of successful conflict negotiation such as the ability to be assertive. However, dealing with patients whose anger has escalated to physical aggression and even violence requires advanced skills and training. The initial focus of this chapter is on those skills that are most basic to meeting difficult and challenging encounters with patients.

Another area that is often challenging for nurses is relating to older people, especially when there are sensory and/or cognitive deficits. As the population ages, encounters with older people are likely to be part of most nursing work.

# CHALLENGING SITUATIONS

While nurses are in a prime position to make interpersonal connections that assist people with successful transitions through health and illness, some circumstances make such connections challenging. These circumstances often involve the expression of strong emotions, for example, when patients become angry or demanding. During these times, nurses often feel frustrated in their attempts to help, and this can lead to nurses themselves feeling angry because their efforts are impeded by the situation. As a result, there may be difficulties in developing and maintaining the patient–nurse relationship; and nurses may perceive the difficulty as residing within the patient rather than in the social context of the relationship. That is, the patient is perceived to be 'difficult'.

## 'Difficult' patients

The behaviours of patients who are considered to be 'difficult' are consistently reported and described in the nursing literature. These behaviours include acting helpless and overly dependent, not cooperating with requests, demanding special treatment, expressing anger towards nurses, making insulting remarks and threatening, even assaulting, nurses (Michaelsen 2012; Pottle & Marotta 2014). In addition, difficult patients are perceived by nurses to be emotionally unstable, highly anxious, depressed, hostile, aggressive, impatient, unappreciative and non-conforming (Vandecasteele et al 2015a). In effect, patients who are regarded as difficult do not readily accept the sick role (see Ch 1); they do not cooperate with healthcare that is offered and fail to accept the rules of the healthcare setting (Koekkoek et al 2011; Vandecasteele et al 2015a). It follows that patients who are considered to be 'good' patients are the opposite; they are friendly, calm, polite, cooperative and accepting of help.

Although documented as 'difficult patients' in the nursing literature, and used by nurses in clinical practice, this term has the potential to stigmatise patients with a label that implies deviance (Pottle & Marotta 2014). The term reflects a general acceptance that the problem or difficulty is located within the patient. Such labelling of patients leads to inadequate care because nurses are inclined to distance themselves, blame the patient and withdraw from interactions (Michaelsen 2012). In addition to withdrawing, nurses may respond to difficult patients by enforcing control over them. Patients who are labelled 'difficult' receive the least supportive care and are generally dissatisfied with that care (Vandecasteele et al 2015b).

Not only is good nursing care challenged by labelling the patient as difficult, but also the nurse's wellbeing may be affected. For example, uncooperative patients who thwart nurses' efforts to help can lead to feelings of distress in the nurse. Therefore, both the patient and the nurse are dissatisfied when the patient is labelled 'difficult' (Pottle & Marotta 2014).

Rather than thinking that the patient is difficult, it is more productive for nurses to interpret situations that are challenging as difficult interpersonal encounters. The difficulty should be recognised as residing within the relationship rather than within individual patients. When viewed as relationship-based, there is acknowledgment of the psychosocial context of the patient's behaviour.

In an effort to understand this social context, Vandecasteele et al (2015a) explored nurses' perceptions of difficult encounters, rather than having them describe which patients were perceived as difficult. Heavy workloads and a focus on task completion were found to be the most important factors in difficult encounters because nurses reported that these factors resulted in time constraints that prevented them from 'knowing the patient' (Ch 1). Therefore, they were challenged in personalising patient care. In addition, nurses in this study recognised that they often resorted to controlling patients rather than engaging them in care, under conditions of tight time constraints.

During difficult encounters, patients and nurses experience interpersonal conflict. Interpersonal conflicts occur when people have goals, needs, wants and desires that are at odds with each other. Difficult encounters between nurses and patients involve conflict because the goals of nursing care seem incompatible with the patient's response. Patients may be in conflict with nurses when they are not cooperative with nursing care. Nurses may experience conflict in relation to being unable to achieve a level of care that they deem professionally desirable.

In order to be successful in managing conflict, nurses must first come to appreciate the nature of conflicts that occur between people.

## Interpersonal conflict

Interpersonal conflicts arise when there is lack of congruence between what people in a relationship want and need. A want is a desire for something, while needs include love, belonging and things necessary for survival (e.g. water and food). Wants and needs give rise to goals and interests. Conflicts of interests exist when the actions of one person attempting to reach their goals prevent, block or interfere with the actions of another person attempting to reach their goals. Although conflicts are a natural part of life, they are especially likely when they involve goals that matter and relationships that are valued.

Interpersonal conflicts are especially likely when people are working together to achieve shared goals and assume complementary roles that involve interdependence (Johnson 2013). How each person behaves in the relationship influences the other (see mutuality and reciprocity in Ch 2), although each person will have different perceptions, desires and needs. The combination of interdependence and differing perspectives makes it impossible for a relationship to be free from conflict (Johnson 2013).

From the context described by Johnson, it is easy to ascertain that a patient–nurse relationship has characteristics that are associated with conflict. First, good nursing care is best achieved when patients and nurses have a mutual understanding of the aims of care (shared goals). Second, patients need help, and nurses are there to help them (complementary roles that are interdependent). Finally, patients and nurses hold different perspectives by virtue of their individuality as people. In the context of the patient–nurse relationship, conflicts are therefore likely to occur.

The outcomes of conflict situations can be destructive or constructive. When constructive, conflicts result in greater understanding between people, as each person better appreciates the viewpoint of the other, no matter how different. Constructive resolution of conflict leaves each person feeling satisfied with the outcome and helps to build a better working relationship between them. Destructive outcomes are those in which differences are not appreciated, anger ensues and the interpersonal relationship between the people involved is harmed if not destroyed (see *Research highlight*).

## RESEARCH HIGHLIGHT How do patients experience difficult encounters with nurses?

*Vandecasteele, T., Debyser, B., van Hecke, A., et al., 2015b. Patients' perceptions of transgressive behaviour in care relationships with nurses: a qualitative study. J. Adv. Nurs. 71 (12), 2822–2833.*

### Background

Most of the research investigating difficult patient encounters that lead to conflict and aggression has focused on patient and workplace characteristics and how 'difficult' patients are perceived by nurses and other healthcare professionals. How patients perceive these interactions has rarely been studied.

### Purpose of the study

The aim of this study was to explore patients' experiences of problematic encounters with nurses that led to aggression in order to ascertain how they perceived nurses' behaviours in these encounters.

**cont.**

*Research Highlight continued*

## Method

Twenty patients in six different units were interviewed in this exploratory study. The authors intentionally did not use the term 'aggression' to allow individual interpretation of how nurses violated their expected standards of care. Grounded theory methods were used to analyse the interview data.

## Key findings

Patients expected that they would receive competent care while in hospital and that nurses would make human contact with them and treat them as a person. Transgressions occurred when these expectations were not met. Patients described nurses' behaviours that indicated such transgressions. These behaviours included being ignored, for example, when nurses talked over them as if they were not present. They also described the feeling of not being heard, especially when nurses were overly focused on completing tasks and fixated on keeping to their routine. They made excuses for these behaviours because they could see the nurses were busy. They adjusted their expectations and behaviour to accommodate the nurses.

## Implications for nursing practice

Patients feel ignored and treated as a number when nurses are extremely task-focused and routine-driven. Nurses need to be mindful that patients have individual needs that may require flexibility in order to meet these needs. Focusing on tasks alone results in patients feeling that they are not being cared for as a person, but rather a number.

# Conflict in the patient–nurse relationship

From the above description, it is clear how conflicts of interest can occur within the nursing context. Patients may want and even demand more of the nurses' time than they have to offer due to a heavy workload. Nurses may want patients to become independent in their healthcare when patients prefer to remain dependent and want nurses to do everything for them. Patients may want to decide the course of their care while nurses want them to just 'do as they are told'. When patients are controlled in this manner, the difficulties often get worse instead of better.

Nurses often try to avoid further contact with patients who are seen as difficult. While avoidance is one way of coping (i.e. emotion-focused) with the distress experienced when encountering 'difficult' patients, this manner of responding can result in neglecting the patient. Furthermore, avoidance as a coping strategy is associated with increased stress in nurses (Chang et al 2007; Kato 2014). Therefore, avoiding these patients not only compromises good nursing care but can actually result in greater distress for nurses.

While it is desirable for patients to negotiate conflict successfully, it is the nurse who is professionally accountable for managing conflict situations. The nurse must assume responsibility for learning the successful conflict negotiation skills. This requires a basic understanding of the nature of interpersonal conflict and negotiation of conflict resolution through effective problem-solving strategies.

Strategies that are successful in dealing with difficult patient encounters include: getting to know the patient; demonstrating respect for the patient; focusing on the issue at hand; moving towards solutions rather than focusing on the problem; avoiding becoming emotionally immersed in the situation; and keeping feelings such as anxiety in check. Employing strategies such as this will help to resolve conflict that is likely to arise during difficult encounters between nurses and patients.

# STRATEGIES TO RESOLVE CONFLICT

There are two major considerations in resolving conflict: achieving goals and maintaining a relationship with the other person (Johnson 2013). These characteristics of conflict resolution are synonymous with the basic aspects of communication competence discussed in Chapter 3. Nurses who are competent communicators are able to meet goals of patient care while maintaining good working (i.e. therapeutic) relationships with patients. Achieving these goals requires skills of assertion, and maintaining relationships requires responsiveness to the needs and feelings of others. Responsive skills are covered fully in Chapter 6 and termed 'understanding'. This chapter focuses on the skills of assertion. Directly related to communication competence as they require the skills of both assertion (meeting goals) and responsiveness (maintaining relationships), conflict-handling strategies have been classified by Johnson (2013) in the following way:

- **Withdrawing**. People who use this strategy neither meet their goals nor maintain their relationships with other people. Quite simply, they try to 'bury their heads in the sand' whenever conflicts arise. They avoid conflict and deny there is a problem. In relation to communication competence, this style is considered incompetent (see Ch 3).

- **Forcing**. People who use this strategy will meet their goals at all costs, including their relationships with others. They demand that other people cooperate with their goals and are quite authoritarian in their approach. In relation to communication competence, this style is considered overly domineering and aggressive (Ch 3).

- **Smoothing**. People who use this strategy will ignore achieving their own goals in an effort to maintain the relationship. They relinquish what they want in order to 'keep the peace'. In relation to communication competence, this style is considered to be overly accommodating (Ch 3).

- **Compromising**. People who use this strategy are willing to give up part of their goals and sacrifice part of the relationship in order to reach an agreement. In relation to communication competence, this style is considered competent (Ch 3); however, a compromise may leave both parties in the conflict unsatisfied and not be constructive to either goals or the relationship.

- **Problem solving or collaboration**. People who use this strategy initiate negotiation so both people in the conflict meet their goals and maintain a good working relationship. With this strategy, agreements are achieved that benefit each person, and negative feelings engendered by the conflict are dissipated. In relation to communication competence, this style is characteristic of competent communicators, as goals are met and relationships maintained in a mutually beneficial way (Ch 3).

People who are successful in resolving conflicts are able to use all five strategies, as each can be effective depending on context. While 'forcing' may be effective when buying a used car, it is not recommended in encounters with people with whom there is an ongoing relationship. If the goals are not important, yet the relationship is valued, then smoothing over the conflict by letting the other person have their way may be effective. However, if personal goals are sacrificed just to 'keep the peace', then smoothing may not effectively resolve the conflict. When the relationship is of moderate importance and the goals of each person cannot be met, or when time is short, compromising may be the best solution to a conflict (Johnson 2013).

Nonetheless, problem solving through negotiation is the strategy that produces the best resolution to conflicts, as this approach reaches goals and maintains relationships (Jordan & Troth 2007; Kaitelidou et al 2012). It is the work of true collaboration. This strategy takes the most time and requires skills of both assertiveness and responsiveness (Ch 3). In addition, success in collaboration has been linked to emotional intelligence (Morrison 2008) because it involves emotional regulation of oneself as well as the ability to understand the feelings of others. Emotional intelligence is particularly relevant because conflicts often involve the expression of intense feelings such as anger, anxiety and depression.

Each nurse will enter the profession with preferred and sometimes ritualised ways of addressing conflicts in their interpersonal interactions with others. Most people tend to use one strategy most of the time and usually have a 'fall back' strategy when this is not effective (Johnson 2013). The strategies used often reflect the interpersonal skills of the person using them. A high degree of self-awareness and reflection (Ch 3) on how they manage conflict enables nurses to understand their preferred strategies. This facilitates them to work on developing skills in the use of other, less preferred, strategies.

Studies that have explored the strategies used by nurses have demonstrated that they often prefer to use the technique of avoiding conflict (Iglesias & de Bengoa Vellejo 2012; Kaitelidou et al 2012; Mahon & Nicotera 2011). Avoidance of conflict and withdrawal may work for a short period of time, but in the long term it results in having conflicts left unresolved. While nurses are not likely to confront conflict in a direct manner, when they do it is done constructively, for example, advocating on a patient's behalf (Mahon & Nicotera 2011).

# Process of negotiation

The process of negotiation is necessary to successful collaboration. There are identifiable steps that, when followed, will result in successful negotiation. Johnson (2013) has described them as follows:

1. **Describe what you want** by using 'I' statements. For example, 'Sam, I want you to stop shouting at me', 'I would prefer if we could work together in your care', and 'I want you to try to do this for yourself'. In describing what you want, it is important to be specific in your communication.

2. **Describe how you feel**, again by using 'I' statements. For example, 'I am afraid when you shout at me' (rather than 'You are frightening me'), 'I am much happier when I am able to work with patients' (rather than 'You need to start cooperating with me') and 'I am more pleased when patients can do things for themselves'. Recognising feelings requires reflection and self-awareness (see Ch 3) on the part of the nurse. Quite often, feelings are hidden in a conflict situation, so bringing them out helps with its resolution.

3. **Exchange the reasons for your position** by explaining what you want rather than assuming an unwavering stance. For example, 'It is difficult for me to help when you shout at me' (rather than 'I do not tolerate shouting from anybody'), 'Working together will help you get better faster' (rather than 'We will get nowhere if you don't cooperate with me') and 'Doing this for yourself will help your recovery' (rather than 'With an attitude like that, you will never get well').

4. **Understand the other person's perspective** by listening with understanding and encouraging the other person to express their ideas (Chs 5, 6 and 7).

5. **Initiate options for mutual gain** by suggesting how to resolve the conflict. For example, 'We can discuss this further in a quiet way', 'Let's discuss what you want from your recovery' and 'Perhaps if I explained what I want you to do, you can tell me the difficulties you are experiencing'.

6. **Reach a constructive agreement** by being flexible and adaptable in finding a mutually agreeable solution.

Like communication competence (Ch 3), the process of negotiation involves both the ability to express one's ideas and opinions, as well as listening and understanding the ideas and opinions of others. The former requires skills of assertion and is task- or goal-focused, while the latter requires skills of responsiveness and is relationship-focused (Ch 6). The skills of assertion are reviewed below.

# The skills of assertion

The skills of assertion are those in which a person expresses their needs and wants without denying the rights of others to express their needs and wants.

Acting assertively is sometimes confused with being aggressive (i.e. a 'forcing' strategy of conflict management). Aggressive behaviour tramples on the feelings of others and ignores their right to be heard.

Assertiveness is in contrast to being passive (i.e. avoiding or withdrawing) and using smoothing-type strategies of conflict management. Passive people do not express their ideas but allow others to dominate in their opinions. The person does not stand up for their own rights to be heard and respected.

The 'I' messages outlined in steps 1 and 2 of the negotiation process are the backbone of assertive communication, as these focus on the issue at hand and the facts of the situation. An 'I' message does not impart blame on the other person but assumes responsibility for actions and responses. In contrast, a 'you' message, such as 'You are being unreasonable', 'You are just plain uncooperative' or 'You are just not that interested in helping yourself', blames the other person and will probably fuel the conflict further.

In addition to 'I' messages, there are two other useful assertive techniques that can be employed in the process of negotiation. First is the use of the 'broken record' (i.e. to keep repeating what you want and how you feel). The use of repetition can be effective when feelings are strongly expressed. Next, it is important to keep focused on the issue at hand through the use of 'fogging over', as this prevents getting sidetracked by other issues. For example, if a patient states that 'You are just one of those nurses who doesn't care', rather than engaging in a conversation to the contrary (e.g. 'Yes, I do'), it is more useful to simply fog over by saying, 'That may be the case, but I still want you to try to get out of bed by yourself'. In this example, it is irrelevant whether the patient thinks the nurse cares, and engaging in a conversation about this does not progress the resolution of the conflict.

It is often difficult for nurses to be assertive in their workplace. They tend to be accommodating and submissive in responding to conflict (Iglesias & de Bengoa Vallerjo 2012; Kaitelidou et al 2012; Mahon & Nicotera 2011) because this is consistent with their image of nurses as 'nice people'. Being assertive is not incompatible with being caring. However, maintaining an attitude of 'being for the patient' implies that assertive skills are necessary because nurses need to be open and state what they think is in the patient's best interests.

## ACTIVITY 10.1 Becoming assertive

### Process

1. Think of a time in your life, preferably at work, when you felt that your right to be respected was violated and you responded by being passive. Consider why you responded in this way. Describe this situation to another participant.

2. Working in pairs discuss each participant's situation and decide what assertive technique would have been useful in this situation and how it could have been employed.

3. Role-play each situation in front of all participants.

**Discussion**

1. After each role-play participants should identify how rights to be respected are violated, especially in the workplace.

2. Discuss why participants behaved passively when they felt their right to be respected was violated.

3. Determine what assertive strategies were used in the role-plays and what effect they had on the interaction.

# RESPONDING TO ANGER

There are times when strong emotions make interactions with patients particularly challenging. One emotion that can create much anxiety and distress is anger. Patients can become angry for a variety of reasons. They could be extremely frustrated with their circumstances; they could be worried about their future or concerned about the welfare of their loved ones; they could be distressed because they don't understand what is happening; or they could be upset by the way they are being treated.

Sensitive handling of patients' anger requires skill, particularly because their anger could escalate to some type of aggression. Aggression is a hazard for all healthcare professionals, but nurses are more likely than other professionals to be on the receiving end of aggression (Arnetz et al 2015; Hahn et al 2008). When a patient's anger takes the form of aggression it can be both psychological and physical. Verbal abuse is the most common way that patients express anger and aggression, but there are also instances when anger escalates to physical assault and even violence.

## Factors that can trigger anger in patients

In a review of the literature Hahn et al (2008) identified contextual factors that are associated with patient violence and aggression in general hospital settings, with the first two days of admission being the most likely time for aggression to occur. In addition, there are factors related to a patient's health status that are associated with aggression. Some of these include: recovering from an unconscious state; intoxication from drugs or alcohol; and cognitive impairment that leads to confusion and an inability to understand current circumstances. While timing of admission and actual health status are not in the control of nurses, there are other factors that are associated with patient aggression in general hospital settings that can be addressed.

Factors that can be addressed are associated with actual patient care and how the patient is relating to others and the hospital system. These include misunderstandings, disagreements and dissatisfaction with treatment and care, as well as physical contact during care that produces pain or violates privacy from the view of the patient. Patients can also become angry about having to wait for attention or not having a doctor available when wanted. They can also become angry if they perceive their concerns are not being taken seriously by hospital staff. In addition, they can take issue with hospital policies and rules (Hahn et al 2008).

One important area that creates anxiety and possible anger in patients is when they are not fully informed about care or when aspects of treatment and care have not been fully explained. Unfamiliarity with hospital routines, procedures and policies also contribute to anger and potential violence (Luck et al 2007). This highlights the need to share relevant and timely information and explanations to patients (see Ch 8).

As is the case with patients considered to be 'difficult', patient anger and aggression should be viewed in an interactional light. Nurses recognise that actions of staff members, such as being condescending and authoritarian, feeling rushed and pressured and providing insufficient attention, are factors that can lead to patient aggression (Chapman et al 2009). The underlying processes that lead to patient anger and aggression are a combination of the context, the environment and how people are relating to the patient.

## Observable behaviours that indicate potential aggression

One of the keys to averting patient anger from turning to aggression is by observing behavioural cues. Such cues include: intense staring (or lack of eye contact depending on culture); a sarcastic, demeaning tone of voice; raised volume of speech; signs of anxiety; mumbling under the breath but loudly enough to be heard; and pacing (Luck et al 2007). In addition, heightened emotional states such as fear and frustration, being overly assertive and confrontational and having difficulty explaining what is needed are also behaviours that alert nurses to the potential for aggression (Chapman et al 2009). These behavioural cues should alert nurses that actions must be taken in an effort to prevent a patient's anger from escalating into aggression or violence.

How these cues are interpreted by nurses and the meaning they ascribe to them will determine how they respond. In an emergency department study nurses responded to patients' aggressive behaviour with understanding and tolerance, thus averting violence, when they perceived there were mitigating factors such as cognitive impairment, confusion or disorientation (Luck et al 2008). In addition, when they considered that the patient's presentation to the emergency department was legitimate and that the patient's behaviour was not a personal attack but rather frustration with the healthcare system, they responded with empathy.

## Effective approaches to patient anger

Nurses can use a number of interpersonal strategies when responding to a patient's anger in an effort to avert that anger from turning into aggression and violence.

First, it is important to recognise early signs of impending aggression, such as verbal assaults, as most nurses do not respond until the patient's behaviour has escalated (Hardin 2012). When signs of impending aggression are observed, nurses can employ a number of 'de-escalation' techniques (Price & Baker 2012), which are well documented in the mental health nursing literature. While pertinent to mental healthcare contexts, where a patient's aggression can be an aspect of an illness or a response to treatment, these techniques are useful for all nurses (Luck et al 2009), especially as the rise in patient aggression has been documented (Hardin 2012).

It is understandable that nurses may respond to a patient's anger by becoming defensive or angry themselves, but this is not a useful approach because it will most likely heighten the patient's anger. More importantly, reactions such as these send a message that the nurse feels threatened and potentially out of control, thus adding to the anxiety of the patient. Rather, it is better to stay calm and in control and focus on what the patient is communicating, not on how the nurse is feeling. Remaining calm is perhaps the most important aspect of responding to a patient's anger and potential aggression; doing so sends a message to the patient that the nurse is willing to listen, thus building trust.

Active listening (see Ch 5) is essential when responding to a patient's anger because it enables the nurse to assess the root of the patient's feelings. The patient should be encouraged to express their anger, and listening provides the most helpful means of doing so. Engaging with the patient through active listening facilitates understanding of the patient's problem and what can be done to address it. Therefore, the skills of understanding (Ch 6) are important. While some element of exploring through questioning (Ch 7) may be useful, it is best not to interrogate the patient or ask them to justify their anger.

The main goal in addressing a patient's anger is to understand what has triggered the anger and whether something can be done. If the patient is angry about having to wait for attention or to see a doctor, it is not helpful to explain that other patients also need attention or that the doctor is busy and will be there later. These are defensive responses that may only fuel the anger. It is better to express empathy (Ch 6) about the patient having to wait and also to say that the situation of waiting is a regrettable one. Doing so acknowledges and validates the patient's anger. This has a tendency to reduce the intensity of the feeling (although the patient may still be angry), as contrasted with a defensive response.

The atmosphere of 'zero tolerance' and related policies may lead some nurses to respond to a patient's anger with an authoritarian, controlling approach such as 'I will not tolerate such language', which is not useful in the first instance. As an initial response, this approach is likely to lead to escalation. That is not to say that taking control and setting limits is not warranted; for example, patients cannot be permitted to physically assault nurses. However, a balance between support and control is an effective approach to de-escalating patient aggression (Price & Baker 2012).

Consider the following nurse's story.

## A Nurse's Story

As I came on duty to begin my night shift in the paediatric ward, I noticed two distraught women in the nursery. They were engaged in what appeared to be a heated discussion. One of the women was Eve, the nurse who was finishing her evening shift. The other woman was Tracey, the mother of one of the babies in the nursery. Tracey's child was hospitalised for respiratory problems. I caught only the tail end of their conversation and, although I couldn't understand the content, I sensed hostility and anger in both of them. Tracey was walking away from Eve as I entered the nursery. I sat down to receive the handover report from Eve, and she began to tell me of her frustration with Tracey. 'It seems that I can't do anything to make her happy,' Eve said. She then went on to tell of the numerous complaints made by Tracey. I listened to Eve, knowing in the back of my mind that I would have to listen to Tracey as well. I told Eve I would try to sort out the situation and would see her the next day. She seemed relieved.

After the report I went to find Tracey. She was packing her baby's belongings and informed me that she was taking her baby home. I knew from the report that Tracey's baby had not taken any fluids by mouth during the previous shift and was at risk of dehydration. I was quite concerned about Tracey's plan to leave. Slowly I said, 'I know you are upset ...', but was cut off mid-sentence by Tracey.

'That nurse is typical of everything here, just typical. You bet I'm upset.' She continued to pack her belongings. 'And I don't want to discuss it. I'm going home with my baby.'

At this point I felt at a loss but also knew I had to try to make contact with Tracey, even though she was shutting me out.

'Look,' I said in an almost pleading manner, 'I want to help, but I don't know what's going on. I don't know what's wrong.'

Tracey picked up her belongings and her baby and said, 'Well, it's too late to start worrying now.'

I protested, 'I am worried, even if it is too late. I'm concerned for you and your baby.'

'Don't give me that; nobody cares around here, not you or any of the other nurses,' she said.

I blurted out, 'Oh, is that what's wrong?'

She looked straight at me for the first time, 'Yes, that's exactly what's wrong.'

I knew I had to think fast. The contact that I'd made with her seemed tenuous and I wanted to strengthen it. I didn't want this mother to leave. 'Please, let's talk,' I said. 'I was just about to have a cup of coffee. Come with me and I'll get you one too.' To my relief, she agreed. I added, 'And I'll get a bottle for your baby.'

We went together into the kitchen area where I prepared coffee for us and a bottle for Tracey's baby, who had been crying the entire time we had been talking. I didn't want to take over but thought it essential to get the baby settled. Her distressed baby could have been half of Tracey's problem. When the bottle was ready I asked Tracey if she would like to feed her baby.

She replied, 'Look, that's what I've been trying to do all evening. He just won't take anything. I can't do it.'

I sensed her anger and frustration, which was now starting to escalate again. 'Okay,' I said, 'I'll feed the baby and you drink your coffee.' I noticed how directive I'd become but decided that Tracey needed some concrete assistance in settling her baby. Besides, it was becoming increasingly difficult to carry on a conversation in the presence of the crying baby.

'Nobody has been able to feed him today and they said he may need a drip. They expect me to feed him but what can I do when he keeps fussing and refusing to suck?' she asked. She felt useless and helpless while at the same time responsible. She was trapped by the circumstances.

I decided to take over a bit more. In proceeding to feed her baby, I explained how his respiratory problems were interfering with his ability to suck. Thankfully, Tracey's baby began to feed and settle. At this point I turned to Tracey and said, 'You must be so frustrated and angry. I know I would be if I were you.' I held my breath, hoping that this statement would connect with Tracey. She nodded and looked at me; some of her anger was dissipating. I continued, 'Sometimes it's hard for us to know exactly when to take over and when to let mothers care for their own babies.'

I really didn't expect her to have much sympathy for the plight of the nurses, but fortunately I had struck a chord with Tracey. She responded by saying, 'Right now, I do need for you to take over and care for my baby. I can't bear the thought that he'd get a drip because I can't feed him.' With this statement I began to understand what this mother was going through.

Eventually, Tracey's baby settled and I managed to put him to bed and get him off to sleep. Tracey also prepared to settle for the night. She was lying down in the bed next to her baby's cot and I prepared to leave the nursery. As I began to exit, she called me over and whispered, 'Thank you'. Even though I now had what seemed like a hundred other chores to complete, I knew I had spent my time wisely. I looked at my watch. Twenty minutes was all that it had taken to turn these events around. I had taken the time to become involved in what might have been a most unfortunate situation. I had taken the time to understand. I felt satisfied.

Situations like this are demanding of nurses. They must contain their natural instincts to defend themselves, their colleagues and their nursing care. Tracey was distressed because she felt unable to care for her baby. She felt responsible for her baby's deteriorating condition and blamed the nurses for not assuming what she perceived to be their responsibility.

When this nurse arrived on the scene, the situation was almost out of control. By involving herself in a non-defensive, concerned manner she was able to make contact with Tracey and begin to see the situation through her eyes. She was assertive in expressing her concerns for both Tracey and her baby. She stated how she would feel under similar circumstances. She offered practical support in offering to feed the baby. All of this took effort, energy and time, all of which she knew were well spent in the end. She offered both practical assistance and an understanding ear, balancing support and control. More importantly, she identified the trigger for Tracey's anger. This took time, acceptance and understanding.

Often nurses believe that no time exists to listen to and understand what patients are experiencing. While this is sometimes the case, lack of time can become an easy excuse for not becoming involved in difficult and emotionally draining interactions. The work involved in managing one's own emotions in this way is referred to as 'emotional labour' (Ch 3).

# RELATING TO OLDER PEOPLE

Most nurses will interact with older people as a result of an ageing population and the complex health needs that ensue. It is for this reason that nurses need to develop interpersonal skills that are specific to older people, and they may be challenged in doing so. This is not to say that older people are challenging but that the challenge lies in the interaction between them and the nurse.

Young nurses may be challenged in their interactions with older people whose life experience has been different from their own. Adults who are a lot older than the nurse may have worldviews that have been developed by experiences that for the nurse are nothing more than a page in a history book. Young adults are likely to be looking forward to a life yet unknown, yet eagerly anticipated. Taking stock and making meaning of one's life through looking back are aspects of growth in late adulthood. Such different perspectives can create a generational gap in understanding each other.

Human growth and development does not end with young adulthood. Physical, psychological and spiritual growth occurs throughout the whole of the human life span; older adulthood is no different. Results of an extensive, seminal study of adult development, conducted for more than half a century, reveal that psychological and spiritual growth occur long after the physical body peaks in the early 20s. Referred to as the Harvard study (Vaillant 1977), participants were surveyed from late adolescence to old age (Vaillant 2002).

Healthy ageing is associated with the capacity to meet the developmental tasks of generativity (Erikson 1963) – the ability to 'pass the baton' to the next generation. People who meet the task of generativity take pleasure and pride in the wisdom that comes with ageing. They willingly share this knowledge with the next generation and achieve a sense of integrity and peace in their final years. Generativity seems to be the key (Vaillant 2002).

Unless there are health and social resources deficits, it has been demonstrated that a sense of coherence, comprehending, managing and finding meaning in life (see Ch 9) increases continuously in old age (Silverstein & Heap 2015). In a survey of 692 adults from New Zealand and the United States it was reported that the majority considered themselves to be ageing successfully (Gasiorek et al 2015). Those who were 'engaged' with ageing by discussing issues and topics related to ageing reported more positive outcomes such as managing the ageing process and maintaining a positive affect than those who were 'disengaged'. Nonetheless, most perceived that they were ageing well.

While most people are capable of healthy ageing, societies that revere youth and longevity may stereotype older people as useless. Such a view is culturally dependent, with some social groups holding their older members in great reverence.

## ACTIVITY 10.2 The generation effect

### Process

Consider the following brief life sketches.

### Elizabeth Eden

Elizabeth was 86 years old in 2004. She had lived through a series of major world crises. She was born in the period following World War I, when people were enjoying life to the full, believing that peace and prosperity were their birthright. These hopes were dashed by the Great Depression, which occurred when she was a teenager, and World War II, which occurred when she was in her 20s. Like many others who lived through the Depression of the 1930s, Elizabeth suffered extreme economic privations. Her father was out of work. She managed to do some casual piecework, which was very poorly paid, but she was, nevertheless, grateful for it. She learned to scrimp and make the most of limited amounts of food and clothing, and to waste nothing. She married Tom when she was 20.

Then World War II started. Tom, along with many other young husbands, went to war. Many soldiers' wives, including Elizabeth, were forced to work outside the home, taking on the work that the men had to leave. Elizabeth and Tom's first child was conceived during Tom's military leave. She had to manage the child virtually as a single working mother while at the same time coping with her anxiety about Tom, who had been taken as a prisoner of war. Tom did not meet his child until he returned from a prisoner-of-war camp in 1945. After the war, their two other children were born.

When the war was over, Elizabeth gratefully retreated to the home to finish bringing up her children, and Tom returned to his former occupation. When the women's movement gained momentum in the 1970s, Elizabeth had little sympathy for the aim of equal employment opportunities for women and felt that women were better off not working outside the home.

### Mark Yates

Mark was born in 1952, during the postwar baby boom. His childhood was spent during a period of economic affluence and full employment. He took economic security for granted and expected to walk straight into a job when he completed his education.

In contrast to Elizabeth, whose life spanned a number of major world crises, Mark has been beset by a number of more indefinite concerns about the future of the world. The Cold War between the Soviet Union and the United States was at its peak during his youth and, as he grew up, Mark became increasingly aware of the possibility of the world being devastated by nuclear war. He was a teenager during the period of Australia's involvement in the Vietnam War and became accustomed to news reports of the suffering and devastation suffered by the Vietnamese. During his adolescence,

*cont.*

*Activity 10.2 continued*

there was increasing public discussion of the effects of overpopulation on the world and the environment. Drugs were rife in schools, and the crime rate was increasing at a rate that was causing public alarm. The revolution in sexual attitudes and freedom was well under way.

Many of his friends, having grown up with security, shunned the advice of their parents to get 'a steady job'. They were vocal in their cynicism about national and international leaders.

**Discussion**

1.  Divide into small groups and discuss how Elizabeth's and Mark's views of life might differ. List these differences on large sheets of paper and display them around the room.

2.  In a large group, discuss how world events may have shaped the views of people who are now in their 60s and 70s. How might they be different from people who are in their 20s and 30s?

3.  What do you fear most about growing old? What do you look forward to most?

4.  How can nurses reduce interaction difficulties that are due to a generation gap?

# Losses associated with ageing

The process of ageing is associated with many losses including the death of loved ones and the realisation that one's own death is closer. These are social in nature. Some, such as the reduction in social roles and social status, are a direct result of negative social attitudes towards older people. Many older people face a decline in economic status as they retire from paid employment and become dependent on a government pension or superannuation.

The most obvious losses are sensory, with loss of vision and hearing being most pronounced. They are the most common health concerns in old age; the loss of hearing has been shown to affect more than 50 per cent of older people, and vision impairment around 30 per cent, negatively affecting their quality of life (Zhang et al 2016).

# Interacting with a person with a hearing impairment

A number of guidelines can be applied to facilitate interactions with patients who experience hearing difficulties. Most people can lip-read to some extent if they can see the speaker's mouth, so nurses should stand where the patient can see them. It is important to speak clearly, articulating the words well and refraining from shouting. If the patient does not understand, the nurse probably needs to try rephrasing sentences, using different words and shorter sentences. Soft-sounding consonants such as 'p' and 'f' are difficult to detect; therefore, using words that avoid these might be helpful. Nurses can be creative in using any means at their disposal to communicate meaning including using pictures or gestures, or writing or drawing.

When nurses are interacting with patients who wear hearing aids, additional techniques are necessary to promote effective interaction. Hearing aids assist people with specific types of hearing impairments; they do not restore normal hearing. They are much more sensitive to background noise than natural hearing. When conversing with a patient with a hearing aid, nurses should try to find a quiet room where there are no other conversations going on in the background. Just hitting a glass on a table or clicking a pen can be a source of interference. Using hearing aids effectively requires perseverance on the part of the user and cooperation on the part of others.

# Interacting with a person with a vision impairment

When communicating with a person who has a vision impairment, it is important to speak and act naturally; visual impairment does not mean loss of hearing. It is important that nurses identify themselves by name as the person may not recognise people by their voice alone. It is equally important to address the person by name so they understand that they are being spoken to. Standing in their line of vision and using body language will enable them to better understand what is being communicated. When exiting a conversation, it is important to let them know because they may not realise that they are speaking to someone who is no longer there (Vision Australia 2016).

When giving verbal directions it is important to be specific and accurate. 'Your telephone is on your right, sitting on the stand next to your bed, at eye level' is better than 'Your telephone is sitting on the stand next to the bed'. If written directions are being used, then inadequate or poor lighting can exacerbate the visual loss. Ample lighting is essential; optical devices and vision aids used for magnification are also useful for reading. If the person uses corrective eye glasses, assure that the lenses are clean and clear.

## ACTIVITY 10.3 Experiencing sensory deficits

**Process**

1. Find an old pair of sunglasses. Cut out a piece of clear contact adhesive (the kind that is used for covering books) and attach it to the lens of the glasses. This should have the effect of allowing in some light but reducing visual acuity. Wear a pair of thin cotton gloves to simulate loss of skin sensation. Wrap elastic bandages firmly around your knees and ankles to simulate a feeling of stiffness in your joints. Place cotton wool plugs in your ears.

2. Spend at least one hour trying to carry out your normal daily activities.

*cont.*

*Activity 10.3 continued*

**Discussion**

1.  How difficult was it to carry out your usual activities with impaired sensory input and impaired mobility?

2.  How much do you think the vagueness of old people could be attributed to difficulties in sensory perception?

# Interacting with a person with a cognitive impairment

Cognitive impairment, such as poor attention and concentration and poor memory and retention of information, is often present in older people. It is important that nurses do not expect all older people to be cognitively impaired, yet it is likely that they will care for people in this state. Impairment of this type affects the person's ability to communicate because they are frequently confused. Cognitive impairment can be the result of dementia or delirium, and these are specific clinical conditions that require advanced skills and training. Nonetheless, there are a few approaches that all nurses need to know in caring for people who are cognitively impaired.

First, it is important to remember that the person has feelings, and their affective self often stays intact. They are easily frightened and can become quite distressed when their confusion increases. Therefore, recognising their feelings (see Ch 6) is often helpful in establishing interpersonal contact. Eye contact, a calm manner, addressing the person by name and speaking slowly are essential to making such contact (Bulechek et al 2013).

It is also important to avoid frustrating the person by quizzing them, especially about their orientation to time and place, as this may increase their frustration. Likewise, their ability to retain new information is impaired, so nurses should not expect people who have a cognitive impairment to be able to easily recall events and conversations. They should never be confronted with their memory loss (e.g. by saying, 'I just told you that'). Most importantly, when a patient is confused, a nurse should never argue with the patient's faulty thinking. Rather, a nurse should listen to the underlying feeling being expressed. For example, if a patient says to a nurse, 'That doctor is out to get me', it might be tempting to counter this thought by saying, 'That is not so'. Rather, the nurse should reflect the feeling that is being expressed – for example, by saying, 'That sounds really frightening'.

Nurses need an enormous amount of patience when patients are cognitively impaired, especially when being asked the same questions over and over again. Answer the questions in a matter-of-fact manner and avoid confronting the person with their losses. It is far better to focus on their feelings and perceptions than to confront them with reality.

As much as possible, the nurses who care for cognitively impaired people should be consistent, as new people and faces only add to their frustration. Consistency in caregivers also aids in the ability to 'know the patient' (Ch 1) and understand their unique life history. This makes family involvement essential when caring for older people with a cognitive impairment.

Consider the following scenario.

## SCENARIO

Maria, an 86-year-old woman, was brought into the emergency department of a busy metropolitan hospital by her daughter and husband. Although diagnosed with dementia, her behaviour over the past day had become markedly different. She was more confused than usual, slurring her speech and dismantling all of her favourite flower arrangements in her home.

While in the emergency department, she was left alone on a stretcher in the hallway while she waited for diagnostic tests to be completed. Her daughter and husband were told to wait elsewhere. Maria perceived that she was left 'for hours' and that no one was there to assist her. She ran up and down the corridor looking for help.

Maria became quite anxious and agitated about this situation; her family members could have anticipated this reaction. They would have preferred to be able to remain with her in order to reassure and orient her, especially because she had not been left alone for a number of years. By the time they returned to her bedside, Maria was in a state of near panic. While her perceptions were not real, the associated emotions were very real, and avoidable in their opinion.

After the tests were completed, Maria was admitted to hospital with a suspected stroke. She was placed on routine neurological observations, which included questions about her orientation and recollection of facts such as her age and number of years married. Prior to her hospitalisation, she was having difficulty remembering these facts, thus rendering any findings of the mental status examinations invalid. Had there been an assessment of her baseline functioning (prior to hospitalisation) in the form of history-taking from her family members, staff would have realised that routine testing in this would not yield accurate results.

The continuous neurological observations were anxiety-provoking for Maria, as she realised that she was being 'tested' and was failing because she could not remember facts such as her age. She expressed her concerns to her family on numerous occasions, and became increasingly anxious about all the questions she was being asked. Had the nursing staff involved the family in Maria's care, they would have realised she had a fear of being alone. More importantly, they would have realised that the results of their neurological testing were invalid as Maria had not been able to remember her age, how many years she had been married or the current date for a number of years. Quizzing her in this manner not only produced invalid results, but added to her distress.

# SUMMARY

Challenges in helping people transition through illness have been presented as difficulties that result in conflict within the social context of the patient–nurse relationship. Conflict has been reviewed, and strategies for successfully resolving conflict have been presented, with an emphasis placed on collaboration through negotiation. Skills necessary for collaboration have placed particular emphasis on assertion, as these have not been previously reviewed in other chapters. The particular challenge of interacting with patients who are angry and possibly aggressive has been highlighted as an area requiring particular attention. In addition, a brief review of some of the factors related to ageing that affect and possibly challenge interpersonal interactions has been undertaken.

# REFERENCES

Arnetz, J.E., Hamblin, L., Essenmacher, L., et al., 2015. Understanding patient-to-worker violence in hospitals: a qualitative analysis of documented incident reports. J. Adv. Nurs. 71 (2), 338–348.

Bulechek, G.M., Butcher, H.K., Dochterman, J.M., et al., 2013. Nursing Interventions Classification (NIC), sixth ed. Mosby Elsevier, St Louis.

Chang, E.M.L., Bidewell, J.W., Huntington, A.D., et al., 2007. A survey of role stress, coping and health in Australian and New Zealand hospital nurses. Int. J. Nurs. Stud. 44, 1354–1362.

Chapman, R., Perry, L., Styles, I., et al., 2009. Predicting aggression against nurses in all hospital areas. Br. J. Nurs. 19 (8), 476–483.

Erikson, E.H., 1963. Childhood and Society, second ed. Norton, New York.

Gasiorek, J., Fowler, C., Giles, H., 2015. What does successful aging sound like? Profiling communication about aging. Hum. Commun. Res. 41, 577–602.

Hahn, S., Zeller, A., Needham, I., et al., 2008. Patient and visitor violence in general hospitals: a systematic review of the literature. Aggress. Violent Behav. 13, 421–441.

Hardin, D., 2012. Strategies for nurse leaders to address aggressive and violent events. J. Nurs. Manag. 42 (1), 5–8.

Iglesias, M.E.L., de Bengoa Vellejo, R.R.B., 2012. Conflict resolution styles in the nursing profession. Contemp. Nurse 43 (1), 73–80.

Johnson, D.W., 2013. Reaching out: Interpersonal Effectiveness and Self-Actualization, eleventh ed. Allyn and Bacon/Merrill, Boston, MA.

Jordan, P.J., Troth, A.C., 2007. Emotional intelligence and conflict resolution in nursing. Contemp. Nurse 13, 94–100.

Kaitelidou, D., Kontogianni, A., Galanis, P., et al., 2012. Conflict management and job satisfaction in paediatric hospitals in Greece. J. Nurs. Manag. 20, 571–578.

Kato, T., 2014. Coping with interpersonal stress and psychological distress at work: comparison of hospital nursing staff and salespeople. Psychol. Res. Behav. Manag. 7, 31–36.

Koekkoek, B., Hutschemaekers, G., van Meijel, B., et al., 2011. How do patients come to be seen as 'difficult'? A mixed methods study in community mental health care. Soc. Sci. Med. 72, 504–512.

Luck, L., Jackson, D., Usher, K., 2007. STAMP: components of observable behaviour that indicate potential for patient violence in emergency departments. J. Adv. Nurs. 59 (1), 11–19.

Luck, L., Jackson, D., Usher, K., 2008. Innocent or culpable? Meanings that emergency department nurses ascribe to individual acts of violence. J. Clin. Nurs. 17, 1071–1078.

Luck, L., Jackson, D., Usher, K., 2009. Conveying caring: nurse attributes to avert violence in the ED. Int. J. Nurs. Pract. 15, 205–212.

Mahon, M.M., Nicotera, A.M., 2011. Nursing and conflict communication: avoidance as preferred strategy. Nurs. Adm. Q. 35 (2), 152–163.

Michaelsen, J.J., 2012. Emotional distance to so-called difficult patients. Scand. J. Caring Sci. 26, 90–97.

Morrison, J., 2008. The relationship between emotional intelligence competencies and preferred conflict-handling styles. J. Nurs. Manag. 16, 974–983.

Pottle, J., Marotta, J., 2014. Promoting better care for stigmatised patients. Nurs. Stand. 29 (16–18), 50–59.

Price, O., Baker, J., 2012. Key components of de-escalation techniques: a thematic analysis. Int. J. Ment. Health Nurs. 21, 310–319.

Silverstein, M., Heap, J., 2015. Sense of coherence changes with aging over the second half of life. Adv. Life Course Res. 23, 98–107.

Vaillant, G., 1977. Adaptation to Life. Little Brown, Boston, MA.

Vaillant, G., 2002. Ageing Well. Scribe, Melbourne.

Vandecasteele, T., Debyser, B., Van Hecke, A., et al., 2015a. Nurses' perceptions of transgressive behaviour in care relationships: a qualitative study. J. Adv. Nurs. 71 (12), 2786–2798.

Vandecasteele, T., Debyser, B., van Hecke, A., et al., 2015b. Patients' perceptions of transgressive behaviour in care relationships with nurses: a qualitative study. J. Adv. Nurs. 71 (12), 2822–2833.

Vision Australia, 2016. Communicating effectively with people who are blind or visually impaired. http://www.visionaustralia.org/living-with-low-vision/family-friends-and-carers/communicating-effectively-with-people-who-are-blind-or-vision-impaired, (Accessed 6 December 2016).

Zhang, S., Simon Moyes, S., McLean, C., et al., 2016. Self-reported hearing, vision and quality of life: older people in New Zealand. Australas. J. Ageing 35 (2), 98–105.

# CHAPTER

# 11

# Building a supportive workplace

## CHAPTER OVERVIEW

- There is growing awareness and mounting evidence that organisational environments and culture have an impact on patient safety and quality.

- The characteristics of an ideal healthcare milieu are based on the evidence from decades of research into 'magnet' hospitals.

- Interprofessional communication is a key characteristic and includes both spoken word and written documentation.

- Ideal environments not only promote quality and safety for patients but also foster nurses' wellbeing and job satisfaction.

- Job-related stress in nursing include the work itself, the organisational environment and professional relationships.

- Two potential consequences of nurse stress are burnout and compassion fatigue.

- Nursing leadership in developing and sustaining supportive colleague relationships is essential in minimising such consequences.

- Coping with job-related stress includes using colleagues as an effective coping resource.

- Dealing with workplace conflict requires the use of assertive skills.

- Building resilience, including mindfulness, self-compassion and clinical supervision, are additional coping resources.

℮ Visit the Evolve site for video content to support the themes and skills explored in this chapter: http://evolve.elsevier.com/AU/Stein-Parbury/patient/

# INTRODUCTION

The central tenet of this book is that effective communication and therapeutic relationships between patients and nurses are at the heart of good nursing care. This is because care can be personalised as a result of the process of 'knowing the patient' through communicating and relating. Delivering personalised care is a long-held value in the nursing profession, and nurses recognise that interactional processes such as comforting, supporting and enabling patients are primary ways that nurses make a difference to patients.

Current workload task demands, such as administrative duties not directly related to nursing care, often prevent nurses from having time to interact meaningfully. When time spent with patients is in short supply, the quality of care suffers, and so do nurses. In the absence of a work environment that supports patient interaction as an essential nursing activity, even the most interpersonally skilled nurses will find it difficult to 'know the patient'. Therefore, consideration must be given to the organisational environment of nursing care.

Organisational arrangements are in place so complex systems such as hospitals for acutely ill patients can operate smoothly. Such arrangements may impact on patient–nurse relationships. For example, when nursing work is organised in such a way that the patient and nurse rarely see each other on more than one occasion in the course of a health event, then the depth of mutual understanding may be restricted by limited opportunity to get to know each other. The patient in this situation may need continuity of interaction with a nurse. For example, for a young woman needing assistance in order to cope with life after having a mastectomy, her needs would be best served by organisational arrangements that enable nurses and patients to get to know each other on more than a clinical level.

Not only might such arrangements impact on the capacity of nurses to form therapeutic patient–nurse relationships, but there is mounting evidence that organisational arrangements may also affect, for better or worse, nurses' wellbeing and the quality of healthcare in general. The emphasis of this chapter is just such arrangements, with a focus on developing effective working relationships with colleagues in healthcare in an effort to support therapeutic relationships with patients. Developing good working relationships requires the same skills as those of therapeutic interactions, especially those of listening, understanding and exploring.

# PRODUCTIVE NURSING ENVIRONMENTS

Healthcare environments influence nurses' commitment and job satisfaction; more importantly, better patient outcomes are obtained in an environment that supports nurses to deliver quality care. Such environments provide the framework for nurses to envision their practice, stay true to their professional values and communicate their practice (Slayter et al 2016). The relationship between organisational characteristics and quality nursing care that results in job satisfaction, nurse retention and quality patient outcomes has been investigated over decades in institutions that are known as 'magnet' hospitals. There is a formal system for credentialling to achieve recognition of Magnet® status.[1] However, the discussion of the body of research regarding these institutions is included here, not in an effort to seek and promote official recognition, but to highlight a conceptual understanding of productive nursing environments. There is much to be learnt from the story of magnet hospitals that extends beyond the formal system.

# The magnet hospital story

A crisis of nurse recruitment and retention in the 1980s sparked a novel investigation into the problem. Rather than focusing on further description of the problem, which had already been subjected to lengthy analyses, the American Academy of Nursing commissioned an investigation into those hospitals without nurse staffing shortages. This initial study investigated hospitals to which nurses were attracted (recruited) and in which they remained employed (retained). They became known as 'magnet hospitals' for these reasons.

The original investigations into the magnet hospitals revealed striking similarities in their organisational arrangements and operations (Kramer & Schmalenberg 1988a, 1988b; McClure et al 1983). In addition to an adequacy of staffing, there were other features of the work environment that typified these institutions. One prominent organisational feature was the professional autonomy of nurses in assuming responsibility for quality patient care. The care was based on a nursing philosophy of holistic and individualised care, based on patient-centred values.

Management structures and attributes of nursing leaders were also similar in the original magnet hospitals. Organisational structures were conducive to participatory decision making and nursing self-governance, with decisions made at a local level. Nursing leaders in these organisations were highly visible and accessible to nursing staff. They demonstrated enthusiasm and commitment to nurses and nursing and conveyed a vision and value system for the profession. These structures and leader attributes, originally observed in the first magnet hospitals, have continued to be associated with high nursing job satisfaction and quality nursing care (Kramer et al 2011; Kutney-Lee et al 2015; Schmalenberg & Kramer 2008; Witkoski Stimpfel et al 2014).

Ongoing investigations into magnet hospitals have produced results that go beyond this description of organisational distinctiveness. There is also evidence that these institutions not only attract and retain nurses but also have been shown to provide a higher standard of care and better patient outcomes than those institutions without magnet characteristics. The evidence of better patient outcomes has been demonstrated over a number of years (Kazanjian et al 2005;

---

[1] Developed by the American Nurses Credentialing Center, the Magnet Recognition Program® recognises healthcare organisations for quality patient care, nursing excellence and innovations in professional nursing practice (American Nurses Credentialing Center 2017).

Kramer et al 2011; Kutney-Lee et al 2015; Laschinger & Leiter 2006; McHugh et al 2013). Outcomes are better for patients even in hospitals with 'some' magnet characteristics (Aiken et al 2009). The outcomes are better because nurses are able to make professional judgments about patients and autonomously act on those judgments. That is, patients and nurses are better off when nurses are able to practise their profession to the full scope of their knowledge and ability.

Three key attributes have emerged that support nursing practice at this level and have become defining organisational characteristics of magnet hospitals. They are professional autonomy, control over nursing practice and good collegial relationships between nurses and doctors.

## Professional autonomy

The first characteristic is professional autonomy of the nursing staff. This means that nurses can practise nursing in a way that they judge is best; they have authority in relation to clinical decisions about patient care. With autonomy comes the freedom to be self-defining and self-governing – characteristics associated with professional status. In describing autonomy, nurses working in magnet hospitals refer to clinical decision making and action that is free from bureaucratic constraints that have little to do with patient care. They are free to act in the best interests of patients. In addition to such freedom, nurses need to be clinically competent and knowledgeable in order to practise autonomously (Kramer & Schmalenberg 2008).

## Control over nursing practice

Related to professional autonomy, which is at an individual clinical decision-making level, control over nursing practice involves wide participation in decision making at the organisational level. Control over practice involves the responsibility to set standards for nursing care and having commensurate authority to meet those standards. Such control is not possible unless organisational structures include nurses at the highest decision-making level. When nurses have legitimate authority, status and recognition, they have influence and control. Organisations that are structured in such ways engender a culture in which nurses take pride in themselves as a professional group (Kramer et al 2008).

## Collaboration with doctors

The third characteristic of the magnet hospitals is good collaboration between nurses and doctors. Such collaboration is marked by shared decision making and mutual respect for each other's contribution to clinical problem solving. An unequal power distribution between nurses and doctors hampers collaboration, as equality of contribution is implied. Nurses in magnet hospitals do not see themselves as subservient to the power of doctors and build cooperation with each other. There is recognition that both nursing and medical knowledge are needed in making sound decisions about patient care (Schmalenberg & Kramer 2009).

## Implications of magnet hospital research

The body of research into magnet hospitals indicates that work environments that are supportive of professional nursing practice are associated with better nursing and patient outcomes. This support includes manageable nursing workloads in the form of adequate nurse-to-patient ratios because nurses cannot cope without adequate resources to meet the demands of nursing work. Adequate staffing is a critical variable to the success of the magnet hospital story. Other characteristics of magnet hospitals relate to this variable. For example, control over nursing practice involves influencing decisions about nurse staffing levels. That is, the organisational characteristics that distinguish magnet hospitals are interrelated.

The three defining characteristics of magnet hospitals are interrelated in other ways. For example, leaders in magnet hospitals were able to provide learning resources and opportunities for nurses to develop their clinical competence, a necessary requisite for clinical autonomy. Professional development opportunities are a central aspect of productive nursing practice models (Slayter et al 2016), as such opportunities promote autonomous clinical practice. And, autonomous practice is synergistic with teamwork. Even when able to practise autonomously, there was a great deal of interprofessional group cohesion in magnet hospitals. Building supportive colleague relationships is an aspect of the magnet hospital research that relates directly to the interpersonal work environment.

# INTERPROFESSIONAL COMMUNICATION

An area that currently is a focus of improving quality and safety in healthcare is the promotion of effective teamwork among healthcare professionals. Improving teamwork communication is receiving so much attention because breakdown in communication between healthcare professionals and fragmentation of care has been cited as a major cause of adverse patient outcomes (Brock et al 2013; Pannick et al 2014). Furthermore, improving teamwork has the potential to have greater effects than other measures to increase safety and quality in healthcare (Barrow et al 2015).

Healthcare teams are multiprofessional in nature; they comprise a variety of different disciplines such as medicine, nursing, physiotherapy and social work. It is equally important to remember that patients and their families arc also members of the healthcare team and should be actively involved in decision making.

There is now a move from conceptualising such teams as multiprofessional to a preference for the concept of interprofessional teamwork. Multiprofessional or multidisciplinary implies that each member of the team develops goals that are based on their unique disciplinary perspective. It is often a doctor who determines the overall goal for a patient, with other professionals following that lead. Interprofessional or interdisciplinary teamwork differs in that the various team members formulate shared goals, with each then working towards discipline-specific goals to meet the common goals. Not only is interprofessional teamwork more interactive and collaborative but it is also linked to improved quality of care and patient safety, job satisfaction and cost savings (Krörner et al 2015).

There are challenges to interprofessional teamwork and the group cohesion necessary for smooth collaboration. The first is that, unlike other 'teams' such as sports team, membership in healthcare teams is fluid in nature, with membership likely to change daily (Barrow et al 2015). They are formed in an 'ad hoc' manner that leads to instability (O'Leary et al 2012). The second is the traditional hierarchy in which doctors are the decision-makers (Matziou et al 2014), with biomedical discourse dominant (Barrow et al 2015). The last is that doctors view collaboration as less important than nurses, yet they are more satisfied than nurses with the quality of collaboration (O'Leary et al 2012; Tang et al 2013). Each of these factors affect the quality of interprofessional communication and collaboration.

Effective communication among healthcare team members is necessary for interprofessional teamwork. Like communication with patients, the aim of effective teamwork communication is to develop a shared understanding. Therefore, collaborative decision making requires that each team member not only understands their own perspective but also that of other team members. In developing shared goals, each member of the team brings a different piece of the puzzle in decision making, based on their understating of the patient. Putting together the puzzle results in a 'shared mental model' (McComb & Simpson 2013) of what the patient needs and the goals for treatment and care. When mental models are shared, all team members understand how the goals will be met and their role in meeting them.

# Shared mental models

Shared mental models arise through negotiating meaning in order to develop mutual understanding among team members. Achieving such understanding may take a great deal of time and communicative effort. In high-stress and emergency clinical situations there may not be sufficient time to develop a shared mental model. The use of standardised protocols that serve as mental models are effective and efficient in such circumstances. Such protocols structure the communication among team members.

A standardised protocol that is used universally and is familiar to healthcare professionals is the SBAR framework. SBAR is a mnemonic in which 'S' is for the situation, 'B' is the background to the situation, 'A' represents the clinician's assessment of the situation and 'R' includes recommended actions. In the Australian context ISBAR is added to the framework, with 'I' representing the introduction of clinicians as well as the patient (Australian Commission on Safety and Quality in Health Care 2016).

The SBAR framework has been shown to enable more focused and efficient communication, with priorities and essential information clearly identified (Cornell et al 2014). In addition, teamwork is improved when the framework is employed (Martin & Ciurzynski 2015). More importantly, its use has been shown to be associated with improved patient outcomes (deMeester et al 2013).

Regardless of whether a standardised protocol is used, communication between healthcare professionals works best when it is structured, for example, during occasions of patient handover or transfer from one clinical setting to another. Structuring the communication is a means of assuring that vital information is not omitted and irrelevant information is not included. Because most healthcare professionals work under some degree of time pressure, structuring communication promotes efficiency.

In addition to standardised protocols, shared mental models are also formulated during interprofessional interactions. Interprofessional rounds, during which all members are involved in decision making regarding patient treatment goals and care, provide an opportunity for such interactions (Tang et al 2013). Interprofessional rounds should also include patients and their families, not just healthcare professionals. Conducting rounds in such a way has been shown to improve patient outcomes and job satisfaction among healthcare professionals (Terra 2015).

The challenge in formulating a shared mental model lies in that different professionals bring their unique perspective and knowledge to the decision-making process. In formulating their judgments, nurses are likely to use what is termed 'subjective' information about the patient's circumstances (patient and person knowledge, see Ch 1), while doctors rely on what are considered to be 'objective' facts and figures (case knowledge, Ch 1). Doctors rely on standardised knowledge – for example, selecting an intervention that has been shown to be effective in the majority of cases. Nurses take into consideration that which is idiosyncratic and specific to a particular patient through coming to know the patient as an individual. Conflicting perspectives may arise under such circumstances because nurses and doctors operate from different knowledge bases (Stein-Parbury & Liaschenko 2007). Doctors do understand that nurses are more likely than them to understand the patient's personal experience of healthcare, yet the traditional hierarchy of healthcare services means that doctors assume ultimate responsibility for clinical decisions (Barrow et al 2015; Burford et al 2013) (see *Research highlight*).

## RESEARCH HIGHLIGHT Interprofessional experiences of recent healthcare graduates

*Thomson, K., Outram, S., Gilligan, C., et al., 2015. Interprofessional experiences of recent healthcare graduates: a social, psychological perspective on the barriers to effective communication, teamwork and patient-centred care. J. Interprofess. Care 29 (6), 634–650.*

### Background

Effective communication among professional members of a healthcare team is central to quality and safety in care delivery. How team members view each other in relation to their professional role and perspective has an impact on their communication, for better or worse.

### Purpose of the study

The aim of this study was to explore attitudes and experiences of recent healthcare graduates in relation to their views of interprofessional communication and teamwork in their education and their recent clinical experience.

### Method

This was a descriptive, qualitative study in which data were collected through 12 focus group interviews with 68 pharmacy, nursing and medicine graduates in three Australian states. The interviews focused on the graduates' reflections of their experience of interprofessional education and how this impacted on their teamwork communication after graduation. Data were analysed using the Social Identity and Realistic Conflict framework.

### Key findings

While the participants acknowledged the importance of team communication and had an understanding of each other's role, there was a consistent pattern of being profession-focused rather than patient-focused. In addition, the findings revealed negative stereotypes such as the perception that doctors think they are superior to other professionals. Participants perceived communication as hierarchical in nature and that team members competed for time with patients.

### Implications for nursing practice

While nurses need to have a clear professional identity, they must also understand the professional identities of other healthcare team members. In addition, they should challenge professional stereotyping of their colleagues. Rather than seeing that they are in competition with other professionals, they need to work towards collaboration and cooperation.

# Written communication

Interprofessional communication not only occurs during face-to-face interactions but also through information that is transmitted in writing that captures and disseminates patient information. Each member of a healthcare team provides written entries into patients' health records in relation to the care of those patient. Doing so provides comprehensive and permanent documentation of the patient journey that is used to plan and evaluate care. All members of the team have access to the information obtained by other members and the care that they have provided, thus ensuring consistency of care.

Documentation is a matter of professional accountability for nurses, providing evidence that care was provided. Maintaining a timely, accurate and comprehensive record of care is embedded in professional standards and codes (Nursing and Midwifery Board of Australia 2006; Nursing Council of New Zealand 2007). Furthermore, patient healthcare records are legal proof of patient care; they can be summoned in a court of law as evidence. The time-honoured adage of 'if it isn't written, it wasn't done' applies in such cases.

In addition to accountability, accurate and reliable documentation affects patient safety and quality of care (Braaf et al 2011; Buus & Hamilton 2016; Jefferies et al 2011). The quality of the documentation is considered to be a reflection of the quality of care (Kim et al 2011). Poor documentation – for example, not recording when a patient is deteriorating – can lead to adverse outcomes and patient harm. While most nurses appreciate the accountability aspect of documentation, they place less emphasis on its safety and quality aspects (Prideaux 2011).

## Documentation guidelines

Nurses' entries into a patient's healthcare record should be patient-centred and include what the person is experiencing; they should not simply be a record of what routine and technical actions have been undertaken. Including the patient's perspective is in keeping with the focus of nursing care, understanding the unique circumstances of each person. Most of the time nurses' notes are focused on physiological matters, such as nutrition and elimination, and do not include social and psychological matters such as how the person is managing their health event and how they are coping (Buus & Hamilton 2016; Kim et al 2011; Paans & Müller-Staub 2015).

Clear and concise information is essential because there is no opportunity to clarify or negotiate meaning – written communication is one-way. Ambiguous language such as 'eating well' is open to interpretation. To maintain clarity and convey meaning, approved abbreviations should be used; for example, 'BIB RP HBD' may be understood at a local level as meaning 'Brought in by Rockdale police, has been drinking' but not convey reliable information to outsiders. Each institution will have a set of approved abbreviations.

In addition there are general rules about making entries into a patient's notes, and these include:

- Entries into the record should be sequential and chronological and made as soon as possible after the event.
- All interventions and patient outcomes need to be included.
- The nursing process should be used – this enables the entries to be structured and logical.
- Writing should be legible, using formal sentence structure, correct grammar and punctuation.
- Patient identification needs to be included on each page.
- Each entry should include a date and a time, as well as the signature, name and designation of the writer.
- No blanks should be left because entries could be made in them at a later date.
- If an error is made, it should have a single line struck through it with the initials of the writer.

Increasingly, electronic records are being introduced in healthcare. They provide a uniform structure to documentation, are legible and can be retrieved any time by members of the healthcare team. They provide up-to-date information that can be accessed at the point of care. In addition, clinical guidelines can be embedded into the record, for example, a clinical protocol appears when a dangerously low blood pressure is entered. While they contain more information than paper records, electronic records do not always convey the patient's story, thus information can remain fragmented (Clynch & Kellett 2015).

## Nurse–doctor interaction

In what is now a classic article on the subject of nurse–doctor interaction, Stein (1967) described a system of communication between nurses and doctors that he termed 'the doctor–nurse game'. When abiding by the rules of the 'game', nurses are only able to express their own ideas and judgments about patient care in a way that appears that they do have an opinion of their own. For example, rather than directly requesting a change in analgesic medication, the nurse playing the game would suggest that the doctor may want to consider reviewing the patient's medications. This is because the doctor has to appear all-knowing, at all times. More importantly, the approach used in the game avoids any possibility of conflict between the nurse and the doctor.

Not only did the game perpetuate a myth of the omnipotent doctor but it also stifled nursing knowledge from finding direct expression about patient care. Twenty-three years after the original article, Stein et al (1990) claimed that the 'game' was played to a lesser extent than originally observed because of the increasing professional status of nurses. Nevertheless, the idea of the doctor–nurse game has retained attention in the literature over a number of years, with claims that vestiges of it still exist (Burford et al 2013; Larson 2012; Reeves et al 2008).

Nurses need to be mindful not to play the 'doctor–nurse game' because it prevents collaboration due to inequality of status and authority. Nurses who 'play the game' unwittingly stifle and oppress the voice of nursing. Stein et al (1990) point out that freeing the oppressed will free the oppressor from the destructive discourse of the doctor–nurse game. The 'perceived' omnipotence of medical authority, embodied in the form of the 'doctor knows best' (i.e. the 'doctor–nurse game'), can be a burden for doctors who are then expected, sometimes by patients, to have all the answers. When no answers are forthcoming or immediately obvious, doctors may turn to nurses for information about the best course of action to follow in relation to their wellbeing.

Developing collaborative relationships with doctors and other healthcare professionals is not merely a matter of individual actions. Structural and organisational arrangements need to be in place that support quality nursing care. The environment and culture of the healthcare organisation must be one that enables nurses to fulfil their professional obligations while being as productive as possible. In doing so they need to cope with the work stress that is inherent in nursing work, even when the most productive organisational arrangements are in place.

# STRESS IN THE WORK ENVIRONMENT

Pressure related to workload and staffing is a major source of stress in nurses because of having to do more and more for patients, with inadequate resources to meet the demands (McVicar 2016). Staff shortages and increasingly ill patients are part of this stressor, as are work–family conflicts, often related to staffing issues. A demanding workload can result in nurses being torn between that which is most important in a professional sense and that which is most urgent and pressing in an organisational sense. For example, nurses on a busy surgical unit might find themselves transporting patients to and from the operating theatre instead of teaching patients and their families how to care for themselves postoperatively. Transporting patients is an organisational demand, while teaching and counselling patients are professional demands. When these demands come into conflict, the organisational demands often take precedence. Nurses become increasingly stressed by management tasks that take them away from the bedside. Job-related stress results because nurses are not able to fulfil their professional role and uphold the values and standards of the profession (Bridges et al 2013; Riahi 2011).

Lack of time to fulfil a professional role has been termed 'moral stress' and 'moral distress' (Musto & Rodney 2016; Oh & Gastmans 2015). This type of stress results from internal conflicts experienced by nurses when institutional constraints prevent nurses from acting in what they believe is the best interests of patients. When workloads are such that nurses are unable to deliver the kind of care they deem of high quality, they experience stress.

Stress in nursing is not only generated from the work itself, including workload, but also from factors related to the work environment. Other than workload, various sources of stress have been documented over a number of years including: dealing with death and dying; lack of professional autonomy and control; conflict relationships with colleagues; lack of leadership support; and poor group cohesion in the workplace (Chang et al 2007; Gardiner & Sheen 2016; Happell et al 2013; McVickar 2016; Sharafi et al 2016). Organisational factors that contribute to nurse satisfaction are primarily related to less-than-supportive professional interactions with colleagues, as well as a lack of professional autonomy. That is, interpersonal relationships in the workplace contribute to nurse stress, and these include relationships with nursing colleagues and other professionals.

## Consequences of work stress

One reason for the continued interest in work stress in nursing is that stress is associated with job satisfaction; higher levels of stress are linked with lower levels of satisfaction and higher job turnover (Zangaro & Soeken 2007). Workload stress – along with disempowering leadership, poor colleague relationships and lack of autonomy – have all been implicated in poor job satisfaction and subsequent turnover in nursing staff (Coomber & Barriball 2007; Lu et al 2012). Current structural arrangements in many healthcare facilities can be at odds with nursing values of patient-centred care, placing the true meaning of 'caring' in nursing (see Ch 1) at risk. Such conditions generate discontent among nurses because the delivery of quality patient-centred care is an enduring value in professional nursing and a major contributor to job satisfaction (Schmalenberg & Kramer 2008).

# Burnout

'Burnout' is a term used to describe an accumulation of work stress over time. It is a phenomenon that is particularly relevant to people service professions such as nursing. In nursing, burnout is often due to the demanding and emotional nature of the relationships between nurses and their patients (Maslach & Schaufeli 1993). People who hold high ideals and standards are at most risk of burning out because they may never be able to achieve the standards they set for themselves. Once burnout occurs, nurses feel as if there is 'nothing left to give', and this is described as emotional exhaustion. In addition, nurses experiencing burnout treat patients like objects, not because they are being deliberately uncaring but because they are protecting themselves from further stress through acknowledging patients' subjective realities and needs. They can tend to the tasks without making reference to the idiosyncratic ways of individual patients. That is, they function in a disengaged manner as a way of protecting themselves from further stress. Finally, burnout is characterised by a loss of job satisfaction.

Nurses who experience a high degree of job-related stress over a period of time are at risk of being lost to the profession through burnout. This is sad, as these are the very nurses who uphold the highest standards of care for their patients. There is an irony that, in the midst of a worldwide shortage of nurses, those who would do their best to embody the values of the nursing profession are at most risk of leaving it behind.

In contemporary healthcare, burnout is fuelled by circumstances in which there are increasing job demands, insufficient resources, lack of collegial support and performance feedback, and limited participation in decision making (control/influence). As such, burnout, as a consequence of nurse stress, is as much an organisational matter as it is an individual nurse problem. While nurses need to develop individual coping strategies (e.g. through stress management courses), there is equal evidence to suggest that organisational attributes and arrangements also affect nurse stress.

# Compassion fatigue

A concept related to burnout is that of compassion fatigue. While these concepts are similar, compassion fatigue is sometimes discussed in the literature as separate and other times as the same phenomenon (Ledoux 2015). Compassion fatigue is considered to be the result of prolonged exposure to traumatic events such as witnessing suffering and death. It is directly related to caring for and being compassionate towards patients. Burnout, on the other hand, is considered to be related to prolonged work-related stress that may or may not involve actual caring for patients. Compassion fatigue results in anxiety and sadness and can leave nurses emotionally drained and detached.

The notion that nurses can become fatigued by being compassionate raises some interesting dilemmas, such as 'Can nurses care too much?' thereby exhausting their emotional resources, and whether compassion fatigue is the cost of caring. In her analysis of the concept Ledoux (2015) concludes that compassion fatigue is not the price that nurses pay for caring but the result of circumstances in which they cannot care and relieve suffering. Fatigue is experienced because they cannot practise as they wish. In this regard compassion fatigue is similar to moral distress.

# COLLEAGUE INTERACTION AND WORK STRESS

The relationship between colleague interaction and stress in nursing is complex because co-workers function both as a resource for handling or modifying this stress and as a source of stress (e.g. conflict with colleagues and lack of performance feedback). Relationships with colleagues can be considered flip sides of the same coin in that they both add to and diminish work stress. Supportive interactions and relationships with colleagues have potentially positive effects; colleague interactions and relationships that lack support can add to work stress, creating negative effects.

## Nurse–nurse interaction

Strained relationships and open conflict add stress to any working environment, but it is an absence of support, especially from nursing leaders (Riahi 2011), rather than the presence of conflict, that often creates strain in colleague relationships in nursing. More often than not, it is that which is missing in colleague relationships that contribute to stress in nursing. Lack of support from supervisors, lack of feedback, withheld information, lack of understanding in response to mistakes and lack of peer cohesion are all reported as factors that positively correlate to stress in nursing (Hussain et al 2012; Riahi 2011; Spence Laschinger et al 2012). Nurses create stress for other nurses largely by failing to provide support when it is needed.

The sad irony is that work-related stress is exacerbated when colleague support is absent, and colleague support is lacking when it is needed most – during times of increased stress. What is most disturbing is that colleague relationships add to stress, not necessarily by creating overt conflict but by failing to provide needed support.

The following nurse's story, told by a recent graduate, highlights this lack of support:

### A Nurse's Story

I chose theatre nursing because of the challenge of working in a high-tech environment, an interest in anatomy and physiology and the order and structure of the day's work. I also take my responsibility to patients very seriously. Their protection, privacy and safety are foremost in my mind as I work. In the year I worked in the operating theatre I became fairly competent. I enjoyed my work there, except when working with one particular surgeon.

This was not because of his skills as a surgeon but because of the way he treated nursing staff. He could be flirtatious and sometimes made lewd comments to women. Although uncomfortable, I tried to ignore the conversation. I never made eye contact with him in response to his inappropriate sexual comments. I ignored his behaviour and got on with the work at hand.

Being a fairly private person, I never said much about my discomfort in working with this particular surgeon. That was, until the day he crossed the line. I was preparing for a case and scrubbing my hands when this surgeon came up to me, from behind, and placed his hands on my breasts. I resisted my impulse to slap his face, and instead firmly asked him to remove his hands from my body. Although quiet and reserved most of the time, I can be quite assertive. He mumbled something about my sense of humour and walked away. The case for which we were preparing proceeded as planned.

Just as well that the surgical procedure went quickly because I couldn't wait to get out of the operating room. Once I knew the patient was safely on his way, I went straight to my nursing supervisor to report, in detail, the incident with the surgeon. I calmly told her what happened, expressed my anger at the situation and requested to not be rostered to work with that surgeon again.

It was my supervisor's reaction that really got to me. She calmly stated that she had a very busy operating theatre to run and that requests such as mine could not be accommodated. When I became visibly upset by her response, she suggested that I calm down. 'After all,' she told me, 'you certainly must be aware that this sort of thing has always occurred in the operating theatres. You will figure out your own way of dealing with it – like we all have. That is how you survive in this environment. You are still young. You will learn.'

I was appalled by what she said, yet helpless to take any further action. The surgeon in question was a powerful force in the organisation. Although I knew that my supervisor's response was in direct violation of hospital policy in relation to workplace behaviour, I was also not going to take that issue further. She was known for her vindictive streak if you crossed her. Instead, I resigned and found an environment where I knew I would feel safe coming to work.

I never really told anybody the reasons I left that job. My friends thought I was happy there and were surprised to hear I took a position in the theatres of another hospital, which was further from my home. I told them I thought it was a good career move. In hindsight it was; I haven't looked back. I knew my personal survival was of most importance and chose to leave the incident behind in that hospital.

This situation illustrates the potentially disastrous effects of an environment that is lacking support for other nurses. This nurse coped with the situation by altering the immediate situation, through changing her work location, but avoided the main cause of the problem. Not only did the supervisor in this situation fail to support this newly graduated nurse but she violated workplace policies that mandate reporting the surgeon's behaviour because it amounts to harassment. Most workplaces have policies that require supervisors to report such instances. Not only should the instance have been reported but the nursing supervisor also lacked understanding of the new graduate's distress.

The lack of colleague support between nurses raises questions about why and how this happens in a caring profession. Nurses risk losing their credibility as caring people when caring for other nurses is not apparent and active in their work environment. Nurses should be able to demonstrate support for colleagues and cultivate a nourishing work environment. Sadly, there are aspects of nursing culture that work exactly against the creation of such environments.

## Culture of horizontal violence

A potential explanation of how colleague interaction is troubled in nursing is the phenomenon termed 'oppressed group behaviour'. Observed in nursing many years ago (Roberts 1983), this interpersonal dynamic continues to receive research interest in studies that have been conducted across a variety of cultural contexts (Castronovo et al 2016; Roberts 2015; Trépanier et al 2016). Sometimes termed 'horizontal or lateral violence', members of oppressed groups are often unsupportive and in conflict with their peers. Horizontal violence creates a climate of divisiveness within nursing groups and pits nurses against each other, thus destroying camaraderie. As such, it can create a breeding ground for interpersonal conflict among nurses. Understanding the dynamics of groups that are oppressed is essential if this negative phenomenon is to be reversed in nursing.

Behaviours of oppression often stem from feeling powerless against a dominant force. Nurses often perceive themselves as powerless against a system that dominates them, shouldering great responsibility within healthcare organisations without a commensurate degree of authority. The dominant culture reveres technology, devalues caring and places curing as superior to caring. This oppression results in feelings of inferiority and creates the myth that the dominant value system and culture is 'right' and superior. In oppression, there is an internalisation of the dominant group's view of the world and a tendency within the oppressed group towards self-blame and rejection of their own values and culture as inferior. This leads to developing a collective poor self-esteem within the group and has the potential to result in poor peer relationships (Roberts 2015; Trépanier et al 2016).

There are frustrations and complaints about the oppressor and the oppression, yet no direct action is taken. Frustrations are directed at each other because the 'system' excludes nurses and silences their voice (Roberts 2015). The anger that builds as a result of oppression is released on members of the group rather than on the oppressor because there is less risk of consequences in fighting each other than there is in fighting the dominant group. The lateral violence within the group keeps the group divided, prevents cohesion, causes psychological harm, decreases job satisfaction and negatively affects retention in the workforce; more importantly, this phenomenon also poses threats to patient safety (Castronovo et al 2016). Threats to patient safety occur as a result of errors due to stress and nurses being reluctant to ask questions when they are uncertain about patient care.

Examples of horizontal violence include withholding information, undermining, back-stabbing and snide remarks. Blaming and scapegoating other nurses are also evidence of the behaviour of oppression in nursing work environments. As long as blame can be found, and it usually is found within the oppressed group, real issues are not addressed because the culprit, another nurse, has been targeted, and there is no need to delve further into what is behind the cause of the problem.

Often horizontal violence is levelled at the most junior of nursing staff, including newly graduated nurses and students of nursing (Wilson 2016), who experience being discredited and put down, as well as feeling humiliated in the presence of others. Termed 'eating our young', this phenomenon of lack of support for those new to the profession is one form of horizontal violence that pervades many nursing cultures.

Bullying, perhaps the most extreme example of horizontal violence in nursing, is a matter of increasing concern internationally, with research into the phenomenon having increased over the past decade (Roberts 2015). Bullying involves persistent and negative acts towards an individual or group in which there is a power imbalance between the perpetrator and the victim.

The behaviours of bullying include such things as personal attacks, intimidation, belittling, calling into question professional abilities and actually obstructing work. The intent is to demean or devalue others. The presence of such acts not only creates hostility and conflict within the work environment but also affects the health of victims and work productivity. Unfortunately, most will be victims or bystanders of such behaviour.

Perhaps most importantly for nursing is the evidence that bullying is a learnt behaviour in the work environment (Trépanier et al 2016). Bullying is not simply a product of individual behaviour; there are factors in the workplace that contribute to, and even sustain, bullying. These include: misuse of legitimate authority; organisational tolerance and reward; and informal alliances. In addition, workload and lack of control in the workplace, which leads to frustration and aggression, has been shown to be factors that lead to uncivil behaviours in nurses (Trépanier et al 2016).

## Reversing the culture of horizontal violence

Nurses can easily remain victims of oppression and horizontal violence if they continually focus on negative characteristics within the culture of nursing. Raising awareness of horizontal violence provides an opportunity for nurses to reverse its negative effects.

Oppressed groups such as nurses often remain submissive to those who dominate them because members of the group are unaware of their behaviour. As a result, horizontal violence stifles the development of support between nurses in an insidious manner. Nurses often unconsciously collude in their own subordination (e.g. by unknowingly diminishing the importance of nursing knowledge). In reversing the culture of oppression, nurses need to challenge internal beliefs that nursing is less valuable than others' contributions to patients' wellbeing.

Instead of identifying with the dominant authority, which is one characteristic of leaders who emerge from oppressed groups, leaders of the magnet hospitals were able to articulate a nursing perspective on patient care and provide strong advocacy for nursing practice. In the magnet hospitals, nursing knowledge assumed authority, as nurses were able to practise their profession in an autonomous, yet collaborative, way. Having recognised professional status enables nurses to engage in interprofessional decision making.

## Nursing leadership

Nursing leaders who demonstrate pride in their profession and project a 'positive professional identity' are critical aspects in reversing a culture of oppression. They hold a strong vision about nursing care that they could articulate to others. In the magnet hospitals, leaders remained visible and accessible to the nursing staff. Focusing on mistakes, referred to as 'management by exception' (i.e. when things go wrong), is likely to increase nursing stress. Magnet hospital leaders were available, offering feedback not only when things went wrong but also when they went well.

By understanding and articulating a nursing perspective on healthcare and providing strong advocacy for nursing, magnet hospital leaders were able to assist in clarifying work roles and reducing role conflicts and associated stress. Effective leaders are pivotal in promoting a positive practice environment for nurses (Slayter et al 2016). They are skilled communicators who not only profess the value of caring in nursing practice but are also able to live these values in their interactions with colleagues.

In this sense they display the behaviours of authentic leadership (Laschinger et al 2014). These types of leaders are oriented towards forming good relationships with nurses. They are empathic listeners who respond to the needs and concerns of those whom they lead. More importantly, authentic leaders create an atmosphere in which nurses are less likely to experience burnout and engage in bullying behaviour. The latter is because authentic leaders are effective in managing workplace conflict.

# COPING WITH WORK STRESS

As reviewed in Chapter 9, there are two types of coping efforts to deal with stress: efforts aimed at meeting or altering the demands of the situation through problem-focused coping; and efforts designed to minimise the impact of stress through emotion-focused coping. Coping efforts that are problem-focused include creative problem solving and reappraisal of the situation. For example, seeking informational support from more experienced colleagues, or locating research evidence to support clinical decision making in situations that are ambiguous and challenging, are effective problem-focused coping efforts. When situations are stressful but cannot be altered (e.g. an untimely death of a young person in a preventable accident), emotion-focused coping may serve best. Emotion-focused efforts, aimed at keeping anxiety in check, include distancing, denial and avoidance.

While both types of coping may be effective in dealing with job stress in nursing, there is research evidence to suggest that problem-focused coping is associated with better mental health and job satisfaction (Chang et al 2007; Kato 2014). Seeking advice and support and 'talking it over with someone who could do something' are both active coping strategies that have been shown to be effective in lowering stress (Chana et al 2014).

## Nursing colleagues as a coping resource

Seeking support from colleagues is an active coping endeavour that can assist in problem solving through practical assistance and advice. That is, colleague support can support problem-focused coping. Likewise, seeking colleague support can also be an emotion-focused coping effort when used to minimise the impact of a devastating situation. For example, using another person as an emotional sounding board for expressing feelings helps to reduce tension.

Colleague support has the potential to positively alter the experience of stress in two identifiable ways. First, support from colleagues can have the direct effect of reducing or preventing stress itself – for example, through encouraging a reappraisal of the situation. An appraisal of death as a natural and expected part of life lessens the likelihood that death will be viewed as a failure. The realisation that nurses are not personally responsible for a patient's death from cancer, for example, is achievable through open, honest interaction with other nurses. The reappraisal of the situation creates a new perception that directly alters the experience of stress.

Second, colleague support can buffer the negative effects of stress in that colleague support reduces the negative effects and consequences of stress. Talking to a trusted colleague, whether through formal or informal channels, can offset a sense of isolation. It is more than likely that nurses are experiencing or have experienced similar feelings and reactions, but sometimes a 'conspiracy of silence' prevents these experiences from being shared. Keeping feelings hidden, especially fears, places nurses in the position of worrying alone and perpetuates the fallacy that 'I am the only one who feels this way' or 'There must be something wrong with me'. There is comfort in knowing one is not alone, and not the only one with fears, worries and negative reactions.

Effective working relationships with colleagues are a necessity in nursing because of the need for collaboration and team effort in most work situations. The interdependence created by this need to pull together has potential to strain colleague relationships and lead to interpersonal conflict with colleagues.

Colleague support has been shown to be correlated with less job stress and strain and is therefore beneficial to nurses' wellbeing (Riahi 2011; Teo et al 2012). Such support is helpful to nurses for the same reasons social support helps patients (see Ch 9). Colleagues provide direct aid, assistance and access to useful and relevant information, in addition to personal affirmation and emotional support.

Such relationships are reflective of an organisational culture and point to the importance of environmental factors in nurse stress. Healthcare organisational structures and work practices contribute to staff conflict and lack of cohesion (Trépanier et al 2016). Effective coping is not simply a matter for an individual nurse; the whole of the nursing work environment comes into play.

# Effective conflict management

Conflict is considered a natural part of social life, and interpersonal conflicts in the workplace are not unique to the nursing environment. This is because nurses work closely with other people with whom there is a high degree of interdependence (i.e. the need to work together towards mutual goals). Differences of opinions and perspectives are inevitable when people work in this interdependent way. Rather than try to avoid conflicts, it is more important to develop skills to manage and resolve them.

In Chapter 10, managing conflict was introduced in relation to interpersonal interactions with patients; in all likelihood, conflicts with colleagues will be encountered more frequently in the workplace. The causes of conflict include: differences in perspectives about patient care; differences in values and opinions; poor or incompetent communication; workload stress; unclear expectations; and incompatible priorities. Successful resolution of conflicts can bring people closer and adds to satisfaction and creativity in the workplace; when handled poorly, conflicts can create extra strain and tension. More importantly workplace conflict affects patients' outcomes and leads to errors (Wright et al 2014).

As in managing conflicts with patients, nurses need to be skilled in the processes of negotiation and collaboration. These processes rely on the skills of assertion and responsiveness because they get the job done (task focus) while maintaining working relationships based on mutual respect (relationship focus). Although the same skills and processes are used in conflicts with patients, the nature of colleague relationships is not the same as therapeutic ones.

In therapeutic relationships, the focus is always on supporting and helping patients, and maintaining the helpful nature of the relationship is paramount. In these relationships, responsibility lies with the nurse to initiate a resolution. In colleague relationships, the responsibility is shared, although often one person will make the first step in finding a resolution.

With patients, it is more likely that conflict will be experienced in an individual interaction or episode and that the relationship will not be ongoing. In colleague relationships, the conflict may be ongoing, as working relationships may last much longer than therapeutic relationships with patients.

In working relationships, the importance of achieving the task may take precedence to focusing on the relationship. While maintaining harmonious working relationships is important, handling conflicts with colleagues requires a focus on the goal or task, and doing so assertively does run the risk of disrupting the relationship (Rakos 2006). For example, advocating for a patient's right to participate in decision making regarding care may cause friction with other members of the healthcare team. The focus on the task of advocacy may disrupt the working relationships because the task of protecting the patient's right is more important. This is not to suggest that treating other members of the team with disrespect is warranted; it means that defending a patient's right may take precedence over the desire to keep colleague relationships running smoothly.

The usual ways of handling interpersonal conflict through withdrawing, forcing, smoothing, compromising and negotiating (reviewed in Ch 10) can be used when resolving workplace conflict. Nonetheless, compromising and negotiating are best suited to working with colleagues in a collaborative manner. Compromising may need to be used when there is little time available for discussion and negotiation. But compromising can lead to less-than-ideal solutions that leave many of those involved less than satisfied with the solution. Negotiating and collaborating, while more time consuming, often leads to mutually agreed solutions. Collaboration is characterised by open dialogue about the problem, thus bringing the conflict actively into the open.

Nurses are likely to meet conflict in the workplace in a passive manner, with avoidance and giving in (withdrawing and smoothing), rather than with active and assertive attempts to negotiate and collaborate (Iglesias & de Bengoa Vallejo 2012; Kaitelidou et al 2012; Mahon and Nicotera 2011). People who use passive strategies, often designed to 'keep the peace', are seen as more likeable (Rakos 2006), and this may be one reason nurses behave this way. Another reason is that nurses are trained to communicate therapeutically; they focus on feelings, rather than finding solutions to conflict. Because they are caring and compassionate towards patients, nurses may suffer under what Street (1992) has termed the 'tyranny of niceness'. That is, they may think that active assertion, which is required for successful negotiation, is not compatible with being a caring person.

Passive strategies, such as avoiding and giving in, are not always successful in resolving conflicts; and, more importantly, they are associated with increased stress and decreased mental wellbeing in nurses (Chang et al 2007; Kato 2014). Therefore, it is important that nurses learn how to deal with workplace conflict by using assertive skills. When used deliberately, compromising and acquiescing can be assertive in their own right; however, more active assertion is often required when dealing with workplace conflict.

## Assertiveness in the workplace

Nurses who behave assertively in the workplace are able to express their own thoughts, feelings and needs to colleagues while maintaining good working relationships.

The use of assertive skills in the workplace is based on the right to be heard and treated with respect. Assertive skills are often viewed as midway between passive and domineering communication. While sometimes confused with assertiveness, domineering or aggressive communication violates the rights of others to be treated with respect. Conversely, people who are usually passive and overly accommodating in their communication violate their own right to be heard.

Nurses who are assertive are able to state their own thoughts in a clear manner, often through 'I' statements (see Ch 10). Such statements are best accompanied by an empathic statement that recognises the obligation to maintain good working relationships. Simply stating a personal view, especially when in conflict with another's view, without acknowledging the perspective of the other person, is likely to be seen as aggressive.

While early definitions of assertiveness emphasised the notion of 'rights', there is now recognition that the assertion of rights carries with it an obligation to others (Rakos 2006). When being assertive, it is vital that nurses take time to try to understand the perspective of the other person or people involved in the conflict.

Although most of the research into assertiveness has focused on conflict and negative encounters, behaving assertively also includes giving and receiving compliments, initiating and maintaining relationships and expressing positive feelings (Rakos 2006). Nurses are often more comfortable with being assertive in positive situations, such as complimenting or thanking a colleague, than they are at expressing their own opinion or to make requests. When they are assertive, it is triggered by a sense of responsibility for a patient. That is, nurses can be assertive in showing care for others but are less likely to act on their own behalf.

Assertiveness involves expressing an opinion that may be different from others and even one that is unpopular. Requesting behavioural change in another person and asking for help are also examples of assertive behaviour. Asking for help involves admitting one's own limitations, which is in itself an assertive act.

Making requests and asking for help are assertive skills that are particularly relevant to a novice nurse. Colleague support, through providing information and opportunities for professional development, is an expectation of professional practice (Nursing and Midwifery Board of Australia 2006); therefore, new nurses should be confident in seeking such support from more experienced colleagues. It is their professional right.

New nurses are often reluctant to ask for help because of the manner in which they have been treated in the workplace. Recognising it and talking about it is helpful; however, developing skills in assertion helps to build coping and resilience.

Here is an example of using assertive skills in the context of colleague interaction. An inexperienced nurse might say to an experienced nurse (who does not appear busy at present): 'Can you please help me with this procedure? I don't have much experience with doing it' (this is being assertive by asking for help). Responses from the experienced nurse to the inexperienced nurse's comments might follow those in the following scenario.

## SCENARIO

Nurse 1: *Don't they teach you anything in university?* (attack that is off the issue)

Nurse 2: *I did learn about it, but I don't have much experience actually doing it and I need help.* (asserting needs and sticking to the issue)

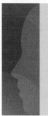

Nurse 1: *That's the trouble with nursing education today – not enough real-world experience, if you ask me.* (continues to focus on another issue)

Nurse 2: *Maybe there isn't enough clinical in basic nursing education, but I still need help with this procedure. Can you help me? If not, I'll find somebody else.* (fogging over a potential sidetrack issue)

As this example demonstrates, it is important to clearly identify the issue at hand and to stay focused on it when dealing with conflicts in the workplace. Staying focused on the issue and separating the person from the problem are essential to successful conflict resolution and assertion. This means not getting sidetracked onto other matters, especially those laden with emotions. In order to do so, it is essential that emotional responses are contained and managed because it is likely to result in collaborative conflict management. Expression of emotions in this way is an aspect of emotional intelligence (Ch 3); collaboration sets the stage for true negotiation, which is the most useful approach in work settings.

The skills of assertion are learnt behaviours and must therefore be rehearsed and practised in the workplace in order to be developed and refined. In practising and using the skills, it is important to be selective about time and place. An assertive confrontation of a co-worker in front of other co-workers is not usually a suitable context; it is better to choose a place where there is privacy. There are also times when nurses will choose not to be assertive, either because they do not have the emotional energy to do so or because the situation does not warrant such an approach. Perceiving the right time to be assertive is a skill in itself. However, lack of assertion should not happen because nurses lack the skills. Like all interpersonal skills, they must be tried and used in order to be effective in resolving conflict.

# CARING FOR SELF: BUILDING RESILIENCE

Because there are a number of reasons that nursing is a stressful profession, it is vital that nurses learn to care for their own wellbeing. Historically there has been more research into the causes of stress in nursing than into how to reduce stress (Irving et al 2009; White 2014). Because workload and lack of resources are major contributors to this stress, individual strategies to reduce stress are limited under such circumstances. Nonetheless there is current interest in helping nurses to manage stress and build resilience in order to meet the demands of the job. The concept of resilience was reviewed in Chapter 9 in relation to coping resources for patients. It is equally relevant to nurses as they too need to adapt and 'bounce back' in the face of adversity. That is, to be resilient.

Nurses who are resilient are able to adapt their coping skills to suit the situation at hand (Rushton et al 2015). They feel in control and demonstrate hardiness and a strong sense of coherence (see Ch 9) (Hart et al 2014). Being self-aware, they are able to reflect on their experiences and 'reframe' situations in a positive light, remain hopeful and optimistic, and manage their emotions (Ch 3). Another hallmark of resilient nurses is that they value and call upon the social support of their colleagues as well as their support systems external to the workplace (Cope et al 2016; Hart et al 2014; McDonald et al 2016; Shimoinaba et al 2015). Resilient nurses not only survive the stress of nursing but are also capable of thriving.

Building resilience is not just a matter for individual nurses. The workplace also affects the capacity for nurses to be resilient (Hart et al 2014; McDonald et al 2016). In fostering resilience, the individual strategies that nurses can use include the practices of mindfulness and self-compassion and formalised workplace systems including clinical supervision. These three serve as examples of nurturing nurse resilience.

# Mindfulness

One way to reduce stress and build resilience that is receiving attention in contemporary healthcare is the practice of mindfulness (Foureur et al 2013; Irving et al 2009; Lamothe et al 2016; White 2014). Mindfulness is a way of being that involves being fully present in the moment and observing one's own thoughts, feelings and actions without evaluating them or trying to change or avoid them. It requires astute awareness of and attention to what is happening 'in the moment'.

Through mindfulness nurses become acutely perceptive of their emotional responses to the situations that they encounter through observation of the self; their self-awareness is enhanced (Ch 3). In addition to this awareness, mindfulness involves the suspension of any judgment related to the emotions. Suspending judgment is a critical aspect of mindfulness, as doing so leads to self-acceptance and self-compassion, which are necessary requisites to self-care and optimum wellbeing.

Unlike many nursing activities, mindfulness is not goal-oriented. It involves being conscious of the present, not the past or the future. White (2014) asserts that the current emphasis on task orientation and evidence-based nursing care has limited other ways of knowing such as the personal and embodied knowledge that is generated through mindfulness.

Mindfulness has been shown to be helpful to all healthcare professionals (Irving et al 2009). Studies demonstrate that mindfulness has the potential to decrease burnout, stress, anxiety and depression in healthcare providers generally (Foureur et al 2013; Lamothe et al 2016). In addition it has the potential to increase empathy for patients and enhance patient-centred care (Dobkin et al 2016; Lamothe et al 2016; White 2014). Participants in these studies undertook a structured training program to learn the art of mindfulness. Therefore, it is a practice that requires support for learning the process – it does not come naturally to most people. Mindfulness requires ongoing commitment and continual development in order to cultivate its success in promoting self-care and wellbeing (White 2014).

# Self-compassion

Mindfulness is a process that leads to self-compassion, as painful thoughts are held in awareness and accepted. However, in their caring role nurses are concerned with alleviating the suffering of others and they are often not attuned to caring for their own distress; they are often lacking in self-compassion. Self-compassion involves being kind and understanding towards the self, especially in times of pain, distress or failure. Self-compassion involves perceiving suffering as part of being human and therefore connected to all of humanity.

Nurses may think that in being self-compassionate they are being selfish. To the contrary. Being self-compassionate is not only compatible with having compassion for others but is a necessary requisite (Mills et al 2015). Rather than detracting from compassion for others, self-compassion has been shown to *contribute* to compassion for others (Gustin & Wagner 2013). More importantly, nurturing the self builds resilience in nurses (Shimoinaba et al 2015) and helps to buffer compassion fatigue (Duarte et al 2016). Self-compassion is closely related to emotional intelligence (Senyuva et al 2014), which is fully reviewed in Chapter 3.

# Clinical supervision

Clinical supervision is a formalised way for nurses to receive support in the workplace and reduce stress, thereby serving as an effective coping resource (Brunero & Stein-Parbury 2008; Francke & de Graaff 2012). It is a process of professional support and learning in which nurses are assisted in developing their practice through regular discussion time with more experienced and knowledgeable colleagues. During clinical supervision, nurses employ the processes of reflection (see Ch 3) in order to identify and meet needs for professional development.

The term 'supervision' is unfortunate because it is associated with management functions and an industrial model in which supervisors are present to spot and rectify workers' mistakes. With an emphasis on learning, clinical supervision has the capacity to enable individual nurses to develop their knowledge and competence.

The interpersonal interaction of clinical supervision can occur either in a one-to-one arrangement (individual supervision) or in a work group (group supervision). Individual supervision is more suited to nurses who practise independently (e.g. community mental health nurses who function as case managers for chronically ill people). Group supervision may be more appropriate in hospital settings where nurses function daily as members of a work team. Team clinical supervision offers opportunities for nurses to engage in mutual problem solving for particularly challenging clinical situations (Francke & de Graaff 2012).

Clinical supervision can pave a path by which nurses can actively share their concerns and emotions generated by the job and be heard and understood by other nurses. Acknowledging another's perceptions through attentive listening can be helpful in and of itself. Colleague support can be requested and received. Another nurse is in a prime position to respond to a need for support. Other nurses already know colleagues, and the nursing work context is familiar. Empathy is easy to demonstrate under these circumstances because colleagues have shared experiences and meanings. Colleagues are also able to provide practical advice and solutions for managing clinical situations that are taxing for an individual nurse. Challenging (Ch 8) is sometimes necessary because of the need to develop new ways of approaching clinical situations. Challenging offers new perspectives, reframes existing perspectives, encourages nurses to improve their work and helps to overcome obstacles to meeting goals.

In order to be effective as a supportive strategy for nursing, clinical supervision must be embedded into organisational structures. When nurses are burdened by workload, 'finding' time for supervision may seem impossible. Clinical nursing leaders need to provide both time and structure if clinical supervision is to be successful as a practice development activity. There must also be organisational clarity about how clinical supervision differs from other types of developmental activities such as educational programs.

---

# SUMMARY

All of the skills described in this book will effectively promote supportive relationships with colleagues because these skills are not exclusive to patient–nurse interactions. Being attentive, responsive, encouraging, understanding and challenging are not skills that can be switched on and off at will, and enactment of these skills on a daily basis in the work environment creates a supportive environment. A necessary backdrop to supportive colleague interaction is an interpersonal work climate that acknowledges and validates nurses as people and is responsive to nurses' reactions, feelings, anxieties and confusions. Nurses cannot be expected to give of themselves without such support from other nurses and the healthcare organisation that employs them because work-related stress is best dealt with in the work environment.

However, colleague support is often lacking in nursing work environments. Reasons for this lack of support have been discussed in relation to the behaviour of oppressed groups and historical subservience of nursing to medicine. The characteristics of magnet hospitals have been described as 'ideal' in creating support for nurses and nursing practice. These characteristics – clinical autonomy, control over nursing practice and collaborative relationships with doctors – not only support nurses but also help develop nursing practice. Most importantly, they are associated with good patient outcomes.

Clinical autonomy, one of the characteristics of magnet hospitals, is evident in patient–nurse relationships. Although levels of involvement between nurses and patients are mutually negotiated (Ch 2), it is within nurses' independent professional domain to develop therapeutically meaningful relationships with patients.

There are a number of ways to manage the occupational stress inherent in nursing. Caring for the self and building resilience is essential in coping with this stress. In addition to coping skills, mindfulness and self-compassion are two effective means of dealing with occupational stress. Through these means nurses can develop and maintain resilience. Furthermore, reflective practice, especially with colleague support, can be effective in dealing with that stress through problem solving and action, or simply a new understanding or perspective on the situation. Clinical supervision has been presented as a formalised process for such reflection.

# REFERENCES

Aiken, L.H., Clarke, S.P., Sloane, D.M., et al., 2009. Effects of hospital care environments on patient mortality and nurse outcomes. J. Nurs. Adm. 38 (5), 223–229.

American Nurses Credentialing Center, 2017. Program Overview. Online. http://www.nursecredentialing.org/Magnet/ProgramOverview. (Accessed 18 January 2017).

Australian Commission on Safety and Quality in Health Care, 2016. ISBAR revisited: identifying and solving barriers to effective handover in interhospital transfer. Hunter New England Area Health Service, Sydney, Australia. Available at: http://www.safetyandquality.gov.au. (Accessed 4 May 2016).

Barrow, M., McKimm, J., Gasquoine, S., et al., 2015. Collaborating in healthcare delivery: exploring conceptual differences at the 'bedside. J. Interprof. Care 29 (2), 119–124.

Braaf, S., Manias, E., Riley, R., 2011. The role of documents and documentation in communication failure across the perioperative pathway. A literature review. Int. J. Nurs. Stud. 48, 1024–1038.

Bridges, J., Nicholson, C., Maben, J., et al., 2013. Capacity for care: meta-ethnography of acute care nurses' experiences of the nurse–patient relationship. J. Adv. Nurs. 69 (4), 760–772.

Brock, D., Abu-Rish, E., Chiu, C., et al., 2013. Interprofessional education in team communication: working together to improve patient safety. BMJ Qual. Saf. 22, 414–423.

Brunero, S., Stein-Parbury, J., 2008. The effectiveness of clinical supervision: an evidenced based literature review. Aust. J. Adv. Nurs. 25 (3), 86–94.

Burford, B., Morrow, G., Morrison, J., et al., 2013. Newly qualified doctors' perceptions of informal learning from nurses: implications for interprofessional education and practice. J. Interprof. Care 27 (5), 394–400.

Buus, N., Hamilton, B.E., 2016. Social science and linguistic text analysis of nurses' records: a systematic review and critique. Nurs. Inq. 23 (1), 64–77.

Castronovo, M.A., Pulizzi, A., Evans, S., 2016. Nurse bullying: review and a proposed solution. Nursing Outlook 64 (3), 208–214. http://dx.doi.org/10.1016/j.outlook.2015.11.008. (Accessed 11 January 2017).

Chana, N., Kennedy, P., Chessell, Z.J., 2014. Nursing staffs' emotional well-being and caring behaviours. J. Clin. Nurs. 24, 2835–2848.

Chang, E.M.L., Bidewell, J.W., Huntington, A.D., et al., 2007. A survey of role stress, coping and health in Australian and New Zealand hospital nurses. Int. J. Nurs. Stud. 44, 1354–1362.

Clynch, N., Kellett, J., 2015. Medical documentation: part of the solution, or part of the problem? A narrative review of the time spent on and value of medical documentation. Int. J. Med. Inform. 84, 221–228.

Coomber, B., Barriball, L., 2007. Impact of job satisfaction components on intent to leave and turnover for hospital-based nurses: a review of the research literature. Int. J. Nurs. Stud. 44, 297–314.

Cope, V., Jones, B., Hendricks, J., 2016. Why nurses chose to remain in the workforce. portraits of resilience. Collegian 23, 87–95.

Cornell, P., Townsend Gervis, M., Yates, L., et al., 2014. Impact of SBAR on nurse shift reports and staff rounding. Medsurg Nurs. 23 (5), 334–342.

deMeester, K., Verspuy, M., Monsieurs, K.G., et al., 2013. SBAR improves nurse–physician communication and reduced unexpected death: a pre and post intervention study. Resuscitation 84, 1192–1196.

Dobkin, P.L., Bernardi, N.F., Bagnis, C.I., 2016. Enhancing clinicians' well-being and patient-centered care through mindfulness. J. Contin. Educ. Health Prof. 36 (1), 11–16.

Duarte, J., Pinto-Gouveia, J., Cruz, B., 2016. Relationships between nurses' empathy, self-compassion and dimensions of professional quality of life: a cross-sectional study. Int. J. Nurs. Stud. 60, 1–11.

Foureur, M., Besley, K., Burton, G., et al., 2013. Enhancing the resilience of nurses and midwives: pilot of a mindfulness-based program for increased health, sense of coherence and decreased depression, anxiety and stress. Contemp. Nurse 45 (1), 114–125.

Francke, A.L., de Graaff, F.M., 2012. The effects of group clinical supervision of nurses: a systematic literature review. Int. J. Nurs. Stud. 49, 1165–1179.

Gardiner, I., Sheen, J., 2016. Graduate nurse experiences of support: a review. Nurse Educ. Today 40, 7–12.

Gustin, W., Wagner, L., 2013. The butterfly effect of caring – clinical nursing teachers' understanding of self-compassion as a source to compassionate care. Scand. J. Caring Sci. 27 (1), 175–183.

Happell, B., Dwyer, T., Reid-Searl, K., et al., 2013. Nurses and stress: recognizing causes and seeking solutions. J. Nurs. Manag. 21, 638–647.

Hart, P.L., Brannan, J.D., De Chesnay, M., 2014. Resilience in nurses: an integrative review. J. Nurs. Manag. 22, 720–734.

Hussain, A., Rivers, P.A., Glover, S.H., et al., 2012. Strategies for dealing with future shortages in the nursing workforce: a review. Health Serv. Manage. Res. 25, 41–47.

Iglesias, M.E.L., de Bengoa Vallejo, R.B., 2012. Conflict resolution styles in the nursing profession. Contemp. Nurse 43 (1), 73–80.

Irving, J.A., Dobkin, P.L., Park, J., 2009. Cultivating mindfulness in health care professionals: a review of empirical studies of mindfulness-based stress reduction (MBSR). Complement. Ther. Clin. Pract. 15, 61–66.

Jefferies, D., Johnson, M., Nicholls, D., 2011. Nursing documentation: how meaning is obscured by fragmentary language. Nurs. Outlook 59 (6), e6–e12.

Kaitelidou, D., Kontogianni, A., Galanis, P., et al., 2012. Conflict management and job satisfaction in paediatric hospitals in Greece. J. Nurs. Manag. 20, 571–578.

Kato, T., 2014. Coping with interpersonal stress and psychological distress at work: comparison of hospital nursing staff and salespeople. Psychol. Res. Behav. Manag. 7, 31–36.

Kazanjian, A., Green, C., Wong, J., et al., 2005. Effect of the hospital nursing environment on patient mortality: a systematic review. J. Health Serv. Res. Policy 10 (2), 111–117.

Kim, H., Dykes, P.C., Thomas, D., et al., 2011. A closer look at nursing documentation on paper forms: preparation for computerizing a nursing documentation system. Comput. Biol. Med. 41, 182–189.

Kramer, M., Maguire, P., Brewer, B.B., 2011. Clinical nurses in Magnet hospitals confirm productive, health unit work environments. J. Nurs. Manag. 19, 5–7.

Kramer, M., Schmalenberg, C., 1988a. Magnet hospitals: part I: institutions of excellence. J. Nurs. Adm. 18 (1), 13–24.

Kramer, M., Schmalenberg, C., 1988b. Magnet hospitals: part II: institutions of excellence. J. Nurs. Adm. 18 (2), 1–19.

Kramer, M., Schmalenberg, C., 2008. The practice of clinical autonomy in hospitals: 20,000 nurses tell their story. Crit. Care Nurse 28 (6), 58–71.

Kramer, M., Schmalenberg, C., Maguire, P., et al., 2008. Structures and practices enabling staff nurses to control their practice. West. J. Nurs. Res. 30 (5), 539–559.

Krörner, M., Wirtz, M.A., Bengel, J., et al., 2015. Relationship of organizational culture, teamwork and job satisfaction in interprofessional teams. BMC Health Serv. Res. 15, 243. doi:10.1186/s12913-015-0888-y.

Kutney-Lee, A., Witkoski Stimpfel, A., Sloane, D.M., et al., 2015. Changes in patient and nurse outcomes associated with Magnet hospital recognition. Med. Care 53 (6), 550–557.

Lamothe, M., Rondeau, E., Malboeuf-Hurtubise, C., et al., 2016. Outcomes of MBSR or MBSR-based interventions in health care providers: a systematic review with a focus on empathy and emotional competencies. Complement. Ther. Med. 24, 19–28.

Larson, E.L., 2012. New rules for the game: interdisciplinary education for health professionals. Nurs. Outlook 60, 264–271.

Laschinger, H.K., Leiter, M.P., 2006. The impact of nursing work environments on patient safety outcomes. J. Nurs. Adm. 36 (5), 259–267.

Laschinger, H.K.S., Wong, C.A., Cummings, G.G., et al., 2014. Resonant leadership and workplace empowerment: the value of positive organizational cultures in reducing workplace incivility. Nurs. Econ. 32 (1), 5–15, 44.

Ledoux, K., 2015. Understanding compassion fatigue: understanding compassion. J. Adv. Nurs. 71 (9), 2041–2050.

Lu, H., Barriball, K.L., Zhang, X., et al., 2012. Job satisfaction among hospital nurses revisited: a systematic review. Int. J. Nurs. Stud. 49, 1017–1038.

Mahon, M.M., Nicotera, A.M., 2011. Nursing and conflict communication: avoidance as preferred strategy. Nurs. Adm. Q. 35 (2), 152–163.

Martin, H.A., Ciurzynski, S.M., 2015. Situation, background, assessment, and recommendation-guided huddles improve communication and teamwork in the emergency department. J. Emerg. Nurs. 41 (6), 484–488.

Maslach, C., Schaufeli, W.B., 1993. Historical and conceptual development of burnout. In: Schaufeli, W.B., Maslach, C., Marek, T. (Eds.), Professional Burnout: Recent Developments in Theory and Research. Taylor and Francis, Washington DC, pp. 1–16.

Matziou, V., Vlahioti, E., Perdikaris, P., et al., 2014. Physician and nursing perceptions concerning interprofessional communication and collaboration. J. Interprof. Care 28 (6), 526–533.

McClure, M., Poulin, M., Sovie, M., et al., 1983. Magnet hospitals: attraction and retention of professional nurses. American Academy of Nursing Task Force on Nursing Practice in Hospitals. American Nurses Association, Kansas City, MO.

McComb, S., Simpson, V., 2013. The concept of shared mental models in healthcare collaboration. J. Adv. Nurs. 70 (7), 1479–1488.

McDonald, G., Jackson, D., Vickers, M.H., et al., 2016. Surviving workplace adversity: a qualitative study of nurses and midwives and their strategies to increase personal resilience. J. Nurs. Manag. 24, 123–131.

McHugh, M.D., Kelly, L.A., Smith, H.L., et al., 2013. Lower mortality in Magnet hospitals. Med. Care 51 (5), 382–388.

McVicar, A., 2016. Scoping the common antecedents of job stress and job satisfaction for nurses (2000–2013) using the job demands–resources model of stress. J. Nurs. Manag. 24, E112–E136.

Mills, J., Wand, T., Fraser, J.A., 2015. On self-compassion and self-care in nursing: selfish or essential for compassionate care? Int. J. Nurs. Stud. 52, 791–793.

Musto, L.C., Rodney, P.A., 2016. Moving from conceptual ambiguity to knowledgeable action: using a critical realist approach to studying moral distress. Nurs. Philos. 17, 75–87.

Nursing and Midwifery Board of Australia, 2006. Registered nurse competency standards – rebranded, Canberra. Online. Available at: http://www.nursingmidwiferyboard.gov.au/Codes-Guidelines-Statements/Codes-Guidelines.aspx#competencystandards. (Accessed 25 May 2016).

Nursing Council of New Zealand, 2007. Competencies for registered nurses. NCNZ, Wellington. Online. Available at: http://www.nursingcouncil.org.nz/Publications/Standards-and-guidelines-for-nurses. (Accessed 24 July 2016).

O'Leary, K.J., Sehgal, N.L., Terrell, G., et al., 2012. Interdisciplinary teamwork in hospitals: a review and practical recommendations for improvement. J. Hosp. Med. 7 (1), 48–54.

Oh, Y., Gastmans, C., 2015. Moral distress experienced by nurses: a quantitative literature review. Nurs. Ethics 22 (1), 15–31.

Paans, W., Müller-Staub, M., 2015. Patients' care needs: documentation analysis in general hospitals. Int. J. Nurs. Knowl. 26 (4), 178–186.

Pannick, S., Beveridge, I., Wachter, R.M., et al., 2014. Improving the quality and safety of care on the medical ward: a review and synthesis of the evidence base. Eur. J. Intern. Med. 25, 874–887.

Prideaux, A., 2011. Issues in nursing documentation and record-keeping practice. Br. J. Nurs. 20 (22), 1450–1454.

Rakos, R.F., 2006. Asserting and confronting. In: Hargie, O. (Ed.), The Handbook of Communication Skills, third ed. Routledge, London, pp. 345–381.

Reeves, S., Nelson, S., Zwarenstein, M., 2008. The doctor–nurse game in the age of interprofessional care: a view from Canada. Nurs. Inq. 15 (1), 1–2.

Riahi, S., 2011. Role stress amongst nurses at the workplace: a concept analysis. J. Nurs. Manag. 19, 721–731.

Roberts, S.J., 1983. Oppressed group behavior: implications for nursing. Adv. Nurs. Sci. 5, 21–31.

Roberts, S.J., 2015. Lateral violence in nursing: a review of the past three decades. Nurs. Sci. Q. 28 (1), 36–41.

Rushton, C.H., Batcheller, J., Schroeder, K., et al., 2015. Burnout and resilience among nurses practicing in high-intensity settings. Am. J. Crit. Care 24 (5), 412–420.

Schmalenberg, C., Kramer, M., 2008. Essentials of a productive nurse work environment. Nurs. Res. 57 (1), 2–13.

Schmalenberg, C., Kramer, M., 2009. Nurse–physician relationships in hospitals: 20,000 nurses tell their story. Crit. Care Nurse 29 (1), 74–83.

Senyuva, E., Kaya, H., Isik, B., et al., 2014. Relationship between self-compassion and emotional intelligence in nursing students. Int. J. Nurs. Pract. 20 (6), 588–596.

Sharafi, M., Nematolahi, S., Fonon, F., et al., 2016. Job stress, causes and treatment of job stress among teachers and nurses: a review. Res. J. Pharm. Biol. Chem. Sci. 7 (1), 656–662.

Shimoinaba, K., O'Connor, M., Lee, S., et al., 2015. Nurses' resilience and nurturance of the self. Int. J. Palliat. Nurs. 21 (10), 504–510.

Slayter, S., Coventry, L.L., Twigg, D., 2016. Professional practice models for nursing: a review of the literature and synthesis of key components. J. Nurs. Manag. 24, 139–150.

Spence Laschinger, H.K., Leiter, M.P., Day, A., et al., 2012. Building empowering work environments that foster civility and organizational trust: testing an intervention. Nurs. Res. 61 (5), 316–325.

Stein, L.I., 1967. The doctor–nurse game. Arch. Gen. Psychiatry 16, 699–703.

Stein, L.I., Watts, D.T., Howell, T., 1990. The doctor–nurse game revisited. NEJM 322 (8), 546–549.

Stein-Parbury, J., Liaschenko, J., 2007. Understanding collaboration between doctors and physicians as knowledge at work. Am. J. Crit. Care 16 (5), 470–477.

Street, A.F., 1992. Inside Nursing. State University of New York Press, New York.

Tang, C.J., Chan, S.W., Zhou, W.T., et al., 2013. Collaboration between hospital physicians and nurses: an integrated literature review. Int. Nurs. Rev. 60, 291–302.

Teo, S.T.T., Yeung, M., Chang, E., 2012. Administrative stressors and nursing job outcomes in Australian public and non-profit health care organisations. J. Clin. Nurs. 21, 1443–1452.

Terra, S.M., 2015. Interdisciplinary rounds: the key to communication, collaboration, and agreement on plan of care. Prof. Case Manag. 20 (6), 299–307.

Thomson, K., Outram, S., Gilligan, C., et al., 2015. Interprofessional experiences of recent healthcare graduates: a social, psychological perspective on the barriers to effective communication, teamwork, and patient-centred care. J. Interprof. Care 29 (6), 634–650.

Trépanier, S., Fernet, C., Austin, S., et al., 2016. Work environment antecedents of bullying: a review and integrative model applied to registered nurses. Int. J. Nurs. Stud. 55, 85–97.

White, L., 2014. Mindfulness in nursing: an evolutionary concept analysis. J. Adv. Nurs. 70 (2), 282–294.

Wilson, J.L., 2016. An exploration of bullying behaviours in nursing: a review of the literature. Br. J. Nurs. 25 (6), 303–306.

Witkoski Stimpfel, A., Rosen, J.E., McHugh, M.D., 2014. Understanding the role of the professional practice environment on quality of care in Magnet and non-Magnet hospitals. J. Nurs. Adm. 44 (1), 10–16.

Wright, R.R., Mohr, C.D., Sinclair, R.R., 2014. Conflict on the treatment floor: an investigation of interpersonal conflict experienced by nurses. J. Res. Nurs. 19 (1), 26–37.

Zangaro, G.A., Soeken, K.L., 2007. A meta-analysis of studies of nurses' job satisfaction. Res. Nurs. Health 30, 445–458.

# APPENDIX

# Notes on the activities

## INTRODUCTION

The information in this appendix supports the book's learning activities by presenting guidelines and suggestions about conducting the activities in a learning group. As such, it is primarily for the benefit of those people who are promoting learning through the activities. These people are referred to as 'facilitators' rather than teachers because this term more accurately reflects the nature of 'teaching' through the use of experiential activities.

The appendix begins with a brief overview of experiential learning, with specific reference to how the skills can actually be used to facilitate this method of learning. Fig. A.1 illustrates the relationship between experiential learning and the skills presented in this book.

Included in this section are some suggestions for facilitators who are using experience-based learning approaches. General guidelines for employing 'role-play' as an experiential learning form of activity follow; and, finally, discussion and material specific to a number of the book's various activities are presented. (Note: each activity referred to in this final section of the appendix is highlighted in its respective chapter by the symbol C.)

## EXPERIENTIAL LEARNING

The activities in this book are designed to stimulate learning of interpersonal skills in nursing and consolidate the theory presented in the text. Some activities trigger learners to reflect on previous experiences, considering theoretical concepts in a 'there-and-then' manner. Other activities enable learners to put into practice interpersonal skills in a 'here-and-now' manner. All are designed to produce

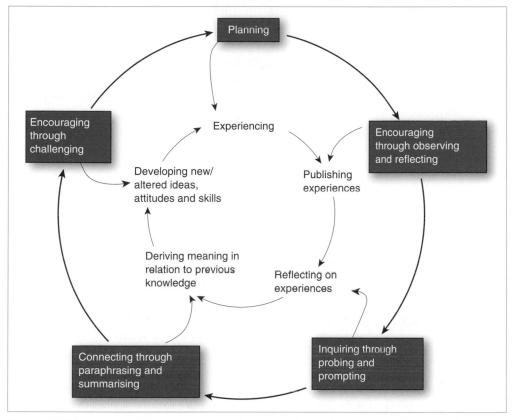

**Figure A.1** The relationship of processing (outer circle) and experiential learning (inner circle)

*Source: Stein-Parbury, J., 1992. Processing skills: enhancing experiential learning. In: Members of the 1991 Teaching Enhancement Team, Quality of Teaching Matters at UTS, Centre for Learning and Teaching, University of Technology, Sydney.*

meaningful learning experiences by actively involving participants in understanding the concepts described in the text.

Learning through experience is one of the most effective ways to integrate interpersonal skills into professional behaviour. While a theoretical comprehension of the skills is essential, they are most effectively understood by participating in experiences that make them 'come to life'. By putting the skills to use in some way through experiential activities, theoretical understanding is developed in conjunction with the technical know-how of employing them.

The majority of the activities are most effective when they are conducted in a learning group led by a knowledgeable and sensitive guide. This guide, the learning facilitator, is a person who not only understands the concepts illustrated in the activity but who is also able to help participants discuss the experience in a meaningful way.

The majority of the activities include a discussion section that focuses on processing the learning experiences. Processing refers to that aspect of experiential learning that enables learners to derive personalised meaning from their experiences.

In processing learning experiences, facilitators respond rather than direct, pull ideas together rather than prescribe what they should be and encourage reflection rather than expect automatic reactions.

When interacting with learners, facilitators who demonstrate the attitudes, skills and knowledge embedded in this book will be most effective if they use an experience-based approach to learning. In addition, facilitators of the method of learning through experience are most productive when they are knowledgeable about experiential learning.

# Suggestions for facilitators of experiential learning

Sometimes experiential learning activities produce lively responses from participants. At other times, experiences designed to facilitate learning may fall flat. Here are some general suggestions for handling some of the more common difficulties that may surface when using experience-based learning:

1.  Because the meaning derived from an experience is personalised, it is difficult to be pedantic about the 'right' or correct way to respond to an experience. This may be uncomfortable for facilitators who are accustomed to presenting material in a step-wise manner. Facilitators of learning through experience need to refrain from using procedural approaches when teaching interpersonal skills. This will allow learners to derive personally relevant meaning from their experiences and allow facilitators to function as a guide on a journey rather than an expert who demonstrates how it 'should' be done. They should be 'the guide on the side', rather than the 'sage on the stage'.

2.  When activities are conducted in a traditional classroom it is sometimes tempting to leave the room while participants engage in an activity. As a general rule, this is not a good idea because participants often need further guidance and assistance during the activity. It is helpful to 'float' around the room, making sure that instructions for the activity are understood. This is also a useful opportunity to discuss the associated concepts with participants.

3.  Sometimes, activities are ineffectual, producing a 'so what?' experience – that is, they fail to enhance participants' learning because no meaning can be constructed from it. An indication that this may be happening occurs when participants do not have much to say in response to the items in the discussion section of the activity. When an activity or its discussion seems to be 'going nowhere', it is often useful to ask a general question such as 'What's happening here?' or 'What's going on?'. When facilitators ask questions such as these, they may be surprised to learn that participants are responding to events other than the presented activity. At other times, there is 'nothing happening', and at this point the activity should be abandoned. Nevertheless, if the

'so what?' experience happens once, it is not enough reason to abandon an activity altogether. Try it again with another group of participants. It may trigger significant learning in another context.

4.  When participants seem hesitant to engage in an activity, make sure they understand the instructions. Most often, reluctance is a result of failure to comprehend what is expected. Do not assume that hesitancy is a result of lack of interest or motivation. Always assume the participants' goodwill. It helps to establish trust.

5.  It is often beneficial to begin formal classes that use an experience-based approach to learning with a 'warm-up' activity. These activities enable participants to get their minds in gear, ready to learn in an active, involved way. Some suggestions for warm-up activities are:

- **Word association.** Have participants say the first word that comes to their mind in response to the theme of the session (e.g. old age).

- **Brainstorm.** Generate as many ideas as possible about a given topic (e.g. reassurance).

- **Touch base.** Have each participant state how they are feeling at the moment.

- **Tell a story.** Begin the session by sharing a personal anecdote about the topic of the session (e.g. 'the time I became overinvolved with a patient').

- **Show a picture.** Display a picture that depicts something of relevance to the session (e.g. a patient who is crying).

These warm-up activities need to be short and snappy in order to be effective. As a general rule, they should consume no more than 10 minutes of a given session.

# GUIDELINES FOR ROLE-PLAY

Role-playing is one of the most commonly used experiential learning methods. Role-playing is a process of acting 'as if' the situation is real. While it does not require formal drama skills, the participants' willingness to behave in ways that may be unfamiliar is essential if the action is to proceed.

Throughout this book, various activities rely on this method. Whenever it is used, it is crucial that the following guidelines be presented to participants (on an interactive whiteboard or by circulating hard copies) who are enacting the role-play. *Remember* that the onus is on the facilitator to present this information to the learners each time a role-play exercise is introduced.

## Before the action

1.  Assume the role. Try not to let personal thoughts and feelings about the role interfere with your ability to adopt the role; accept it for what

it is – an act designed to enhance learning. Take a few minutes before the role-play to 'put yourself' into the role.

2.  Don't be concerned if you think you cannot enact the role because you are not good at dramatising and performing. The purpose of role-playing is to act naturally, although you may be required to adopt a stance that feels different from your usual way of interacting with others.

3.  Once you have assumed the role, let the action flow naturally. Do not overact or exaggerate your actions in an effort to be a good role-player.

4.  During the role-play, invent needed information about yourself or specific details of the situation. Do not let the role-play stop or flounder because you think you should know something; simply make it up in an effort to keep the action going.

5.  It is acceptable, sometimes desirable, to change your ideas and attitudes during the role-play. Even if your role prescribes certain attitudes and feelings, these may change as a result of the progress of the action. When this happens, let it flow naturally; do not cling to your original script.

## After the action

1.  Remain in the role and take a few minutes to discuss how you responded to the role and how it felt playing the role.

2.  Make sure you clarify any information or detail what was fabricated in an effort to keep the action going.

3.  Discuss any concerns you have about what others who participated in the role-play may think or feel about you as a result of the role you have just assumed.

4.  When the time comes, state aloud that you are no longer in the role and are returning to who you really are.

# ADDITIONAL MATERIAL FOR ACTIVITIES
## Chapter 3   Nurse as therapeutic agent
### Activity 3.1   What do I have to offer patients?

This activity can be threatening and frightening to participants if they think they will be expected to reveal their responses. For this reason, it is essential to stress that participants will not be required to disclose the answers to the questions posed in the process section. Participants should be seated in a way that allows their papers to remain in their own view only. The discussion centres on how it felt to complete the activity, not on the answers to personal questions asked during the process.

## Activity 3.3   Beliefs about helping in nursing practice

The questionnaire used in this activity is designed to trigger thoughts about assumptions of personal responsibility for problems and how these assumptions affect approaches to helping. Participants may take issue with some of the items on the questionnaire, especially if their results are not in accordance with what they believe, want to believe or think they 'should' believe. Much time and effort could go into discussing the items, and this may detract from the purpose of the activity. Individual participants' results are therefore not the major issue, and this should be stressed during the discussion of the activity.

It is equally important to emphasise that a mismatch between how patients view their responsibility and how nurses view personal responsibility can create problems in the relationship. For this reason, participants should be encouraged to develop awareness of patients' orientation to helping as well as of their own orientation.

# Chapter 4   Considering culture

## Activity 4.4   Working with an interpreter

See 'Guidelines for role-play' on page 331.

# Chapter 5   Encouraging interaction: listening

## Activity 5.3   Attending and non-attending

See 'Guidelines for role-play' on page 331.

## Activity 5.5   Listening for content

Participants often request to have stories read more than once. Facilitators need to emphasise that doing so would interfere with the purpose of the activity. While nurses may request patients to repeat what they have said (e.g. when nurses cannot hear what has been said or when the patient's speech is garbled), such requests may be interpreted as a failure to listen in the first place.

Participants' responses (the who, what, when and where content) should be reviewed after each story is read, rather than reading all stories, then reviewing the responses. As each story is reviewed, participants become more skilled at listening for content (i.e. the learning is immediate).

In answering the 'who, what, when and where' of each story, participants often become frustrated if the facilitator is pedantic about the 'correct' answers. Rather than giving the impression of right and wrong answers, it is better to focus the discussion on reasons for discrepancies between participants and their answers, and the ones provided at the end of the chapter. The purpose of the activity is to discover the process of listening – not to 'get' the right answers. This may need to be continually reinforced.

## Activity 5.6    Listening for feelings

Participants' responses should be reviewed after each patient statement is read, rather than reading all the statements and then reviewing the responses. There is often great variety between participants in their interpretation of feelings. Because answers are provided at the end of the chapter, these may be perceived as 'correct' and any other answers as 'incorrect'. Take care not to give the impression that responses that are different from those presented at the end of the chapter are 'incorrect'. Rather, focus the discussion on why the interpretations differ between participants. Some of the reasons for these differences include cultural variance, role expectations, personal needs, values and beliefs. Emphasise the importance of self-understanding within the context of listening for feelings.

This activity often highlights problems with the language used to describe feelings; participants sometimes find it difficult to 'find the words' to express emotions. A general discussion about the role of language in discussing feelings is useful and timely in the discussion phase of this activity. It is also beneficial to follow this activity with Activity 6.5: *Building a feeling-word vocabulary*.

## Activity 5.9    Responses that indicate listening

Do not become overly concerned if there is a discrepancy between participants' answers and the ones provided at the end of the chapter. Sometimes such discrepancies indicate different interpretations of the words used in the responses; at other times, different meanings are constructed. Sometimes, participants want to argue about the answers in an effort to determine the correct one, and this can become counterproductive to learning. Rather than arguing, participants should be encouraged to reflect on their interpretation of the given responses and compare these with other participants' interpretations. As a result of this type of discussion, participants are better able to understand that meanings are in people, not words.

# Chapter 6    Building meaning: understanding

## Activity 6.2    Recognising the types of responses

Participants often experience difficulty differentiating between an analysing and interpreting response (A) from a paraphrasing and understanding response (U). It should be explained that an A response 'adds' to what the patient has expressed. When such additions are an accurate reflection of what a patient is experiencing, this is referred to as 'advanced empathy'. Advanced empathy delves into feelings and meanings that are beneath the surface. When such additions are inaccurate, they are often a reflection of the nurse's personal value judgments. A 'U' response remains on the surface and does not delve more deeply into hidden and obscured meaning.

### Activity 6.7    Connecting thoughts and feelings

Sometimes participants are frustrated by using the format 'You feel … when …'. When this happens, encourage them to use their own style of expression, as long as the connection between thoughts and feelings is made. Emphasise that the suggested format is a useful mental aid; it is not a prescription for connecting feelings and thoughts. When adhered to rigidly, the suggested format interferes with the development of a personal style.

# Chapter 7    Collecting information: exploring

## Activity 7.3    Cues and inferences

Some of the inferences presented in this activity could actually be cues. For example, item 2 would be a cue if the patient directly stated that they were uninterested in the interview. This point should be brought out during the discussion phase of the activity.

It should be stressed that inferences can be valid interpretations of cues. Sometimes participants may form the impression that inferences should be avoided at all costs. The discussion phase of this activity provides a useful opportunity to clarify this incorrect impression.

Finally, nurses must take care in supporting inferences with the cues on which they are based. In recording patient data in a chart, for example, it is essential that inferences are not stated, unless their supporting cues are also stated. On the other hand, cues can be recorded on their own – that is, they do not require an interpretation (inference).

### Activity 7.4    Ways of exploring: questions versus statements

See 'Guidelines for role-play' on page 331.

### Activity 7.7    Recognising types of questions

Some participants may not be able to perceive the disguised 'why' question, and further explanation may be necessary to complete the process. 'Why' questions are often hidden behind statements such as 'What made you feel that way?', 'What are your reasons for thinking this way?' and 'How come?'. If the word 'why' can be substituted for a word or phrase in the question without destroying its meaning, then there is a good chance that a disguised 'why' question has been asked.

### Activity 7.9    Patient interview

See 'Guidelines for role-play' on page 331.

# Chapter 8   Intervening: comforting, supporting and enabling

## Activity 8.4   Sharing information

This activity is conducted over two sessions. In the first session, participants are given scenarios for sharing information (developed in steps 1 and 2 of the process). In doing so, they have the opportunity to familiarise themselves with the information they will be sharing. They should come to the next session prepared to share information. Without this opportunity, participants may be caught 'off guard' and feel unable to share information because they do not know enough about a given topic.

See 'Guidelines for role-play' on page 331 and 'Guide for sharing information' (below).

# GUIDE FOR SHARING INFORMATION

Did the nurse …

1.  Identify what the patient wants to know?
    Yes   No
    How?

2.  Clarify what the patient already understands?
    Yes   No
    How?

3.  Assess the accuracy of the patient's current information?
    Yes   No
    How?

4.  Determine the patient's readiness to receive the information?
    Yes   No
    How?

5.  Limit the amount of information shared (about two items at a time)?
    Yes   No
    How?

6.  Use understandable language?
    Yes   No
    How?

7.  Present information clearly?
    Yes   No
    How?

8.  Assess the patient's comprehension?
    Yes   No
    How?

9. Request feedback from the patient?
   Yes   No
   How?

10. Discuss the patient's reaction to the information?
    Yes   No
    How?

# INDEX

Page numbers followed by "*f*" indicate figures, "*t*" indicate tables, and "*b*" indicate boxes.

# D

# E

# F

# S

# U

# Z